Pathology for Urologists

Gregory T. MacLennan, MD

Associate Professor of Pathology, Urology, and Oncology
Case Western Reserve University
University Hospitals of Cleveland
Cleveland, Ohio

Martin I. Resnick, MD

Lester Persky Professor and Chair
Department of Urology
Case Western Reserve University
University Hospitals of Cleveland
Cleveland, Ohio

David G. Bostwick, MD, MBA

Medical Director
Bostwick Laboratories
Richmond, Virginia
Clinical Professor of Pathology
The University of Virginia
Charlottesville, Virginia

Pathology for Urologists

SAUNDERS

An Imprint of Elsevier Science

SAUNDERS
An Imprint of Elsevier Science (USA)

The Curtis Center
Independence Square West
Philadelphia, Pennsylvania 19106

PATHOLOGY FOR UROLOGISTS   ISBN 0–7216–0091–3
Copyright © 2003, Elsevier Science (USA). All rights reserved.

Notice

Medicine is an ever-changing field. Standard safety precautions must be followed, but as new research and clinical experience broaden our knowledge, changes in treatment and drug therapy may become necessary or appropriate. Readers are advised to check the most current product information provided by the manufacturer of each drug to be administered to verify the recommended dose, the method and duration of administration, and contraindications. It is the responsibility of the treating physician, relying on experience and knowledge of the patient, to determine dosages and the best treatment for each individual patient. Neither the publisher nor the editor assumes any liability for any injury and/or damage to persons or property arising from this publication.

The Publisher

Library of Congress Cataloging in Publication Data

MacLennan, Gregory T.
 Pathology for urologists/Gregory T. MacLennan, Martin I. Resnick,
David Bostwick.
  p. ; cm
 ISBN 0-7216-0091-3
  1. Genitourinary organs—Diseases—Atlases. I. Resnick, Martin I. II. Bostwick, David G.
III. Title.
 [DNLM: 1. Urogenital System—pathology—Atlases. 2. Urogenital
System—surgery—Atlases. WJ 17 M164a 2003]
 RC873.9.M33 2003
 616.6–dc21   2003041525

Acquisitions Editor: Hilarie Surrena
Project Manager: Mary Anne Folcher
Book Designer: Ellen Zanolle

EH/RRD

Printed in China

Last digit is the print number: 9 8 7 6 5 4 3 2 1

To our families—

For my wife, Carrol, and my sons, Darren and Grayden

GREG MACLENNAN

For my wife, Vicki, and for Andy, Jeff, Missy, Katie, and Daniel

MARTIN RESNICK

For my wife, Elizabeth, and my children, Kathleen, Daniel, and Brian

DAVID BOSTWICK

Preface

For many years, the residency training program in urology at Case Western Reserve University has included a formal monthly tutorial in urologic pathology. Residents have frequently asked whether a textbook was available to assist them in their study of this often complex and daunting field. Although there are many excellent textbooks dealing with urologic pathology, all such texts have been written primarily for the purposes of instructing pathologists in training and assisting practicing pathologists in their diagnostic work. Until now, none has been written expressly for urologists in training, as well as for practicing urologists.

In composing the text and choosing illustrations for this book, we have tried to include material that we believe is of relevance and interest to urologists. Clearly, there are some very rare entities that we have chosen not to emphasize, or even to include.

We have also drawn from our many years of experience in directing the American Urological Association's Board Review Course in Pathology and, most recently, the Bostwick Laboratories Board Review Course in Pathology and Radiology.

We hope that urologists in training as well as those in practice will find this book helpful in understanding more completely the pathology of the disease processes they treat. It is our firm belief that a strong understanding of pathology is essential to a successful practice in urology.

Gregory T. MacLennan, MD
Martin I. Resnick, MD
David G. Bostwick, MD, MBA

Acknowledgments

Many individuals were extraordinarily helpful in preparing this book, and we wish to extend our sincere thanks:

To Junqi Qian, MD, of Bostwick Laboratories, Richmond, Virginia, for his tireless assistance with image preparation.

To Stephanie Donley, Hilarie Surrena, Mary Anne Folcher, and Norm Stellander, of Saunders, for their very professional management of the project.

To Lisa Dickason and Sheila Hoyle, University Hospitals of Cleveland, for their secretarial and logistic assistance.

To all those who contributed images for this book, with special thanks to Beverly Dahms, MD, and Ray Redline, MD, for allowing us access to their spectacular collections of images, and to the pathology residents at University Hospitals of Cleveland for their diligence in taking many of the excellent gross photographs that were used in the book.

Contents

|||| Chapter 1

KIDNEY 1

|||| Chapter 2

BLADDER, URETHRA, RENAL PELVIS, AND URETER 33

|||| Chapter 3

PROSTATE, SEMINAL VESICLES, AND PROSTATIC URETHRA 81

|||| Chapter 4

TESTIS 121

|||| Chapter 5

SPERMATIC CORD AND TESTICULAR ADNEXAE 151

|||| Chapter 6

with Roy King, MD

PENIS AND SCROTUM 167

|||| Chapter 7

ADRENAL 185

SELECTED REFERENCES 199

INDEX 201

ANATOMY

The kidney is a paired, bean-shaped organ located high in the retroperitoneum averaging 12 cm long, 6 cm wide, and 2.5 cm thick, and weighing between 115 and 170 g. It is enclosed by a thin fibrous capsule that ends at the renal sinus. Fat surrounds the kidney and the blood vessels, nerves, and collecting structures at the hilum. The perirenal fat is enclosed within Gerota's fascia.

Each kidney is composed of 8 to 18 lobes, each of which consists of a conical medullary pyramid capped by cortical tissue. The cortex is normally about 1 cm thick over the pyramids; downward extensions of cortical tissue between the pyramids are called columns of Bertin. Medullary rays of Ferrein extend from the cortex into the medulla; they consist of collecting ducts, straight segments of proximal and distal tubules, and vasa recta (Fig. 1–1). The inner medulla (papilla) drains into a minor calyx through the orifices of the terminal collecting ducts (Bellini's ducts).

A nephron is the functional unit of the kidney. Each kidney contains 1 to 2 million nephrons, each of which includes a glomerulus, proximal tubule, distal tubule, connecting segment, and collecting duct (which actually is derived from the ureteric bud) (Figs. 1–2 and 1–3).

CONGENITAL DISORDERS

UNILATERAL RENAL AGENESIS

This defect occurs about once in every 1000 to 1500 births. Males are more often affected by this anomaly than females, and the left kidney is more commonly absent than the right. The ipsilateral ureter is absent or atretic in 75% of cases.

BILATERAL RENAL AGENESIS

This anomaly occurs approximately once in every 4000 births and is twice as common in males as in females. The condition is incompatible with extrauterine survival and is usually associated with multiple other organ system anomalies.

HYPOPLASIA

Hypoplasia is defined as reduction in size of a single renal unit by more than 50%, or reduction of total renal mass by more than 33%. In unilateral cases, the affected kidney usually has fewer than five minor calyces. In contrast to the gross appearance of a dysplastic kidney, a

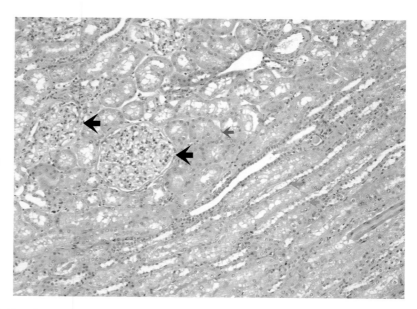

FIGURE 1–1 ▌▌▏▏ Normal kidney. The section is from the corticomedullary junction and demonstrates glomeruli *(black arrows)* surrounded by convoluted tubules *(blue arrow),* and long straight medullary rays of Ferrein *(green arrows).*

Several images in this chapter are courtesy of Mayo Clinic Foundation, Rochester, MN.

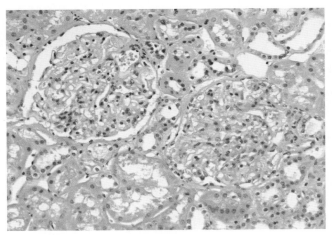

FIGURE 1–2 I▌I I   Normal glomeruli, surrounded by cross sections of convoluted tubules.

hypoplastic kidney, apart from being small, retains grossly normal architecture.

SUPERNUMERARY KIDNEY

A *supernumerary kidney* is a structurally normal renal unit with its own ureter and blood supply in an individual also possessing two normally situated renal units. It is usually smaller than normal and is usually located caudad to the ipsilateral normal kidney. It is believed to be the result of anomalous development of the ureteral bud. Detection of the anomalous renal unit is most often prompted by symptoms related to urinary tract infection.

SIMPLE (INFERIOR) ECTOPIC KIDNEY

This anomaly is noted about once in every 900 autopsies and more often in females than in males. The ectopic kidney is most often located in the pelvis and less often at or just above the level of the sacral promontory. Renal vasculature is variable, but usually it is derived directly from the aorta or iliac vessels. The opposite kidney is normally positioned in 90% of cases. In rare instances, the inferior ectopic kidney is the only renal unit present. An inferior ectopic kidney is usually flat and malrotated anteriorly, and poor urinary drainage is common.

CROSSED ECTOPIC KIDNEY

A crossed ectopic kidney lies on the side opposite to its ureteral insertion, usually below the normally situated kidney. In 90% of cases it is fused with the normally situated kidney *(crossed fused ectopia)*. The renal pelvis of such a kidney is malrotated, so urinary drainage from this unit is commonly compromised. Descriptive terms applied to such kidneys (L-shaped, disc, lump, sigmoid, inferior, and superior) refer to variations in shape and position. Rarely, both kidneys are crossed. Anorectal, skeletal, or genital anomalies are noted in 20% to 25% of patients with crossed ectopic kidneys.

SUPERIOR ECTOPIC KIDNEY

This term denotes a kidney located higher than its expected position. A *cephaloid ectopic kidney* still resides in the retroperitoneum and occurs in association with an omphalocele. A *thoracic kidney* lies above an intact diaphragm, in the posterior mediastinum, usually on the left. In both types of superior ectopia, the ureter and renal pelvis are usually free of anomalies. The frequency of this finding at autopsy has been reported to be 1 in 13,000.

HORSESHOE KIDNEY

This is the most common form of renal fusion, occurring in 1/400 to 1/2000 births. It is twice as common in females as in males. It is composed of two distinct renal masses fused together in the midline (Fig. 1–4). The site and extent of fusion vary, but the lesion always demonstrates caudal ectopia and is usually anterior to the great vessels. The collecting systems face anteriorly and often

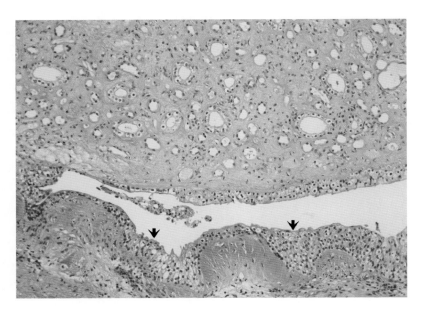

FIGURE 1–3 I▌I I   Normal kidney. In the upper half is the tip of a papilla, with cross sections of collecting ducts. In the lower half is a minor calyx, lined by layers of urothelial cells *(black arrows).*

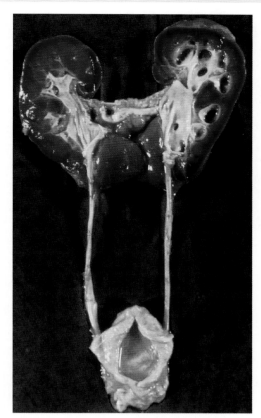

FIGURE I–4 |▮|| Horseshoe kidney. The two renal units are joined at their lower poles. One kidney shows hydronephrotic changes resulting from obstructed drainage. (Courtesy of Beverly Dahms, MD, Cleveland, OH.)

drain poorly because of anomalies of the ureteropelvic junction. Cardiac, skeletal, central nervous system, or gastrointestinal anomalies accompany this disorder in 30% of cases. Horseshoe kidneys also are involved by nephroblastoma and carcinoma of the renal pelvis more frequently than normal kidneys.

RENAL CYSTIC DISEASES

There is a lack of uniformity in the classification of cystic diseases of the kidney. The disorders described in this section are those that we believe are most likely to be encountered in urologic practice. We have elected to group them into heritable diseases, dysplastic conditions, and miscellaneous lesions.

HEREDITARY CYSTIC KIDNEY DISEASES

The hereditary cystic diseases include adult (autosomal dominant) polycystic kidney disease (AD-PKD) and infantile (autosomal recessive) polycystic kidney disease (AR-PKD). Heritable cystic kidney disease may also occur in tuberous sclerosis, von Hippel-Lindau disease, and numerous "glomerulocystic" kidney diseases.

AD-PKD and AR-PKD occur in both children and adults. Each has an associated liver lesion, without other visceral anomalies.

Adult (Autosomal Dominant) Polycystic Kidney Disease

Occurring with an approximate frequency of 1:500 to 1:1000, this disorder is linked to defects in chromosomes 4 and 16, with autosomal dominant inheritance. It is the most common cystic renal disease, as well as the most common genetic disease. Five to 10 percent of dialysis patients have AD-PKD. Hematuria, flank pain, or symptoms related to hypertension or urinary infection arise usually between 30 and 50 years of age. Progressively enlarging hepatic cysts arise in one third of patients, more commonly in women. Hypertensive vascular complications and berry aneurysms afflict up to 15% of patients.

When the disease is fully developed, both kidneys are huge but retain a vaguely reniform shape (Fig. 1–5). The collecting systems remain intact. The renal parenchyma is essentially replaced by myriad cysts measuring up to several centimeters in diameter and filled with serous, opaque, gelatinous, or hemorrhagic fluid. Renal stones are associated with the disorder in about

FIGURE I–5 |▮|| Adult polycystic kidney disease.

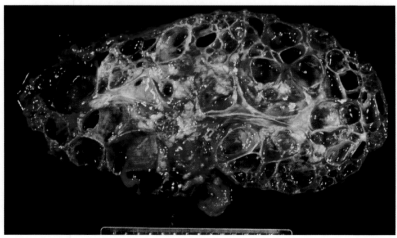

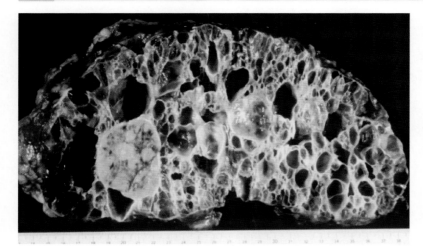

10% of patients, and the incidence of renal cell carcinoma is at least 10 times that of the normal population, occurring in 1% to 5% of AD-PKD patients (Fig. 1–6).

Microscopically, the cysts are usually lined by a layer of flat or low cuboidal epithelium, but some exhibit papillary or polypoid excrescences within the cysts, and papillary renal neoplasms may be present. Atrophic changes, chronic inflammation, and fibrosis are noted in the parenchyma between the cysts.

Infantile (Autosomal Recessive) Polycystic Kidney Disease

This condition, characterized by an autosomal recessive inheritance pattern, is linked to a defect in chromosome 6. In most cases, stillbirth or death in infancy occurs from pulmonary insufficiency. Those infants who survive longer commonly die of congenital hepatic fibrosis.

Both kidneys are massively enlarged (12 to 16 times normal size) and diffusely cystic, often with a "spongelike"

appearance. The cysts radiate through the cortex and medulla (Fig. 1–7). The collecting systems are preserved.

Microscopically, the cysts consist of ectatic dilatations of the medullary and cortical collecting ducts, lined by benign cuboidal epithelium. The uninvolved portions of the nephron unit lying between the cysts show no abnormalities. The liver shows portal fibrosis and bile duct proliferation. In some cases, a less severe degree of cyst formation permits extended survival. In these patients, the parenchyma between the cysts shows atrophic and degenerative changes with fibrosis and chronic inflammation and the progressive fibrotic changes in the liver may result in the clinical features of portal hypertension.

RENAL DYSPLASTIC CONDITIONS

The term *dysplasia* in this context does not imply any relationship to neoplasia. The term implies arrested organ development, with persistence of structures that

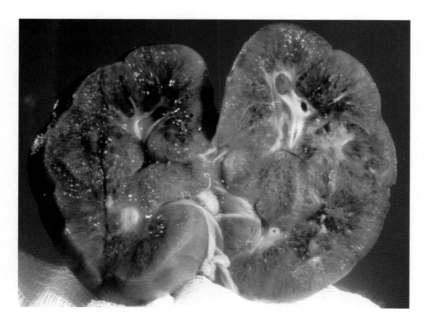

FIGURE 1–7 ▏█▏▏ Infantile polycystic kidney disease. (Courtesy of Beverly Dahms, MD, Cleveland, OH.)

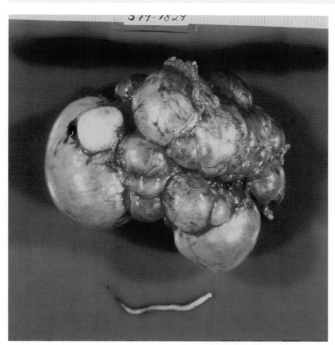

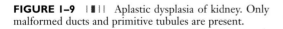

FIGURE 1–8 ▍▊▎▎ Multicystic dysplastic kidney. A short segment of ureter is at bottom; it is narrow and fibrotic at one end. (Courtesy of Beverly Dahms, MD, Cleveland, OH.)

never completely developed. Therefore, dysplastic kidneys show a wide variety of gross and microscopic findings.

There are two theories concerning the etiology of renal dysplasia. One theory holds that the basic flaw is an obstructed drainage system. An alternate theory is that there is impairment of the embryologic interaction between the ureteral bud and the metanephric blastema.

Multicystic and Aplastic Renal Dysplasia

These conditions represent opposite ends of a spectrum, varying only in the degree of cyst formation. Both lesions are commonly associated with contralateral malformations requiring correction. They are usually unilateral and are more commonly observed on the left. Bilaterality results inevitably in renal failure. Obstructed drainage appears to be causative in 90% of cases.

Multicystic dysplastic kidney is the most common renal mass in infancy, is more common in males, and most often presents as a palpable abdominal mass. In contrast, unilateral aplastic dysplasia is usually an incidental finding in later life.

On gross evaluation, the kidney size may range from small (aplastic) to very large (multicystic), with weights up to several hundred grams. The extent of cyst formation is variable. In all instances, the ipsilateral ureter is atretic or obstructed at the level of the ureteropelvic junction (Fig. 1–8).

Microscopic findings vary widely. In most cases, there are malformed ducts encased by spindle cells and lined by columnar epithelium (Fig. 1–9). Cysts of variable size and number, lined by flat cuboidal cells, are commonly observed, as are primitive tubules and malformed glomerular structures. Immature cartilage is often noted. Small components of normal nephron units may also be found.

Renal Dysplasia Associated with Other Obstructive Anomalies

Segmental dysplasia occurs in one segment (usually the upper pole) of a duplex kidney. The affected segment is the one drained by a ureter that is distally obstructed by ectopia or ureterocele (Fig. 1–10).

Dysplasia associated with lower urinary tract obstruction involves both kidneys. Examples include bladder neck obstruction, posterior urethral valves, and urethral stenosis (Fig. 1–11).

Renal Dysplasia Associated with Multiple Malformation Syndromes

Renal dysplasia has been reported as a component in a host of "multiple malformation syndromes," such as

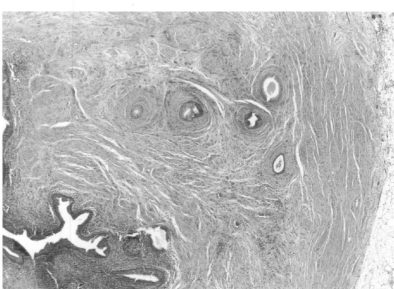

FIGURE 1–9 ▍▊▎▎ Aplastic dysplasia of kidney. Only malformed ducts and primitive tubules are present.

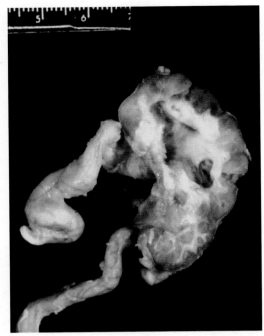

FIGURE 1-10 ▮▮▮ Segmental dysplasia of upper pole. The kidney has a duplex collecting system; the upper pole shows changes consistent with long-standing ureteral obstruction. (Courtesy of Beverly Dahms, MD, Cleveland, OH.)

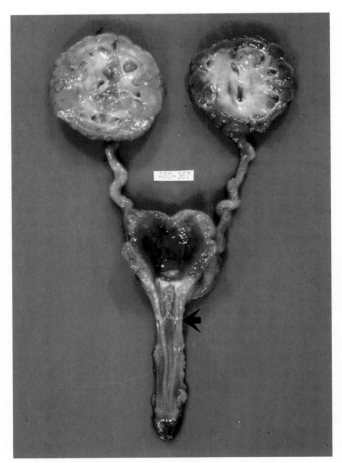

FIGURE 1-11 ▮▮▮ Bilateral renal dysplasia secondary to lower urinary tract obstruction—in this case, posterior urethral valves *(black arrow)*. (Courtesy of Raymond Redline, MD, Cleveland, OH.)

VATER syndrome, prune-belly syndrome, cloacal exstrophy, and urogenital sinus syndrome.

MISCELLANEOUS RENAL CYSTIC CONDITIONS

Acquired Cystic Kidney Disease

This is the progressive nonhereditary development of multiple cysts bilaterally in patients on long-term dialysis. The development of these cysts is independent of the type of dialysis and the original cause of renal failure and is observed in 80% to 90% of patients who have been on dialysis for 10 years. Significant complications are associated with the development of acquired cystic kidney disease (ACKD), including local hemorrhage, infection, and the risk of acquiring renal cell carcinoma.

Kidneys involved by ACKD contain multiple cysts ranging from 0.5 to 3.0 cm in diameter (Fig. 1–12). The cysts are predominantly cortical in early stages, with involvement of the medulla as dialysis continues. Eventually all renal parenchyma is obliterated by cysts. Renal tumors may be grossly identifiable in some cases.

Microscopically, the epithelium lining the cysts is flat, cuboidal, hyperplastic, or dysplastic. Solid or papillary neoplasms may be present; if so, they are bilateral in 10% and multicentric in 50% of cases. Metastasis has been documented in 20% of these neoplasms.

Medullary Sponge Kidney

This disorder afflicts 1:5,000 to 1:20,000 people but is a condition familiar to urologists because of its association with nephrolithiasis. The disorder is most often detected during the radiologic evaluation of patients with suspected nephrolithiasis. The condition is bilateral and most common in adult males, but it has been reported in childhood. Kidney size and function are normal,

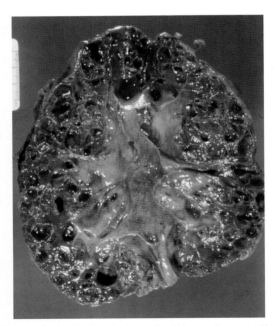

FIGURE 1-12 ▮▮▮ Acquired cystic kidney disease. All renal parenchyma has been replaced by cysts of variable size. (Courtesy of Beverly Dahms, MD, Cleveland, OH.)

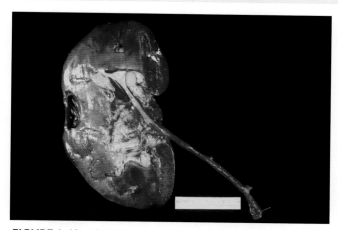

FIGURE 1–13 | ▌| | Simple cortical cyst with a smooth inner wall.

although in some patients a concentrating defect is noted. Intravenous urography shows stones and opacified medullary cysts congregating in the papillary collecting ducts in a distinctive "fan-shaped" array.

Medullary sponge kidneys may appear grossly normal, but 30% of such kidneys have a "spongelike" appearance from the presence of ectatic collecting ducts. In about one half of affected kidneys, small stones are evident in all pyramids bilaterally.

Microscopically, the collecting ducts are cystically dilated and often contain small calculi. The epithelium lining the ectatic ducts is cuboidal, flattened, or columnar. The interstitial tissue of the papillae shows fibrosis and chronic inflammation.

Simple Cortical Cyst

This is the most common renal cystic abnormality. Most are detected after age 40; incidence, multiplicity, and size increase after this age. The etiology of these cysts is uncertain and is probably multifactorial. They are more common in males and more frequently involve the left

kidney. Symptoms related to bleeding, infection, hypertension, or the sheer bulk of the cyst occur but are uncommon.

Simple cortical cyst may be single, multiple, widespread, or localized. It is usually located in the cortex and is filled with clear serous fluid (Fig. 1–13).

Microscopically, the cyst is lined by flattened epithelium. Sometimes no lining epithelium is identified (Fig. 1–14). The wall is commonly thick and fibrotic and is occasionally calcified.

INFLAMMATORY CONDITIONS OF KIDNEY

ACUTE PYELONEPHRITIS

This is an acute renal infection, in most instances caused by coliform bacteria. Bacteria gain access to the kidney usually by ureteral ascent and less commonly via the bloodstream. Patients with diabetes, pregnancy, or anomalous drainage systems are at highest risk for developing this condition.

Grossly, the affected kidney appears swollen and pale. Microabscesses may be visible in the papillae and the renal cortex. If infection breaches the renal capsule, perinephric abscess may develop.

Emphysematous pyelonephritis refers to gas bubble formation in the renal parenchyma or perirenal tissues; it is often accompanied by abscess and cortical infarcts (Fig. 1–15).

Pyonephrosis implies obstructed drainage. The collecting system is a contained abscess, and a variable degree of renal parenchymal destruction is evident (Fig. 1–16).

A kidney involved by acute pyelonephritis commonly shows ulceration of the pelvic and calyceal mucosa and infiltrates of neutrophils in the renal interstitium. Parenchymal destruction and neutrophil aggregation result in abscess formation.

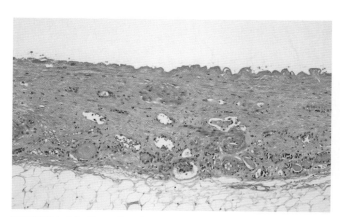

FIGURE 1–14 | ▌| | Simple cortical cyst. The wall is fibrotic. In this example, no lining epithelium is evident.

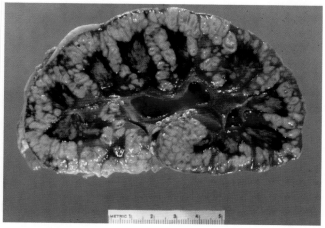

FIGURE 1–15 | ▌| | Acute emphysematous pyelonephritis (autopsy specimen). Tiny gas bubbles are visible with the purulent infiltrates, mainly in the cortex. (Courtesy of Beverly Dahms, MD, Cleveland, OH.)

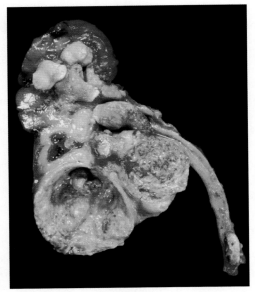

FIGURE I–16 |▌|| Pyonephrosis. An abscess cavity obliterates the lower pole. Drainage was obstructed by calculus material.

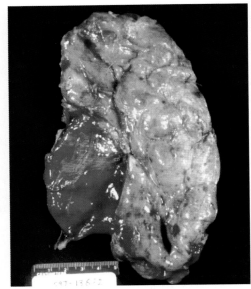

FIGURE I–18 |▌|| Chronic pyelonephritis associated with long-standing ureteropelvic junction obstruction. Renal pelvis is dilated. Much of the cortex is thin and scarred. (Courtesy of Beverly Dahms, MD, Cleveland, OH.)

CHRONIC PYELONEPHRITIS

This is a general term implying chronic interstitial renal infection caused by long-standing obstruction or vesicoureteric reflux, resulting in loss of renal parenchyma with scarring. Chronic pyelonephritis accounts for 5% to 15% of cases of end-stage renal failure. Most patients are asymptomatic until hypertension or uremia develop.

The gross findings in chronic pyelonephritis are variable. If the condition is primarily reflux-related, the affected kidney is usually small (Fig. 1–17). If the condition is obstruction-related, the kidney may be large because of dilatation of the collecting system (Figs. 1–18

and 1–19). In either case, the cortical surface is distorted by irregular scars that are often "saddle shaped." Beneath the scars, the renal cortex is thin and the papillae are scalloped or obliterated, causing the affected calyces to appear dilated. The renal parenchyma adjacent to scarred regions may appear grossly normal.

Microscopically, chronic pyelonephritis consists of interstitial fibrosis, tubular atrophy, and sclerosis of glomeruli, often patchy in distribution. The interstitial inflammation is mixed but is composed mainly of lymphocytes. Tubules usually contain eosinophilic material, a feature known as *thyroidization*. Arteries and arterioles commonly show fibrosis, mural hyalinization, and occlusion (Fig. 1–20).

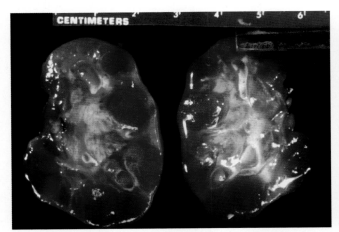

FIGURE I–17 |▌|| Chronic pyelonephritis associated with long-standing vesicoureteric reflux. The kidney is small, the papillae are blunted, and saddle-shaped scars replace portions of the cortex (Ask-Upmark kidney). (Courtesy of Beverly Dahms, MD, Cleveland, OH.)

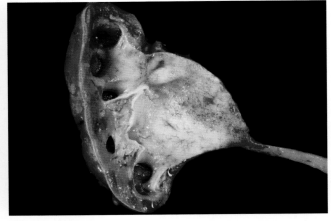

FIGURE I–19 |▌|| Chronic pyelonephritis associated with long-standing ureteropelvic junction obstruction. Calyces are dilated and papillae are blunted. The cortex is thin.

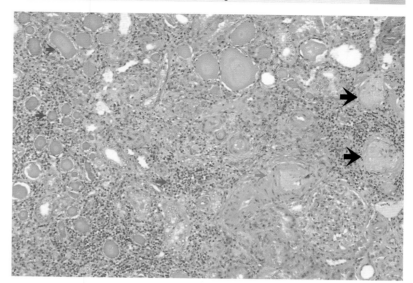

FIGURE 1–20 ▮ ▮ | | Chronic pyelonephritis. The interstitium is extensively infiltrated by chronic inflammatory cells *(red arrow)*. Tubules contain eosinophilic material ("thyroidization") *(blue arrows)*. The walls of blood vessels are thickened *(green arrow)*. Sclerotic glomeruli are seen at far right *(black arrows)*.

PAPILLARY NECROSIS

This is necrosis of a component of the renal medulla, which can result from analgesic abuse, diabetes mellitus, acute pyelonephritis, urinary obstruction, sickle cell disease, hypoxia, or dehydration. The necrosis results from tissue infarction caused by occlusion of vessels supplying the renal papilla. Subsequent sloughing of the papilla is associated with hematuria and renal colic (Fig. 1–21).

A line of demarcation is grossly evident between the congested viable kidney and the pale infarcted papillary tip. After the papilla sloughs, an irregular excavation remains. Granulation tissue and residual necrosis in variable phases of healing at the demarcation site are seen microscopically.

XANTHOGRANULOMATOUS PYELONEPHRITIS

This condition affects all age groups, although most patients are 30 to 60 years old. It is more common in females and mimics renal malignancy clinically, radiologically, grossly, and microscopically. Signs and symptoms include fever, flank pain, anorexia, malaise, and weight loss. There is a history of present or past urinary infection in up to 70% of cases. A tender flank mass may be noted. The majority of affected kidneys (50% to 70%) are nonfunctional, with stones in 20% to 70%.

The cut surface shows multiple golden-yellow nodules ranging up to 3 cm in diameter (Fig. 1–22). The yellow color is caused by the presence of lipid in macrophages. The process may be diffuse, segmental, or focal. The papillae are blunted, and the renal pelvis contains purulent material and, commonly, stones. The inflammatory process often extends into the perirenal fat.

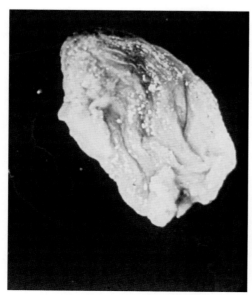

FIGURE 1–21 ▮ ▮ | | Papillary necrosis. This sloughed infarcted papilla caused renal colic and was extracted from the distal ureter with a stone basket.

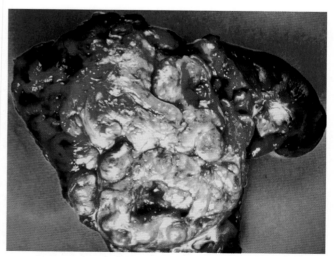

FIGURE 1–22 ▮ ▮ | | Xanthogranulomatous pyelonephritis. The inflammatory process has obliterated much of the kidney and has extended to involve perirenal soft tissues. (From Murphy WM: Urological Pathology, 2nd ed. Philadelphias, WB Saunders, 1996.)

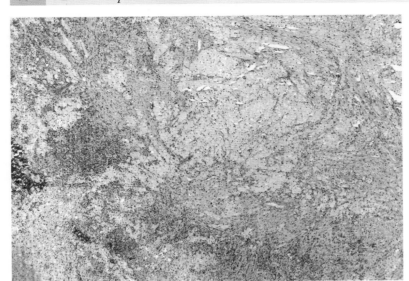

FIGURE I–23 ▮▮▮▮ Xanthogranulomatous pyelonephritis. Fibroconnective tissue is extensively infiltrated by small dark lymphocytes and plasma cells and by numerous pale-staining foamy macrophages. Lipid in the macrophages imparts the golden-yellow color noted grossly.

Microscopically, the nodules consist of necrotic debris and neutrophils centrally, surrounded by a zone of lipid-laden macrophages (which may be mistaken for tumor cells of clear cell carcinoma), plasma cells, eosinophils, and lymphocytes (Figs. 1–23 and 1–24). There is usually a fibrous reparative reaction (granulation tissue) at the periphery of the nodules, which may be difficult to distinguish from a spindle cell neoplasm. Multinucleated giant cells may also be present in the peripheral fibrous tissue.

MALAKOPLAKIA

Renal involvement by malakoplakia is rare; the condition much more commonly affects the urinary bladder. Commonly, the patient is a middle-aged woman with a history of recurrent urinary tract infection.

The cut surface of the kidney shows soft yellow-brown parenchymal nodules. Microscopically, the nodules consist of aggregates of large eosinophilic macrophages (von Hansemann histiocytes), many containing targetoid laminated mineral inclusions (Michaelis-Gutmann bodies). The inclusions are composed of incompletely digested bacteria and contain calcium or iron, demonstrable with special stains. The disorder is related to macrophage dysfunction.

TUBERCULOSIS

Most patients diagnosed with renal tuberculosis are younger than 50 years of age. Renal infection by tuberculosis results from hematogenous dissemination of the infectious agent and occurs in up to 5% of patients with pulmonary tuberculosis. In most instances, clinical or

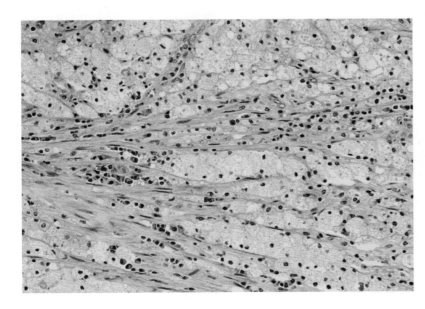

FIGURE I–24 ▮▮▮▮ Xanthogranulomatous pyelonephritis. Foamy macrophages predominate; lymphocytes, plasma cells, and occasional eosinophils are also present.

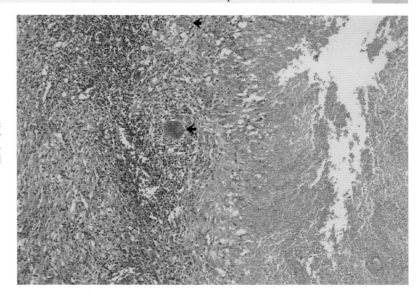

FIGURE 1–25 ▐▌▐▐ Renal tuberculosis. At right is a cavity containing caseous material. The wall of the cavity is densely infiltrated by inflammatory cells, mainly lymphocytes and epithelioid histiocytes. Multinucleated giant cells are also present *(arrows).*

radiologic pulmonary disease is not evident when renal tuberculosis is diagnosed. Symptoms may result from renal medullary necrosis (polyuria due to a concentrating defect), or ureteral obstruction (flank pain), or bladder fibrosis (urinary frequency or dysuria).

The kidney shows caseous necrosis and/or cavitation centered on the medulla, with variable loss of cortical tissue. Fibrosis and stenosis of the renal pelvis and/or ureter may be present, with secondary dilatation of the upper collecting system caused by obstruction.

Microscopically, necrotizing granulomatous inflammation with caseous necrosis is present (Fig. 1–25). Mycobacterial organisms may be demonstrable in areas of necrosis with the use of acid-fast stains. Resolution of the inflammatory process produces local scarring (fibrosis).

BENIGN RENAL EPITHELIAL NEOPLASMS

RENAL ADENOMA

Renal adenoma is usually discovered incidentally, with a frequency of up to 23% in autopsy studies. Lesions smaller than 5 mm are considered benign. Lesions larger than 5 mm in diameter are considered to be potentially malignant and do not qualify for the term *adenoma.*

Renal adenoma appears as a pale gray or yellow well-delineated cortical nodule, often located immediately beneath the renal capsule. Microscopically, it is composed of small cuboidal cells with benign nuclei and little cytoplasm arranged in papillary or tubular arrays. There is usually no fibrosis or inflammation at the interface between the adenoma and normal renal parenchyma (Fig. 1–26).

RENAL ONCOCYTOMA

About 5% of renal neoplasms excised surgically are oncocytomas. This tumor arises in collecting duct epithelium.

The average patient age is 62 years, and males are affected about twice as often as females. Rare cases have been reported in children. Oncocytoma is usually asymptomatic, and most tumors are discovered incidentally. Rarely, it presents with the "classic triad" of hematuria, flank pain, and palpable abdominal mass. Most are solitary, but rare cases of multiple oncocytomas arising in a single kidney (renal oncocytomatosis) occur. In 4% of cases, oncocytoma is bilateral. It is considered benign.

Oncocytoma is classically well circumscribed, mahogany brown, and without gross evidence of necrosis (Fig. 1–27). Hemorrhage is absent or minimal. Central stellate white or gray fibrosis is commonly present.

Microscopically, oncocytoma is composed of round to oval tumor cells with abundant finely granular eosinophilic cytoplasm, forming "organoid" nests in an edematous or fibrous stromal background (Figs. 1–28

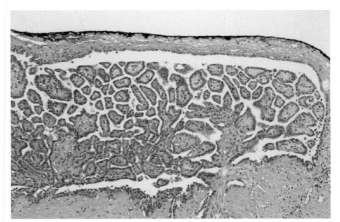

FIGURE 1–26 ▐▌▐▐ Papillary adenoma. This 3-mm papillary lesion was noted incidentally in a nephrectomy specimen containing a clinically evident clear cell renal cell carcinoma.

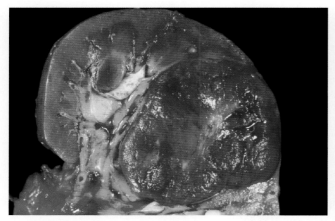

FIGURE 1–27 ▮▮▮▮ Renal oncocytoma. Tumor is mahogany brown, well circumscribed, and contains areas of central scarring.

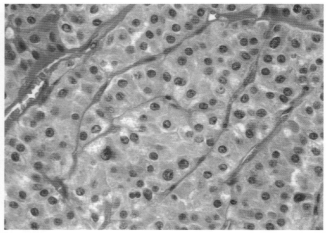

FIGURE 1–29 ▮▮▮▮ Renal oncocytoma. Cells have abundant finely granular eosinophilic cytoplasm and fairly uniform nuclei with small inconspicuous nucleoli. Some degree of nuclear atypia may be seen. Mitotic figures and necrosis are absent.

and 1–29). Tumor cells may also be arranged in diffuse sheets or tubular structures. Necrosis is absent, and mitotic figures are absent or rare. A minor component of cells with enlarged bizarre nuclei is often present. Microscopic extension of tumor into small veins or perirenal fat is observed in some tumors and is considered "atypical."

Oncocytic renal neoplasms with gross vascular invasion or extension into perirenal fat, easily detected mitotic figures, necrosis, papillary architecture, components of clear or spindle cells, or chromophobe-type vesicles evident by electron microscopy are usually excluded from consideration for the diagnosis of oncocytoma. The diagnosis of oncocytoma on a limited specimen (core biopsy or fine-needle aspiration) is perilous.

METANEPHRIC ADENOMA

Metanephric adenoma is a rare tumor that occurs in children and adults. It is twice as common in females as in males. It is usually asymptomatic, and most cases have been discovered incidentally. Some patients have been noted to have polycythemia. Its biologic behavior is benign.

It is gray, yellow, or tan and sharply circumscribed. Focal hemorrhage or necrosis may be grossly apparent. Microscopically, it resembles the epithelial component of Wilms' tumor. It is extremely cellular and lacks a fibrous interface with the adjacent renal tissue. This type of adenoma is composed of small cells with round uniform nuclei and minimal cytoplasm. Mitotic figures are absent or rare. The tumor cells form small acini or tubules, which may be so small that they appear solid. Papillae or glomeruloid structures are sometimes observed (Figs. 1–30 and 1–31).

A variant of this neoplasm, known as *nephrogenic adenofibroma*, is similar morphologically but has a spindle

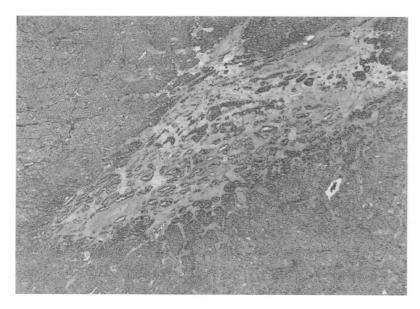

FIGURE 1–28 ▮▮▮▮ Renal oncocytoma. Cells form organoid nests and a few small tubules. Some are dispersed in a fibrous matrix, imparting an "archipelaginous" appearance.

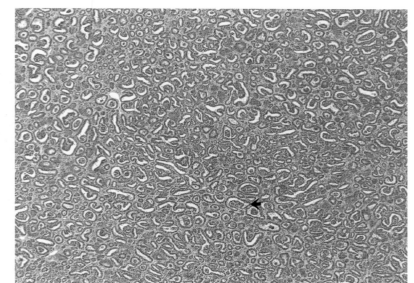

FIGURE 1–30 ▌▌▌ Metanephric adenoma. Densely cellular neoplasm, forming small tubular structures. Focally, the architecture appears "glomeruloid" *(arrow).*

cell stromal component. It is more common in young patients, with a mean age of 16 years, and is more commonly associated with polycythemia.

Cystic Nephroma

Cystic nephroma is not a purely epithelial neoplasm; it is composed of a mixture of epithelial and stromal elements. However, it is included in this section because it is at least partially epithelial and is benign. A discussion of the distinction between cystic nephroma and cystic partially differentiated nephroblastoma is given in the section on renal tumors in children.

The great majority of patients with cystic nephroma are women older than 30 years of age. In most cases, cystic nephroma is discovered incidentally, although some are heralded by flank pain and/or hematuria. An abdominal mass is palpable in some patients. Cystic nephroma is cured by complete surgical excision but may recur if it is incompletely excised. Rarely, sarcoma develops in a background of cystic nephroma.

Cystic nephroma is well circumscribed, with a thick fibrous pseudocapsule (Fig. 1–32). Tumor size is quite variable; average diameter is 9 cm. The tumor consists entirely of cysts ranging up to 5 cm in diameter with no solid nodules. The septa between the cysts are thin enough to be translucent.

Microscopically, the cysts are lined by low cuboidal or "hobnail" epithelial cells, demonstrating no appreciable mitotic activity (Fig. 1–33). The septa between the cysts are composed of myxoid or collagenous tissue; they contain no fat, skeletal muscle, smooth muscle, or blastemal elements.

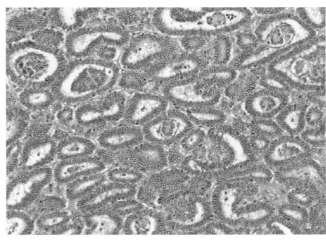

FIGURE 1–31 ▌▌▌ Metanephric adenoma. Very little stroma is present. Tumor cells are small, dark, and uniform, with minimal cytoplasm.

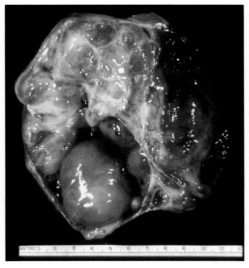

FIGURE 1–32 ▌▌▌ Multilocular cystic nephroma. Cysts are separated by broad fibrous septa.

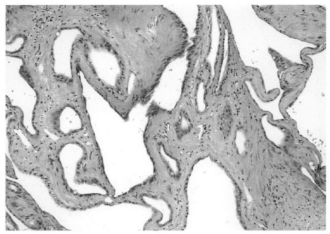

FIGURE 1–33 ▮▮▮ Multilocular cystic nephroma. Collagenous septa of variable thickness are lined by flat, inconspicuous, low cuboidal cells. Note absence of clear cells and absence of any components of nephroblastoma.

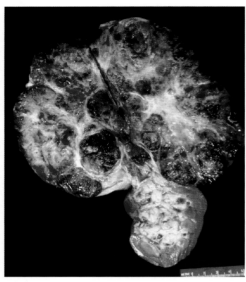

FIGURE 1–34 ▮▮▮ Renal cell carcinoma, clear cell type, Fuhrman nuclear grade 3. Areas of hemorrhage and necrosis are evident.

MALIGNANT RENAL EPITHELIAL NEOPLASMS

RENAL CELL CARCINOMA

About 23,000 new cases of renal cell carcinoma (RCC) are reported each year. Numerous risk factors have been identified, of which smoking, obesity, and acquired cystic kidney disease are most often cited. The vast majority of patients are adults, but patients in the first 2 decades of life with RCC have also been reported. Males are affected twice as often as females. Detection of RCC may result from investigation of local symptoms (hematuria, flank pain), systemic symptoms (paraneoplastic syndromes), or symptoms of metastatic disease, or may be incidental (radiologic imaging for reasons other than renal disorders).

Classification of Renal Cell Carcinoma

Before 1997 there was lack of uniformity in the classification of RCC. At a consensus conference in Rochester, Minnesota, in 1997, the following classification of RCC was proposed. This classification has achieved widespread acceptance since that time.

> Conventional clear cell RCC
> Papillary RCC
> Chromophobe RCC
> Collecting duct RCC
> RCC, unclassified (purely sarcomatoid tumors; tumors with unrecognizable morphology)

Conventional Clear Cell Renal Cell Carcinoma

This neoplasm accounts for about 75% of surgically resected RCC. It is believed to arise from proximal tubular epithelium. Cytogenetically, it is associated with inactivation of a tumor suppressor gene on chromosome 3p. The majority occur sporadically, but the incidence of clear cell RCC is markedly increased in certain geneti-

cally transmitted diseases, including von Hippel-Lindau disease and tuberous sclerosis. In 4% to 13% of patients, multiple clear cell RCC are observed in the affected kidney; bilaterality occurs in 0.5% to 3.0% of patients.

Clear cell RCC is classically solitary, bosselated, well circumscribed, solid, highly variegated, and orange-yellow, with areas of necrosis, hemorrhage, and fibrosis (Fig. 1–34). Satellite lesions are common. Diffuse parenchymal infiltration with obliteration of normal renal parenchyma is observed in a small minority of cases. Cysts are commonly present and vary greatly in size and degree of prominence. Extension of carcinoma into the renal vein is often present (Figs. 1–35 and 1–36).

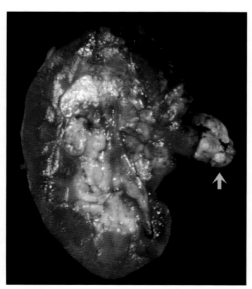

FIGURE 1–35 ▮▮▮ Renal cell carcinoma growing within and protruding from the renal vein *(arrow)*. (Courtesy of Jan Gorniak, DO, Cleveland, Ohio.)

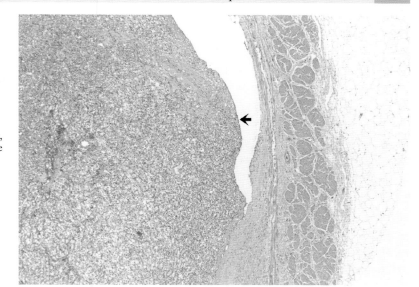

FIGURE 1–36 I ▌ I I Renal cell carcinoma, at left, growing within and adherent to the muscular wall of the renal vein *(arrow)*.

Microscopically, clear cell RCC is composed of cells with abundant clear cytoplasm (Fig. 1–37). Clonal cell populations may have eosinophilic granular cytoplasm or sarcomatoid features. The tumor cells form compact nests, tubules, or cystic structures, interspersed with a rich network of thin-walled blood vessels. Scattered papillary structures may be present. Areas of necrosis, hemorrhage, calcification, and fibrosis are common, and deposits of cholesterol crystals and hemosiderin are often observed. Tumor cell nuclei show variations in size, shape, and degree of nucleolar prominence; these features define the Fuhrman nuclear grading system.

Grade 1   Small round uniform nuclei, up to 10 μm, inconspicuous nucleoli (Fig. 1–38)
Grade 2   Nuclei slightly irregular, up to 15 μm, readily evident uniform nucleoli (Fig. 1–39)
Grade 3   Nuclei very irregular, up to 20 μm, large prominent nucleoli (Fig. 1–40)
Grade 4   Nuclei bizarre, spindle or multilobated, over 20 μm, macronucleoli (Fig. 1–41)

Renal cell carcinoma of any type may contain areas with *sarcomatoid* features—cytologic and architectural findings usually associated with sarcoma (Fig. 1–42). Occasionally, RCC is entirely sarcomatoid, with no recognizable epithelial elements (Figs. 1–43 and 1–44).

A variant of the neoplasm described previously is *multilocular cystic clear cell RCC*, a tumor composed entirely of cysts, without nodules of solid tumor (Fig. 1–45). The clear cell population lines cyst walls and forms small aggregates in the septa between the cysts (Fig. 1–46). Nuclear grade is low. No instance of clinically malignant behavior by this neoplasm has been reported.

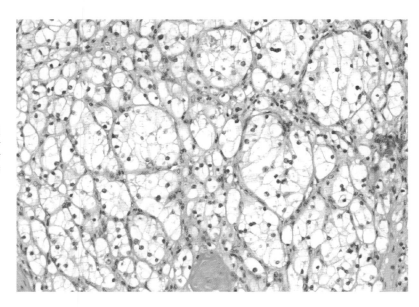

FIGURE 1–37 I ▌ I I Renal cell carcinoma, clear cell type. The tumor cells form small nests, surrounded by delicate blood vessels. The cytoplasm appears optically clear because glycogen and lipids are removed from the cytoplasm by chemicals used in histologic processing.

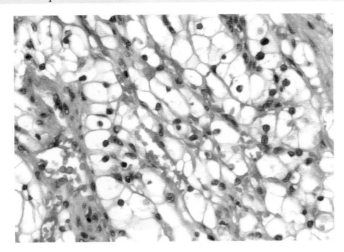

FIGURE 1–38 ▐▌▐▐ Fuhrman nuclear grade 1. Nuclei are barely larger than red cells; nucleoli are absent or barely discernible.

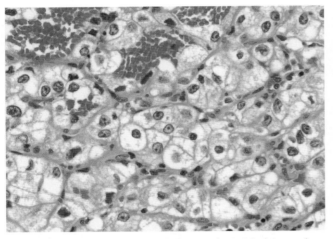

FIGURE 1–39 ▐▌▐▐ Fuhrman nuclear grade 2. Nuclei are about twice the diameter of a red cell; nucleoli are readily identified but are not conspicuous.

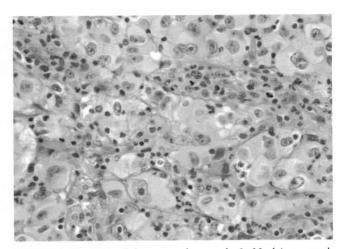

FIGURE 1–40 ▐▌▐▐ Fuhrman nuclear grade 3. Nuclei are much larger than red cells; macronucleoli are present in some cells. Many cells of this clear cell carcinoma are eosinophilic, a common finding in this cancer.

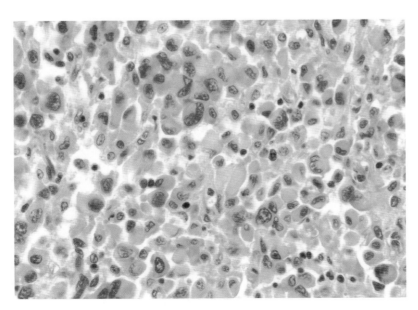

FIGURE 1–41 ▐▌▐▐ Fuhrman nuclear grade 4. Nuclei are large, many contain macronucleoli, and many are markedly distorted or multilobated, that is, "bizarre."

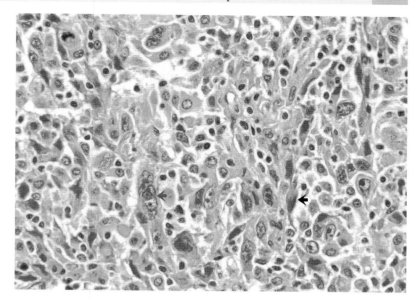

FIGURE 1–42 ▮▮▮ This area of tumor with pleomorphic *(blue arrow)* and spindle cell *(black arrow)* nuclear morphology was noted in a sarcomatoid papillary renal cell carcinoma.

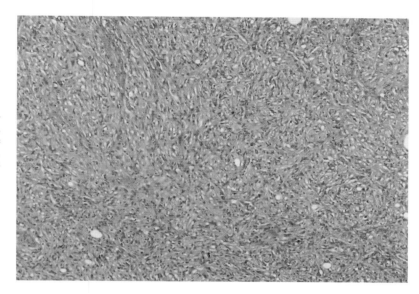

FIGURE 1–43 ▮▮▮ Renal cell carcinoma with exclusively sarcomatoid morphology (renal cell carcinoma, unclassified). The tumor was initially thought to be primary malignant fibrous histiocytoma of kidney; keratin immunostaining (see Fig. 1–44) proved it was epithelial in origin.

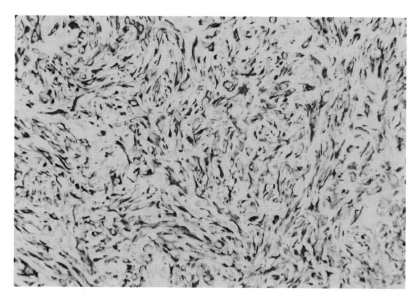

FIGURE 1–44 ▮▮▮ Tumor illustrated in Figure 1–43 immunostained with antibodies against keratin MAK6. The brown cytoplasmic staining indicates the presence of epithelial antigens, confirming that the tumor is carcinoma, not sarcoma.

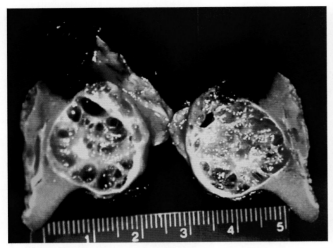

FIGURE I–45 ▮▮▮▮ Multilocular cystic clear cell renal cell carcinoma.

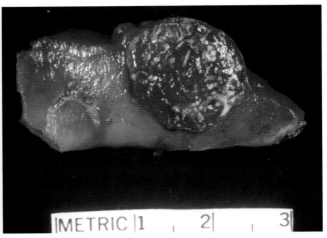

FIGURE I–47 ▮▮▮▮ Papillary renal cell carcinoma.

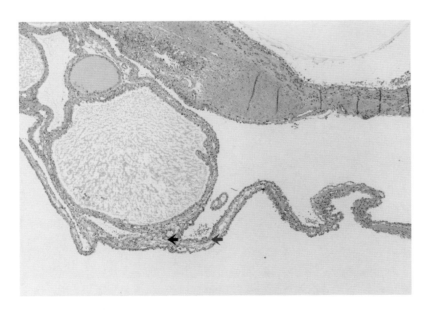

FIGURE I–46 ▮▮▮▮ Multilocular cystic clear cell renal cell carcinoma. In contrast to multilocular cystic nephroma (see Fig. 1–32), cells with clear cytoplasm line the septa *(green arrow)* and also form small aggregates within the septa *(black arrow).*

Papillary Renal Cell Carcinoma

Papillary RCC accounts for 10% to 15% of surgically resected renal carcinomas. It afflicts patients from early adulthood onward (mean age, 50 to 55 years) and occurs twice as frequently in males as in females. Cytogenetically, it is associated with trisomy or tetrasomy of chromosomes 7 and 17 and with loss of the Y chromosome in males. Nearly half of carcinomas arising in kidneys with end-stage disease are papillary RCC.

Papillary RCC is usually pseudoencapsulated and spherical and may be light gray, tan, yellow, or brown (Fig. 1–47). Most tumors have extensive hemorrhage and necrosis. Cystic degeneration is common, and one third have areas of calcification. The microscopic diagnosis of papillary RCC is based on the architecture of the tumor, rather than on the appearance of the tumor

cells, which can be quite variable. Papillary or tubulopapillary structures lined by a single layer of tumor cells are readily evident in 90% of papillary RCC. Abundant foamy macrophages are commonly present in the stroma of the fibrovascular cores (Fig. 1–48). Calcified "psammoma bodies" may be present. In some cases the fibrovascular cores are tightly packed to form "parallel arrays" (Fig. 1–49), and in rare instances the tumor cells are so tightly packed that it is difficult to discern either papillary or tubular structures.

Some papillary RCCs are composed of small basophilic cells with little cytoplasm, whereas others consist of large cells with abundant eosinophilic cytoplasm. In either case, the nuclei tend to be small, uniform, nearly round, and without prominent nucleoli. In a minority of cases, tumor cell nuclei show enlarge-

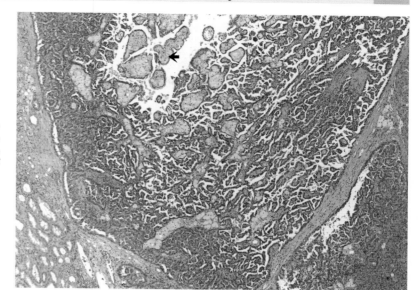

FIGURE 1–48 |▊|| Papillary renal cell carcinoma. The papillary fronds have an "arborizing" appearance. The septa are infiltrated in many areas by large, pale, foamy macrophages, a finding often seen in this tumor (*arrow*).

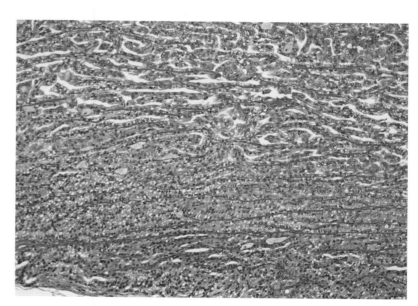

FIGURE 1–49 |▊|| Papillary renal cell carcinoma. In this architectural variant, thin fibrovascular cores are oriented parallel to one another, forming "parallel arrays."

ment, hyperchromasia, and nucleolar prominence, and these tumors have been shown to exhibit more aggressive biologic behavior. Papillary RCC sometimes has a sarcomatoid component.

Chromophobe Renal Cell Carcinoma

Chromophobe RCC was first described in 1985 and accounts for about 5% of surgically resected renal carcinomas. It affects men and women equally. The average patient age at the time of diagnosis is 55 years, with an age range of 27 to 86 years. Cytogenetically, it is characterized by loss of entire chromosomes (1, 2, 10, 13, 6, 21, 17). It arises from collecting duct epithelium. The prognosis for chromophobe RCC is better than that for clear cell or papillary RCC.

Chromophobe RCC is usually solitary, spherical, solid, and well circumscribed. The cut surface is typically gray, beige, or brown, and in most instances necrosis and hemorrhage are minimal or absent (Fig. 1–50). The microscopic findings in chromophobe RCC are distinctive. The tumor cells form solid sheets intersected by thick fibrovascular strands. Tubule formation may be present focally. Tumors are composed of two distinct cell types: typical and eosinophilic. Typical chromophobe RCC is composed of large, polygonal cells of variable size, with prominent cell membranes and pale flocculent or finely granular cytoplasm, admixed with a minor component of small eosinophilic cells (Fig. 1–51). Cell nuclei are generally 10 to 15 μm in diameter and demonstrate moderate pleomorphism and modest nucleolar prominence. In the eosinophilic variant, tubular architecture is more prominent. Tumor cells contain dense granular cytoplasm with pronounced eosinophilia. Cytoplasmic retraction away from the nucleus creates a "perinuclear

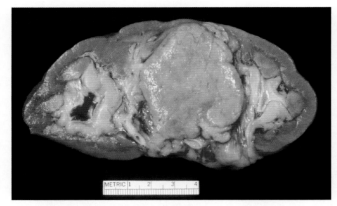

FIGURE 1–50   ▮▮▮   Chromophobe renal cell carcinoma.

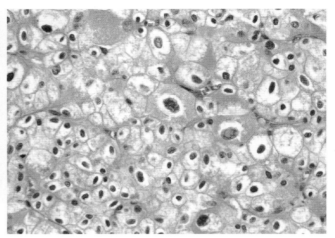

FIGURE 1–52   ▮▮▮   Chromophobe renal cell carcinoma. Cytoplasm is finely granular and eosinophilic. Cytoplasmic clearing around nuclei creates a perinuclear halo effect. Many nuclei appear "raisinoid."

halo effect." The nuclei are often quite irregular, with a "raisinoid" appearance (Fig. 1–52). The distinction of eosinophilic variant of chromophobe RCC from oncocytoma is difficult in some cases.

Ancillary studies can be helpful in diagnosing chromophobe RCC. Tumor cells show positive immunohistochemical staining for epithelial membrane antigen (Fig. 1–53) and for paralbumin and no staining for vimentin. Histochemical staining for Hale's colloidal iron is positive. Electron microscopy demonstrates the presence of distinctive cytoplasmic membrane-bound vesicles, probably derived from mitochondria. Abundant mitochondria are also present in the eosinophilic variant.

Collecting Duct Carcinoma

This neoplasm arises in collecting duct epithelium. It is the least common type of RCC, accounting for about 1% of surgically resected carcinomas. Cytogenetic studies associate it with loss of heterozygosity in chromosomes 1q and 6p. Clinical stage is often advanced at the time of diagnosis, and prognosis is poor.

Because collecting ducts extend from the medulla to the cortex, collecting duct carcinoma (CDC) can originate anywhere in the parenchyma. The cut surface of

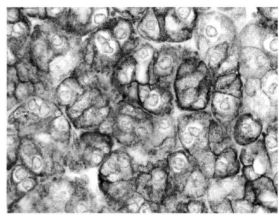

FIGURE 1–53   ▮▮▮   Chromophobe renal cell carcinoma. Immunostaining with antibodies against epithelial membrane antigen demonstrates fine granularity in the cytoplasm, probably corresponding to the cytoplasmic microvesicles seen in this tumor.

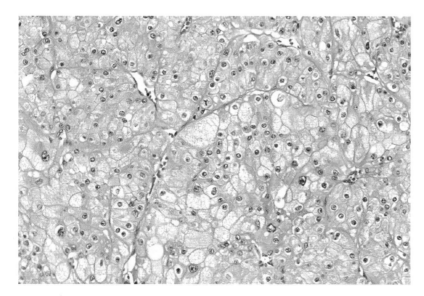

FIGURE 1–51   ▮▮▮   Chromophobe renal cell carcinoma. Some cells are very large, with pale, flocculent cytoplasm; other are small, with compact eosinophilic cytoplasm. Cell membranes are distinct.

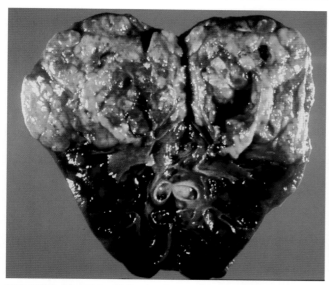

FIGURE 1–54 ▮▮▮ Collecting duct carcinoma. This tumor occurred in a patient with sickle cell trait. Collecting duct carcinoma arising in patients with sickle cell trait is also called *renal medullary carcinoma.* (Courtesy of Howard S. Levin, MD, Cleveland Clinic, Cleveland, OH.)

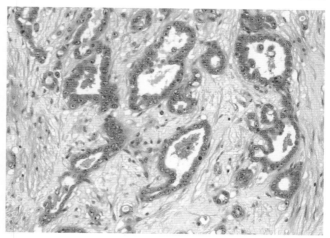

FIGURE 1–55 ▮▮▮ Collecting duct carcinoma. Irregular tubules and ducts lined by malignant cells.

CDC is usually gray-white. In contrast to other types of RCC, the borders of CDC are indistinct. Central necrosis and gross extension of tumor into perirenal tissues are common (Fig. 1–54).

Microscopically, CDC is composed of cuboidal and columnar cells with hyperchromatic and pleomorphic nuclei, forming tubules or ducts or arranged in nests and cords (Fig. 1–55). Cells lining luminal structures may display a "hobnail" appearance. The interface between tumor and the adjacent normal kidney is infiltrative (Fig. 1–56). A prominent desmoplastic and inflammatory response in the stroma around the tumor is commonly present (Fig. 1–57). A sarcomatoid component has been observed in nearly 30% of reported cases, in keeping with the generally poor prognosis of this lesion.

A variant of this neoplasm, designated *renal medullary carcinoma*, afflicts young persons with sickle cell

disease and has an exceptionally bleak prognosis (Fig. 1–58).

An additional rare variant of this neoplasm, designated *low-grade CDC*, has been described. It is often grossly cystic (Fig. 1–59). Findings suggestive of collecting duct origin include architectural features (formation of luminal structures), cytologic features (hobnail cells), mucin production, and immunohistochemical staining characteristics similar to those noted in conventional collecting duct carcinoma (Fig. 1–60). Low-grade CDC does not have an infiltrative interface with the normal adjacent kidney, nor does it incite stromal desmoplasia or inflammation. Stage and nuclear grade are low, and prognosis is favorable.

Renal Cell Carcinoma, Unclassified

Four to 5 percent of all surgically resected renal carcinomas show architectural and/or cytologic characteristics that do not conform to any of the tumor types described earlier. Renal carcinoma with purely sarcomatoid morphology is included in this category.

FIGURE 1–56 ▮▮▮ Collecting duct carcinoma, inflammatory response. Malignant tubules on the right are encroaching on normal renal parenchyma on the left. At the interface between tumor and normal kidney there is a prominent inflammatory infiltrate.

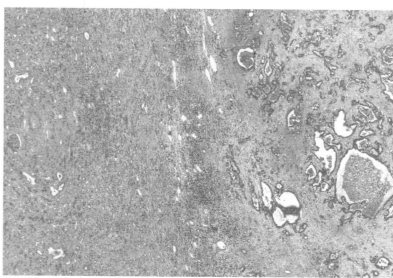

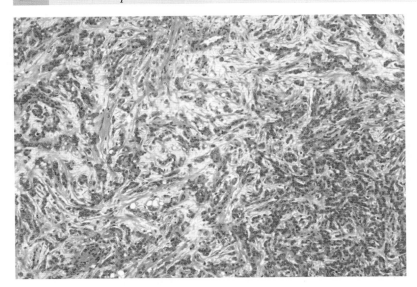

FIGURE 1-57 ▐▌▐▐ Collecting duct carcinoma, desmoplastic response. The malignant infiltrate induces fibroblasts to lay down young collagen.

STAGING RENAL CELL CARCINOMA

Staging renal cell carcinoma requires knowledge of tumor size, extent of local invasion, presence or absence of involvement of large veins or adrenal, lymph node involvement, and metastatic spread of disease. The staging definitions recommended by the AJCC are shown in Table 1–1.

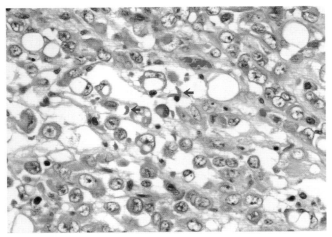

FIGURE 1-58 ▐▌▐▐ Collecting duct carcinoma in a patient with sickle cell trait *(renal medullary carcinoma)*. Section is from the tumor illustrated in Figure 1–54. Sickled red cells are present *(arrows)*.

TABLE 1-1
TNM STAGING OF RENAL CELL CARCINOMA

Primary Tumor (T)

TX	Primary tumor cannot be assessed
T0	No evidence of primary tumor
T1	Tumor 7 cm or less in greatest dimension, limited to the kidney
T1a	Tumor 4 cm or less in greatest dimension, limited to the kidney
T1b	Tumor more than 4 cm but not more than 7 cm in greatest dimension, limited to the kidney
T2	Tumor more than 7 cm in greatest dimension, limited to the kidney
T3	Tumor extends into major veins or invades adrenal gland or perinephric tissues but not beyond Gerota's fascia
T3a	Tumor directly invades adrenal gland or perinephric and/or renal sinus fat but not beyond Gerota's fascia
T3b	Tumor grossly extends into the renal vein or its segmental (muscle-containing) branches, or vena cava below the diaphragm
T3c	Tumor grossly extends into vena cava above diaphragm or invades the wall of the vena cava
T4	Tumor invades beyond Gerota's fascia

Regional Lymph Nodes (N)

NX	Regional lymph nodes cannot be assessed
N0	No regional lymph node metastases
N1	Metastases in a single regional lymph node
N2	Metastases in more than one regional lymph node

Distant Metastasis (M)

MX	Distant metastasis cannot be assessed
M0	No distant metastasis
M1	Distant metastasis

Used with the permission of the American Joint Committee on Cancer (AJCC), Chicago, Illinois. The original source for this material is the *AJCC Cancer Staging Manual, Sixth Edition* (2002) published by Springer-Verlag New York, www.springer-ny.com.

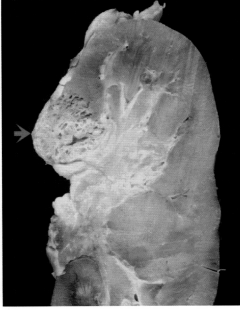

FIGURE 1-59 ▐▌▐▐ Low-grade collecting duct carcinoma. Cystic architecture is common in this tumor.

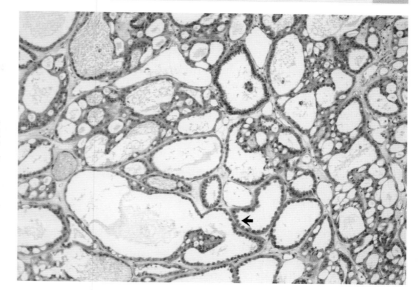

FIGURE 1–60 |▌|| Low-grade collecting duct carcinoma. Tumor is composed of variably sized tubules lined by low columnar cells, some of which have a "hobnail" appearance *(arrow)*. Nuclear grade in these tumors is low (1 or 2).

NEUROENDOCRINE RENAL NEOPLASMS

CARCINOID TUMOR

Primary renal carcinoid tumor is rare. Most patients are older than age 40 years. Symptoms may be absent, may be related to the bulk of the lesion, or may be caused by hormone production. Metastasis occurs in one third of cases.

Renal carcinoid tumor is typically large, solid, well circumscribed, and red-tan, with hemorrhage and necrosis. Microscopically, it resembles its counterparts in more usual locations. Tumor cells are arranged in nests and cords, often with a "ribbon and festoon" appearance (Fig. 1–61).

SMALL CELL CARCINOMA

Although common in the lung, small cell carcinoma originating in the kidney is rare and the differential includes metastasis from an unsuspected lung primary. The prognosis is generally poor.

Primary renal small cell carcinoma is usually large, locally infiltrative, and commonly associated with regional lymph node metastases. The microscopic appearance is similar to that of tumors arising in more usual sites. Tumors consist of sheets of "oat cells" or intermediate cells, with dispersed nuclear chromatin, nuclear molding, absent or inconspicuous nucleoli, abundant mitotic figures, and widespread necrosis.

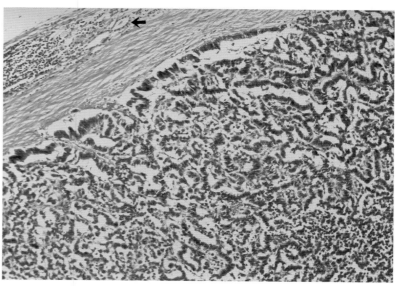

FIGURE 1–61 |▌|| Renal carcinoid tumor, with complex interanastomosing luminal spaces characteristic of this neoplasm, regardless of site of occurrence. *Arrow* indicates atrophic renal tubules.

SOFT TISSUE NEOPLASMS OF THE KIDNEY

In this category, renomedullary interstitial cell tumor is by far the most common but is rarely of clinical significance. Angiomyolipoma is the lesion encountered most often in a clinical setting and is reviewed in the greatest detail. The other soft tissue neoplasms are uncommon and are discussed only briefly.

BENIGN SOFT TISSUE NEOPLASMS OF KIDNEY

Renal Angiomyolipoma

The majority of renal angiomyolipomas (AMLs) arise in female patients. About half occur in patients with tuberous sclerosis and are linked to a heritable genetic trait— loss of heterozygosity on chromosome 16p. The other half arise sporadically. Recent studies have confirmed that AML is a true neoplasm.

Up to 80% of patients with tuberous sclerosis develop AML. Their tumors are most often detected between the ages of 25 and 35 years. Tuberous sclerosis–associated tumors tend to be small, multiple, bilateral, and asymptomatic.

Patients who develop sporadic AML are usually between 45 and 55 years old at the time of diagnosis. Sporadic tumors are more often large and solitary and more likely to cause symptoms (such as flank pain) than heritable AML.

Angiomyolipoma has been associated with a variety of complications, the most common of which is hemorrhage. Hemorrhage is unlikely in tumors under 4 cm in diameter but becomes a risk in larger tumors, particularly in pregnant women. Infiltration of local structures is a rare complication, which has resulted in death in one patient. Sarcoma has developed in a background of AML in two patients. The development of innumerable bilateral tumors in patients with tuberous sclerosis may lead to obliteration of functioning renal parenchyma and subsequent renal insufficiency.

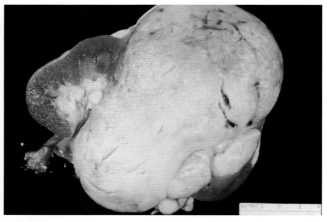

FIGURE 1–62 ▎▌▎▎ Angiomyolipoma. This example resembles mature fat.

Grossly, AML may be intrarenal, capsular, or entirely extrarenal (retroperitoneal) and up to 20 cm in diameter. The border between tumor and adjacent renal tissue is usually indistinct. A tumor extensively composed of fat may resemble lipoma, and one extensively composed of smooth muscle may mimic leiomyoma (Fig. 1–62). Focal hemorrhage is common.

The microscopic findings in AML vary according to the proportions of blood vessels, muscle, and fat comprising the tumor (Figs. 1–63 and 1–64). Smooth muscle may be present in strands or fascicles or may be radially arranged at the periphery of blood vessels, producing a "hair-on-end" appearance. Smooth muscle cells may appear epithelioid, with copious pink cytoplasm. In diagnostically difficult cases, a useful feature of AML is that the smooth muscle cells of this tumor show positive immunostaining for HMB45, a marker traditionally associated with cells of melanocytic origin. Blood vessels are usually thick walled and may have eccentric or very small lumens. Fat cells are of usual morphology; fat necrosis may be present.

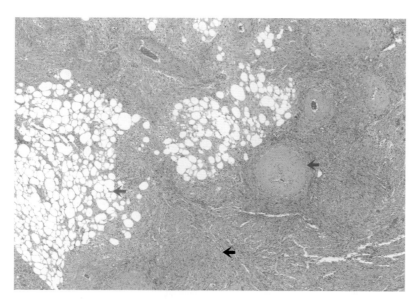

FIGURE 1–63 ▎▌▎▎ Angiomyolipoma. In this section are mature fat cells *(red arrow)*, thick-walled blood vessels *(green arrow)*, and disorganized bundles of spindle-shaped smooth muscle cells *(black arrow)*.

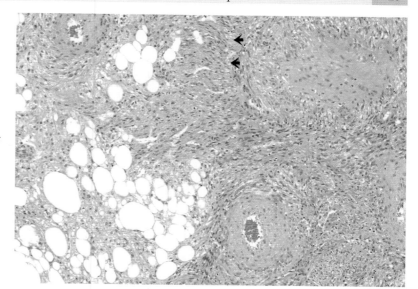

FIGURE 1–64 ▌▍▎ Angiomyolipoma. Smooth muscle cells are often perpendicularly oriented at the periphery of the thick-walled blood vessels, producing a "hair on end" appearance *(arrows)*.

Involvement of regional nodes by foci of AML is thought to represent multicentricity, not metastasis from the renal primary tumor.

Renomedullary Interstitial Cell Tumor

This lesion is extremely common, often noted incidentally at autopsy or in kidneys removed for other reasons. Occasionally it forms a pedunculated intrapelvic nodule, which may cause symptoms of obstruction. Nearly one half of people older than age 20 years have at least one renomedullary interstitial cell tumor. It is composed of renomedullary interstitial cells whose products aid in blood pressure regulation. Whether it is hyperplastic or neoplastic is unclear; it is benign.

Its typical appearance is that of a well-circumscribed white nodule, usually less than 1.0 cm in diameter, localized to the renal medulla (Fig. 1–65). It is a paucicellular tumor composed of small stellate or ovoid cells in a loose matrix of delicate stroma. It commonly encircles normal renal tubules at the periphery of the lesion.

Juxtaglomerular Cell Tumor (Reninoma)

This rare tumor arises from renin-producing smooth muscle cells lying adjacent to the afferent arteriole, so it

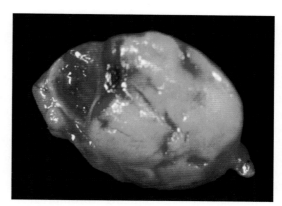

FIGURE 1–66 ▌▍▎ Juxtaglomerular cell tumor ("reninoma").

is not surprising that in all cases hypertension is present. It affects adolescents and young adults, with an average age at onset of 27 years. Females are afflicted twice as commonly as males. It does not metastasize, invade locally, or recur.

Juxtaglomerular cell tumor is tan or gray-white, rubbery, and well circumscribed (Fig. 1–66). Small cysts may be present. It is usually less than 3 cm in diameter and occasionally is so small that very careful dissection is necessary to identify it. Microscopically, it is composed of uniform round to oval cells with modest amounts of eosinophilic or clear cytoplasm. In most, the tumor cells form trabeculae in a loose myxoid background, with abundant vascularity and infiltrates of lymphocytes (Fig. 1–67). Tubules, cysts, or papillary structures may be present. Tumor cells often show positive immunohistochemical staining for renin. Electron microscopy shows unique intracytoplasmic inclusions (rhomboid granules).

Hemangioma

Hemangioma occurs most often in young to middle-aged adults, with an equal male-to-female incidence. The

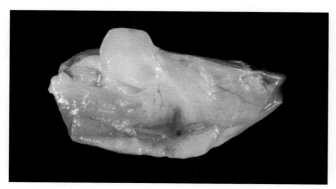

FIGURE 1–65 ▌▍▎ Renomedullary interstitial cell tumor.

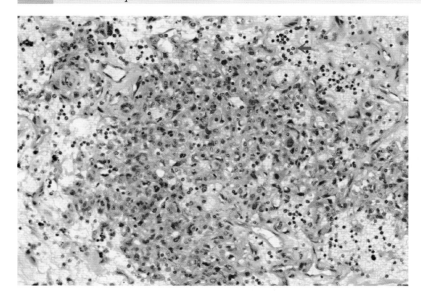

FIGURE 1–67 ▕▊▕▏ Juxtaglomerular cell tumor. Tumor cells have clear or eosinophilic cytoplasm. Background is myxoid, and aggregates of chronic inflammatory cells (*arrow*) are present.

great majority are solitary, but some are multiple and occasionally bilateral. The presenting complaint is recurrent hematuria, often accompanied by anemia.

Hemangioma may arise in any part of the kidney and may be up to 18 cm in diameter. A tumor centered in the medulla and papilla is likely to cause hematuria and to be diagnosed during life. Most are less than 1 cm in diameter and may be difficult to discern grossly. Larger tumors appear spongy red. Hemangioma consists of irregular anastomosing cavernous vascular spaces lined by endothelial cells with benign nuclei without appreciable mitotic activity, features that help distinguish this lesion from angiosarcoma. Organizing thrombi are often present.

Lymphangioma

Fewer than 50 cases of this neoplasm have been reported, the majority occurring in adults, but spanning the entire age spectrum. It is usually peripelvic but may be intrarenal. It consists of a solitary pseudoencapsulated aggregate of cysts containing clear fluid. The septa separating the cysts are composed of fibromuscular tissue. The cysts are lined by benign endothelial cells.

Leiomyoma

Leiomyoma is rarely primary in the kidney, and when present it is rarely symptomatic. The great majority occur in adults.

Tumor location may be capsular or intrarenal. The largest reported renal leiomyoma weighed 37.2 kg. Grossly, the findings are similar to those of uterine fibroid: leiomyoma is white, solid, well circumscribed, and rubbery, with a whorled cut surface. Microscopically, leiomyoma is composed of fascicles of smooth muscle fibers, without mitotic activity, necrosis, or significant nuclear atypia (Fig. 1–68). Areas of hyalinization and

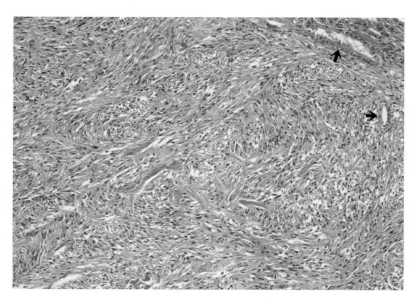

FIGURE 1–68 ▕▊▕▏ Leiomyoma of renal capsule. Tumor is composed of intersecting fascicles of smooth muscle cells. Nuclear atypia, mitotic activity, and necrosis are absent. *Arrows* indicate native renal tubules.

calcification may be noted. Distinction from smooth muscle-predominant angiomyolipoma is aided by detection of HMB45 immunoreactivity in the tumor cells of the latter.

Lipoma

Renal lipoma is rare, and almost all reported examples have occurred in middle-aged females. Grossly, lipoma is circumscribed, yellow, and lobulated and appears fatty. Microscopically, it is composed of mature adipose tissue. Differential considerations include fat-predominant angiomyolipoma and parapelvic lipomatosis.

RENAL SARCOMA

Leiomyosarcoma

Leiomyosarcoma is the most common renal sarcoma and accounts for about half of the neoplasms in this category. It can occur at any age, but most patients are over 40 years of age. Flank pain or symptoms related to mass effect are common at presentation. Prognosis is generally poor.

Leiomyosarcoma may originate in the renal capsule or the wall of the renal pelvis or renal vein. It may be intrarenal, peripheral, or mainly hilar. It is solid, circumscribed, and pale gray, with a cut surface resembling leiomyoma, with the exception that areas of hemorrhage and necrosis are often present. Microscopically, it consists of bundles of spindle cells resembling smooth muscle, and some cases are difficult to distinguish from leiomyoma. Necrosis, mitotic activity, and nuclear atypia are features favoring malignancy.

Malignant Fibrous Histiocytoma

Origin of malignant fibrous histiocytoma (MFH) in the kidney may be difficult to establish, because most originate in retroperitoneal soft tissues. Most patients are adult males. MFH is large and diffusely infiltrative. Two microscopic patterns predominate: the spindle and pleomorphic cell type (which is easily confused with sarcomatoid RCC) and the inflammatory type (which may be difficult to distinguish from xanthogranulomatous pyelonephritis).

Other Rare Sarcomas

Rare cases of hemangiopericytoma, osteogenic sarcoma, chondrosarcoma, and angiosarcoma arising in the kidney have been reported.

OTHER RENAL NEOPLASMS

LYMPHOMA

Renal involvement late in the course of systemic lymphoma is very common. In addition, there are numerous case reports of lymphoma arising in the kidney without evidence of systemic disease at the time of diagnosis. In most instances, systemic disease subsequently becomes apparent. Renal lymphoma is most commonly of large cell type. Rare cases of extramedullary plasmacytoma and Hodgkin's disease localized to the kidney have also been reported.

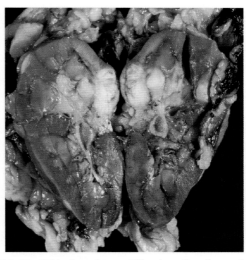

FIGURE I–69 I▊II Lymphoma, diffuse large B-cell type, forming a nodular mass in the kidney. Patient was not known to have lymphoma before surgery. (Courtesy of Wei Yang, MD, Cleveland, OH.)

Renal lymphoma may form a discrete cortical or medullary nodule (Fig. 1–69) or a large mass up to 15 cm in diameter, commonly surrounding hilar tissues. Lymphoma sometimes diffusely infiltrates and expands the renal parenchyma without forming a distinct mass lesion. Microscopically, it consists of sheets of malignant lymphoid cells filling interstitial spaces, often leaving tubules and glomeruli intact (Fig. 1–70).

TUMORS METASTATIC TO THE KIDNEY

Up to 7% of patients dying of cancer have renal metastases. The most common primary sites are lung, skin (melanoma), gastrointestinal tract, ovary, and testis. Occasionally the renal metastasis prompts resection before the primary malignancy is discovered (Fig. 1–71).

RENAL NEOPLASMS IN CHILDREN

NEPHROBLASTOMA (WILMS' TUMOR)

Nephroblastoma accounts for about 8% of solid tumors in children and 80% of pediatric renal tumors. Females are affected slightly more frequently than males, and 75% of patients are between 1 and 5 years old. Occasionally, nephroblastoma occurs in adolescents and adults. Presenting symptoms include pain, anorexia, fever, and/or gross hematuria. Hypertension is noted in some patients. An abdominal mass is palpable in 90% of patients; bilateral tumors occur in 4.4%. Numerous anomalies (cryptorchidism, hypospadias, aniridia, hemihypertrophy) and syndromes (Beckwith-Wiedemann, Drash) have been associated with nephroblastoma. Development of the neoplasm is linked to aberrations on several chromosomes, notably 11p.

Nephroblastoma is usually more than 5 cm in diameter and often weighs more than 500 g. It is usually circumscribed by a distinct pseudocapsule. Its cut surface is

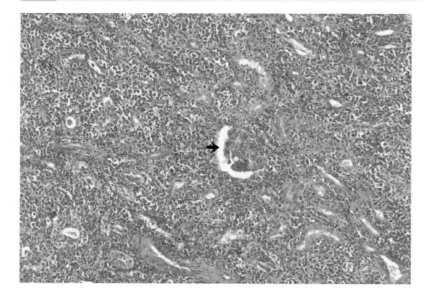

FIGURE 1–70 I I I I Lymphoma, diffuse large B-cell type. Tumor cells diffusely infiltrate the interstitium, leaving tubules and a glomerulus *(arrow)* intact.

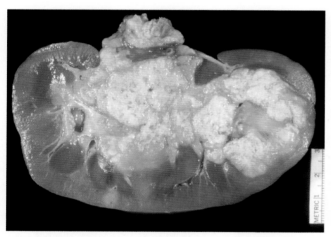

FIGURE 1–71 I I I I Squamous cell carcinoma of lung, metastatic to the kidney.

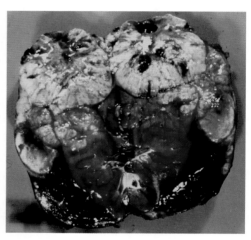

FIGURE 1–72 I I I I Nephroblastoma (Wilms' tumor). (Courtesy of Raymond Redline, MD, Cleveland, OH.)

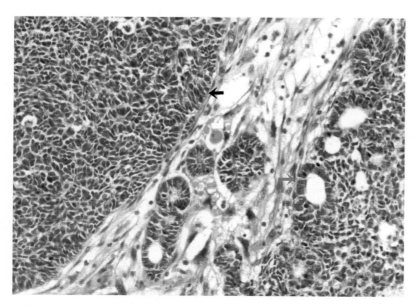

FIGURE 1–73 I I I I Wilms' tumor. Section demonstrates blastema *(black arrow,* primitive tubules *(red arrow),* and malignant stromal cells *(green arrow).*

pink or gray and commonly shows areas of hemorrhage, necrosis, and cyst formation (Fig. 1–72). Extension of tumor into the renal pelvis may impart a "botryoid" appearance. Multicentricity occurs in 5% of cases.

The microscopic findings in nephroblastoma are extremely variable, owing to the possible admixture of three components: blastema, stroma, and epithelial elements (Fig. 1–73). Blastema consists of small cells with scant cytoplasm, dark nuclei, and numerous mitotic figures, forming serpentine arrays, nodules, or diffuse sheets. The stromal component may include any of a number of mesenchymal derivatives, such as fibroblast-like spindle cells, smooth or skeletal muscle, cartilage, fat, or bone. The epithelial component most commonly consists of poorly formed tubules and glomeruli, but epithelial cells with mucinous, squamous, neural, or endocrine differentiation may also be observed.

Anaplasia in nephroblastoma is defined as the combination of cells with large multipolar mitotic figures and cells with very large hyperchromatic nuclei, at least three times the size of typical blastemal nuclei (Fig. 1–74). This feature is found in about 6% of cases, most often in patients older than 2 years old. Its presence determines "unfavorable histology," which worsens prognosis.

CYSTIC PARTIALLY DIFFERENTIATED NEPHROBLASTOMA

Cystic nephroma and cystic partially differentiated nephroblastoma are separate entities. Cystic nephroma is a disease of adults, is a composite neoplasm of stromal and epithelial elements, and has no known link to nephroblastoma. Cystic partially differentiated nephroblastoma occurs in young children and is considered part of the spectrum of Wilms' tumor.

Cystic partially differentiated nephroblastoma affects boys and girls with approximately equal frequency. It is only rarely discovered in children older than 24 months of age. Complete surgical excision of this lesion is curative.

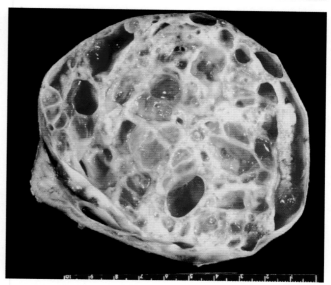

FIGURE I–75 | ▌ | | Cystic partially differentiated nephroblastoma. Tumor is circumscribed and cystic. Papillary excrescences are visible in the cystic space at far right. (Courtesy of Beverly Dahms, MD, Cleveland, OH.)

It tends to be large, measuring up to 18 cm in greatest dimension. It is circumscribed and entirely composed of variably sized cysts (Fig. 1–75). Solid nodules may be present, and papillary excrescences may be evident in the cysts. Microscopically, the cysts are lined by low cuboidal or hobnail epithelium. The septa and the solid nodules contain elements of nephroblastoma (blastema, mesenchymal stromal tissue, and/or epithelial elements) in varying degrees of differentiation.

MESOBLASTIC NEPHROMA

This neoplasm accounts for about 3% of pediatric renal neoplasms but is predominantly a tumor of infancy; two thirds of patients are younger than 3 months old, and few are more than 6 months old. Mesoblastic nephroma is the most common renal neoplasm presenting in the first 3 months of life. An association with polyhydramnios and prematurity has been noted. It is most often discovered by palpation of an abdominal mass in an infant. In rare adult cases, hematuria or hypertension is more likely to lead to the diagnosis. Some cases are unresectable, owing to tumor extension into surrounding structures. Recurrence (7%) and metastases (2%) are uncommon; most adverse outcomes have been experienced by older patients.

Mesoblastic nephroma is always unilateral and may be up to 14 cm in diameter. It is solid, bosselated, and light tan, with a trabeculated or whorled cut surface resembling uterine leiomyoma (Fig. 1–76). It infiltrates the adjacent normal parenchyma, with the result that the line of demarcation between tumor and normal kidney is indistinct. Tumor extension into perirenal fat may be evident grossly, and renal vein invasion is sometimes present. Cysts, hemorrhage, and necrosis are sometimes noted.

Two morphologic patterns are recognized microscopically and are respectively designated classic and

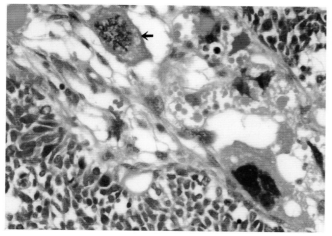

FIGURE I–74 | ▌ | | Anaplasia in Wilms' tumor. A very large hyperchromatic nucleus is at lower right (*green arrow*), and an abnormal mitotic figure is at upper left (*black arrow*).

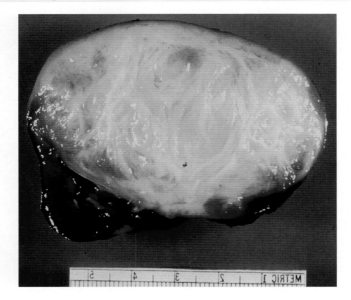

FIGURE 1–76 ▮▮▮ Mesoblastic nephroma. Tumor has a whorled and trabeculated cut surface. (Courtesy of Beverly Dahms, MD, Cleveland, OH.)

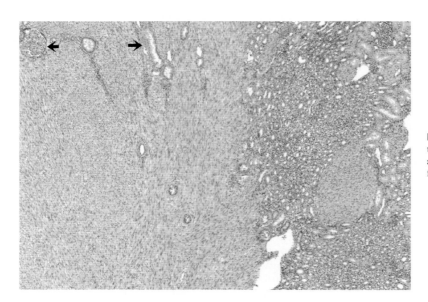

FIGURE 1–77 ▮▮▮ Mesoblastic nephroma, classic type. Fascicles of spindle-shaped tumor cells infiltrate around native glomeruli and tubules *(arrows)* at the interface between tumor and normal kidney.

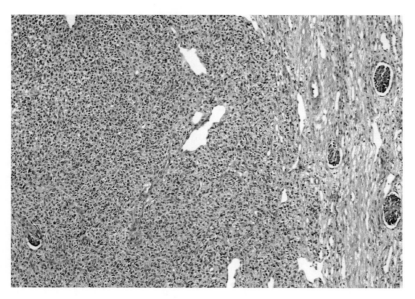

FIGURE 1–78 ▮▮▮ Mesoblastic nephroma, cellular type. Spindle and polygonal cells form a "pushing front" at the interface between tumor and normal kidney, rather than infiltrating between native structures, as seen in classic mesoblastic nephroma.

cellular mesoblastic nephroma. The classic pattern consists of interlacing fascicles of spindle cells resembling smooth muscle or fibrous tissue. Nuclei are elongated, bland, and uniform, and mitotic figures are infrequent. Tumor cells infiltrate around tubules and glomeruli at the interface between tumor and normal parenchyma (Fig. 1–77). This classic morphology is almost always present in adult tumors. Sections from the more common cellular mesoblastic nephroma show densely packed short spindle-shaped or polygonal cells with up to 30 mitotic figures per 10 high-power fields and less propensity to infiltrate normal renal structures at the interface between tumor and normal kidney (Fig. 1–78). Necrosis, hemorrhage, and cyst formation may be present. The morphologic pattern seems to have little influence on prognosis, which seems more dependent on patient age and completeness of surgical excision.

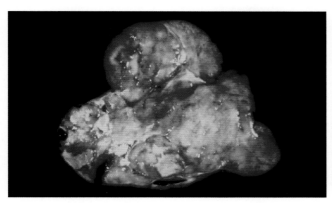

FIGURE I–79 | ▌ | | Clear cell sarcoma.

CLEAR CELL SARCOMA OF KIDNEY (BONE-METASTASIZING RENAL TUMOR OF CHILDHOOD)

This tumor accounts for about 6% of pediatric renal neoplasms. It affects children in the same age group affected most often by nephroblastoma (12 to 36 months). About two thirds of patients are male. Its name is reflective of the fact that it metastasizes to bone 10 times more often than other pediatric renal malignancies. It is resistant to treatment regimens proven to be effective for nephroblastoma, but responds to doxorubicin-based chemotherapy.

Clear cell sarcoma is always unilateral. It is well circumscribed and often weighs over 500 g. About one third contain cysts of variable size. On sectioning, some are gray and homogeneous and others are gray-tan with soft pink areas (Fig. 1–79). The cut surface may appear shiny, owing to mucin production. Microscopically, it is composed of cells with pale cytoplasm and small round to oval nuclei with dispersed chromatin and inconspicuous nucleoli (Fig. 1–80). Tumor cells are arranged in nests and cords, which are separated by septa consisting of delicate blood vessels and dark spindle cells. The degree of septal prominence varies from inconspicuous to wide and hyalinized. The interface between tumor and adjacent kidney is infiltrative, in contrast to the pushing border of nephroblastoma.

RHABDOID TUMOR OF KIDNEY

Rhabdoid tumor comprises about 2.5% of pediatric renal neoplasms. It affects males more often than females, and the vast majority of patients are younger than 3 years old, with a median age of 11 months at the time of diagnosis. Rhabdoid tumor carries the worst prognosis of any pediatric renal neoplasm; at least 80% of patients die within 1 year.

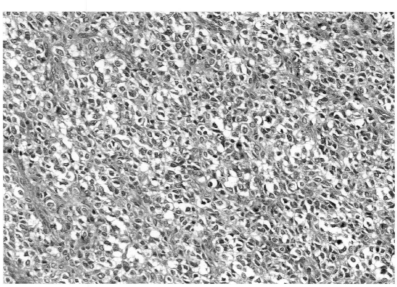

FIGURE I–80 | ▌ | | Clear cell sarcoma. Tumor consists of sheets of tumor cells with clear or lightly eosinophilic cytoplasm.

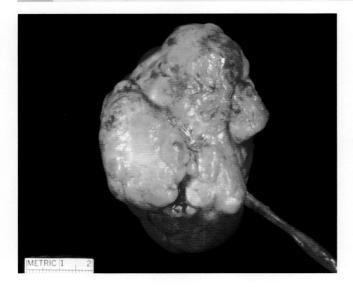

FIGURE 1–81   ▮▮▮   Rhabdoid tumor.

Rhabdoid tumor is diffusely infiltrative, particularly in the hilar region. Its cut surface is yellow-gray or light tan and friable, with areas of hemorrhage and necrosis (Fig. 1–81). It usually weighs less than 500 g. It is composed of monotonous sheets of large polygonal cells with abundant darkly eosinophilic cytoplasm (Fig. 1–82). Nuclei are vesicular, with prominent nuclear membranes and conspicuous nucleoli. Many tumor cells contain a globular eosinophilic paranuclear inclusion, which displaces the nucleus to an eccentric location. Ultrastructurally, these paranuclear inclusions are composed of whorled intermediate filaments. Despite the resemblance of the tumor cells to differentiating rhabdomyoblasts, the tumor is not of skeletal muscle derivation.

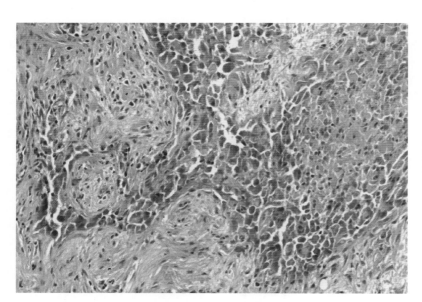

FIGURE 1–82   ▮▮▮   Rhabdoid tumor. Tumor cells have eccentric nuclei and darkly eosinophilic cytoplasm; they resemble differentiating rhabdomyoblasts.

Chapter 2

BLADDER, URETHRA, RENAL PELVIS, AND URETER

The renal pelvis, ureter, bladder, and urethra are muscular structures, are all lined by urothelium, and are all involved in the collection and expulsion of urine. Many pathologic conditions are common to all these sites.

ANATOMY AND HISTOLOGY

The renal pelvis is the site of convergence of the minor and major calyces and drains into the ureter, which averages 30 cm in length. The renal pelvis and ureter consist of intricately arranged bundles of smooth muscle with an inner lining of lamina propria and urothelium and an outer sheath of fibrous tunica adventitia, which invests these structures from the renal capsule to the urinary bladder (Figs. 2–1 and 2–2).

The urinary bladder is a hollow muscular organ with an inner lining of lamina propria and urothelium three to six cell layers thick (Fig. 2–3). The surface layer of urothelium consists of large "umbrella cells" with eosinophilic cytoplasm and large, often double nuclei.

The urothelial cells beneath the surface are uniform and much smaller than umbrella cells. They have modest amounts of pale or clear cytoplasm. Their nuclei are central, ovoid, uniform, and oriented roughly perpendicular to the basement membrane. The nuclei have dispersed chromatin and inconspicuous nucleoli. The trigone in postpubertal females is commonly covered by nonkeratinizing glycogenated squamous epithelium; this is almost certainly a normal variant (Fig. 2–4). Between the basement membrane of the urothelium and the underlying detrusor muscle is the lamina propria, consisting of loose connective tissue, scattered inflammatory cells, vascular channels, and wisps of discontinuous muscularis mucosae (Fig. 2–5). The lamina propria also normally contains invaginated aggregates of urothelial cells, called von Brunn's nests. Small aggregates of fat may be seen normally within the bladder wall, and adipose tissue covers the external aspect of the detrusor muscle.

The male urethra has prostatic, membranous, and penile segments. The prostatic urethra is surrounded by prostate tissue and receives drainage from prostatic ducts

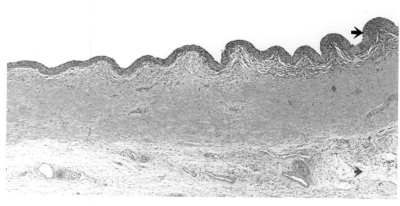

FIGURE 2–1 ❙▮❙❙ Renal pelvis, normal histology. Layers include urothelium (*black arrow*), lamina propria (*yellow arrow*), muscularis propria (*green arrow*), and adventitial soft tissues (*blue arrow*). Renal parenchyma is seen at upper right.

Several images in this chapter are courtesy of Mayo Clinic Foundation, Rochester, MN.

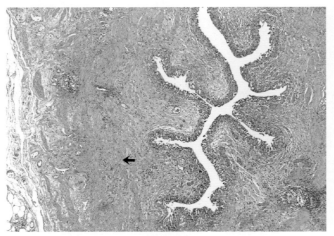

FIGURE 2–2 ▮▮▮ Ureter, normal histology. The anatomic structures are similar to those of the renal pelvis. The muscularis propria *(black arrow)* consists of interlacing smooth muscle fascicles arranged in a spiral fashion; no distinct muscle layers are evident.

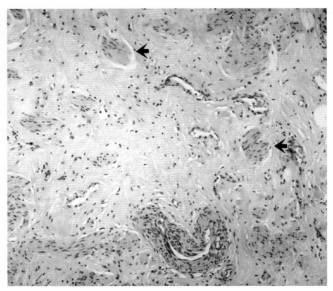

FIGURE 2–5 ▮▮▮ Lamina propria of the bladder. Loose connective tissue containing blood vessels and wispy bundles of discontinuous muscularis mucosae *(arrows)*.

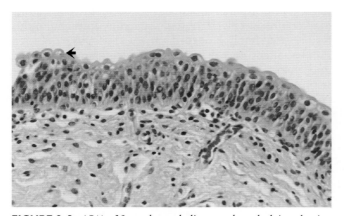

FIGURE 2–3 ▮▮▮ Normal urothelium and underlying lamina propria in the bladder. The *arrow* indicates a layer of umbrella cells at the surface.

and ejaculatory ducts. The membranous urethra traverses the urogenital diaphragm and receives secretions from Cowper's glands. The penile urethra is surrounded by corpus spongiosum and receives secretions from bulbourethral glands and mucus-secreting periurethral glands (glands of Littré). The prostatic urethra is lined by urothelium, the membranous urethra and most of the penile urethra are lined by pseudostratified columnar epithelium, and the fossa navicularis and urethral meatus are lined by nonkeratinizing squamous epithelium.

The proximal third of the female urethra is lined by urothelium, and the distal third is lined by nonkeratinizing squamous epithelium. Paraurethral (Skene's) glands empty into the distal portion of the female urethra.

BLADDER

CONGENITAL ANOMALIES

Urachal Anomalies

In early fetal development, the urachus connects the apex of the bladder to the allantois, located at the umbilicus. Failure of obliteration of the urachus (which usually occurs by the fourth month in utero) results in several malformations, which may be complicated by abdominal pain, chronic drainage from the umbilicus, infection, abscess formation, or stone formation (Fig. 2–6).

Completely patent urachus denotes free communication between the bladder and the umbilicus, with efflux of urine via the umbilicus. The condition is evident at birth. *Alternating urachal sinus* is a variant of completely patent urachus, in which loculated infections developing in potential spaces along the course of the urachus even-

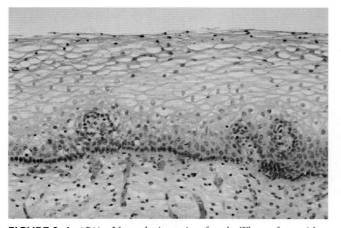

FIGURE 2–4 ▮▮▮ Normal trigone in a female. The surface epithelium is nonkeratinizing glycogenated squamous epithelium.

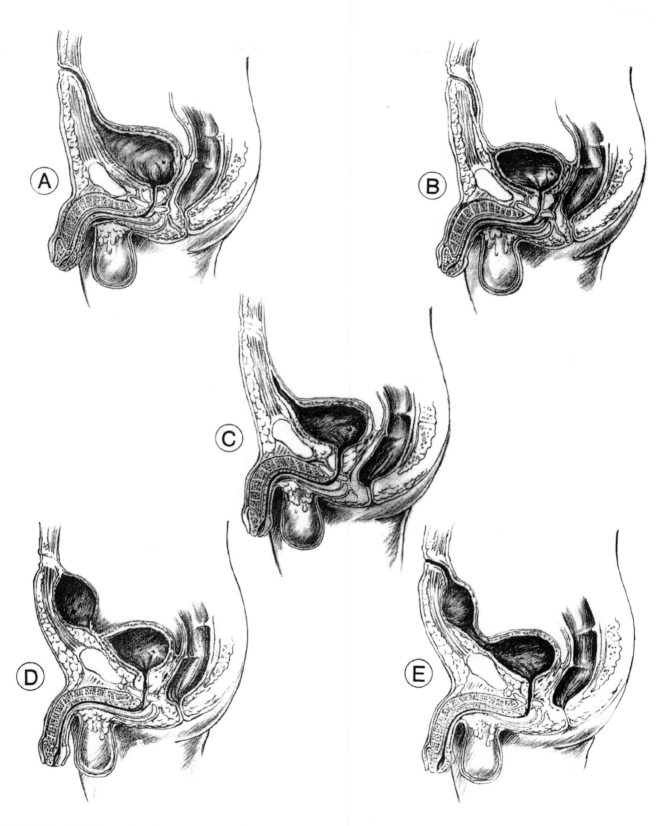

FIGURE 2–6 |▌|| Types of persistent or patent urachus. Complete patency *(A)*; umbilicourachal sinus *(B)*; vesicourachal sinus *(C)*; blindly patent urachus *(D)*; alternating urachal sinus *(E)*. (From Bostwick DG, Eble JN: Urologic Surgical Pathology. St. Louis, Mosby, 1997.)

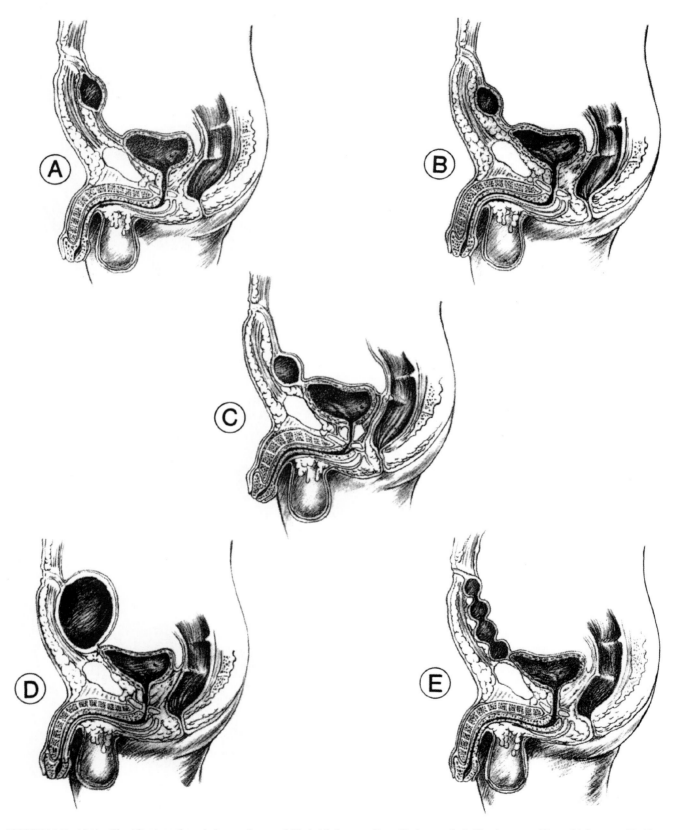

FIGURE 2-7   ▮▮▮▮   Classification of urachal cysts. Juxtaumbilical *(A)*; intermediate *(B)*; juxtavesical *(C)*; giant cyst *(D)*; multiple cysts *(E)*. (From Bostwick DG, Eble JN: Urologic Surgical Pathology. St. Louis, Mosby, 1997.)

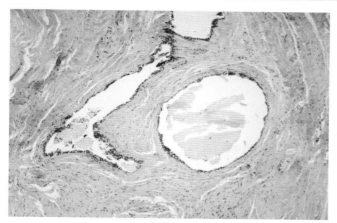

FIGURE 2–8 ▮▯▮▯ Intramural segment of urachus with mild cystic dilatation, found incidentally at autopsy.

tually drain into the bladder and via the umbilicus; the condition becomes apparent after the neonatal period.

Incompletely patent urachus may manifest as a *blind urachal cyst* (Fig. 2–7), formed by closure of the urachus at each end, an *umbilicourachal sinus*, closed at the bladder end and patent at the umbilical end, or a *vesicourachal sinus or diverticulum*, patent at the bladder end and closed at the umbilical end (Figs. 2–8 and 2–9).

Exstrophy

Exstrophy is the result of anomalous cloacal membrane development during fetal life, occurring much more commonly in males. Defective closure, including diaphysis of the symphysis pubis and abdominal wall musculature, may extend from the urethral meatus to the umbilicus; epispadias and unfused labia are commonly present (Fig. 2–10).

The exposed bladder mucosa develops acute and chronic inflammation, ulcerations, squamous metaplasia, and cystitis glandularis. Intestinal metaplasia supervenes if surgical closure is delayed. In untreated patients there is an increased risk of developing bladder carcinoma, especially adenocarcinoma.

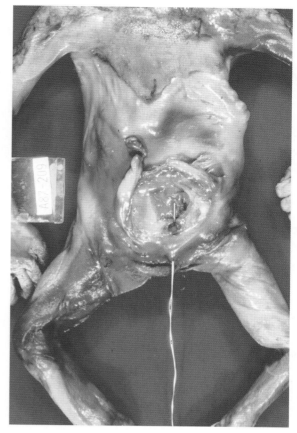

FIGURE 2–10 ▮▯▮▯ Autopsy photo of a fetus with exstrophy of the bladder. Metal probe indicates the path of the urethra.

INFLAMMATORY AND REACTIVE CONDITIONS

Cystitis

The term *cystitis* is nonspecific. It is applied to a wide variety of benign conditions, some of which are defined by pathologic findings and some of which are defined mainly by their clinical characteristics.

The urinary bladder is an unsophisticated organ with a limited set of responses to various pathologic conditions. As a result, there is considerable overlap in the symptoms elicited by these conditions, which may include urinary frequency, lower abdominal discomfort, urgency, urge incontinence, hematuria, obstructive voiding symptoms, or constitutional symptoms.

Von Brunn's Nests, Cystitis Cystica, and Cystitis Glandularis

Von Brunn's nests are round to oval aggregates of normal urothelium located in the lamina propria. They represent normal histology (Fig. 2–11).

Cystitis cystica is the term used to describe the formation of central cystic spaces within von Brunn's nests. The cystic spaces may be up to 5 mm in diameter and may be detected as submucosal cysts endoscopically. They contain clear yellow fluid. Microscopically, they are lined by urothelium or flat cuboidal epithelium and contain acidophilic fluid (Fig. 2–12).

Cystitis glandularis of the typical type is the descriptive

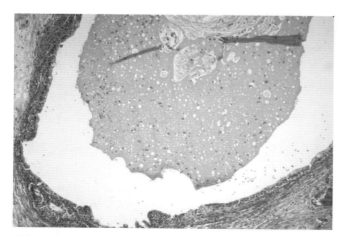

FIGURE 2–9 ▮▯▮▯ Symptomatic urachal cyst with marked luminal dilatation.

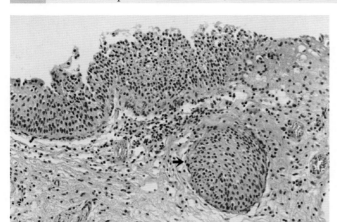

FIGURE 2–11 ❙❚❙❙ von Brunn's nest of urothelial cells in the lamina propria *(arrow).*

term applied when the luminal spaces within von Brunn's nests are lined centrally by columnar cells supported by urothelial cells. There is little or no mucin production, and goblet cells are absent. This finding is so common that it is considered normal histology.

Cystitis glandularis of the intestinal type may coexist with the typical type or may be the dominant finding in patients with chronic bladder inflammation. Histologically, goblet cells and mucin production are evident (Fig. 2–13). It may be focal or diffuse (in which case it is termed *intestinal metaplasia*) (Fig. 2–14). Chronically infected neurogenic bladders and bladders chronically irritated by stones or an indwelling catheter are at risk for the development of intestinal metaplasia. Extensive diffuse intestinal metaplasia is considered a risk factor for the development of adenocarcinoma.

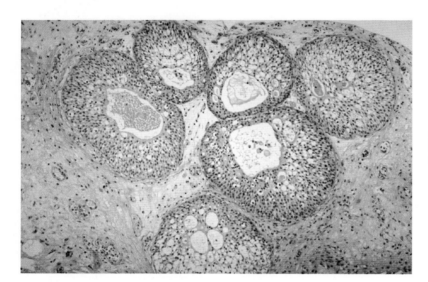

FIGURE 2–12 ❙❚❙❙ Cystitis cystica. Nests of urothelial cells with central luminal spaces, lined by urothelial cells or flat cuboidal cells.

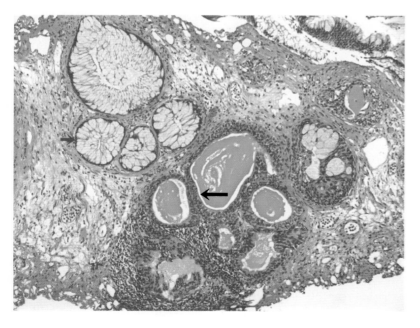

FIGURE 2–13 ❙❚❙❙ Cystitis glandularis. The cystic spaces of cystitis glandularis of the typical type are lined by columnar cells *(black arrow);* those of cystitis glandularis of the intestinal type are lined by mucin-producing goblet cells *(blue arrow).*

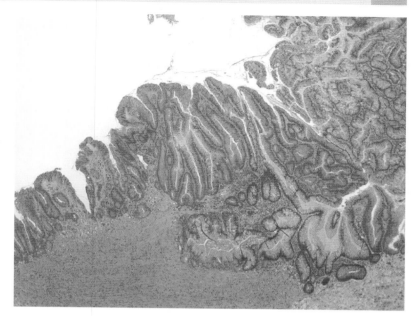

FIGURE 2–14 |▌|| Intestinal metaplasia of bladder mucosa in an elderly woman with a 40-year history of recurrent bladder infections. No normal urothelium is present; it has been replaced by intestinal-type epithelium without significant cytologic atypia.

Acute Cystitis

Clinically, these conditions are characterized by abrupt onset, with associated irritative bladder symptoms and a variable degree of hematuria.

In bacterial cystitis, the lamina propria is edematous, neutrophil infiltration of lamina propria and urothelium is prominent, and urothelial ulceration may be apparent.

In certain settings (e.g., diabetes, neurogenic bladder), bacterial cystitis may be accompanied by gas formation, with creation of mucosal "blebs"—clinically, "emphysematous cystitis."

Cystitis caused by chemotherapeutic agents, such as metabolites of cyclophosphamide, is characterized by extensive hemorrhage in the lamina propria and by urothelial ulceration (Fig. 2–15).

Chronic Cystitis

Chronic cystitis includes many clinicopathologic entities, all of which are characterized histologically by accumulation and persistence of chronic inflammatory cells in the lamina propria, often accompanied by varying degrees of edema and fibrosis. In early acute cystitis, the lamina propria commonly shows vascular dilatation and congestion, hemorrhage, and edema. Polypoid or bullous cystitis may develop, sometimes with ulceration. The urothelium may be hyperplastic or metaplastic and, when ulcerated, is replaced by fibrinopurulent exudate. Granulation tissue may be conspicuous in the early stages of chronic inflammation and may be replaced by scar. Persistent chronic inflammation may lead to mural fibrosis, which may be transmural and may sometimes involve perivesical tissue.

Follicular cystitis is most often associated with bladder cancer or a history of recurrent urinary infection. Endoscopically, the bladder mucosa appears studded with tiny nodules. Microscopically, the lamina propria contains lymphoid follicles with germinal centers (Fig. 2–16).

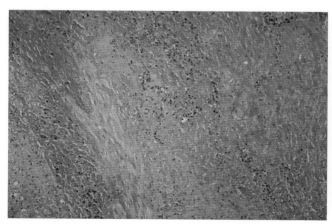

FIGURE 2–15 |▌|| Hemorrhagic cystitis after cyclophosphamide therapy. Extravasated blood extensively infiltrates the soft tissues.

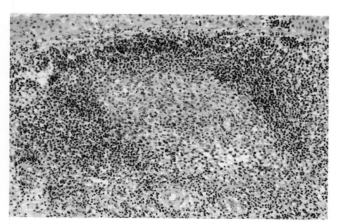

FIGURE 2–16 |▌|| Follicular cystitis. A thin urothelium overlies a large benign lymphoid follicle with a germinal center.

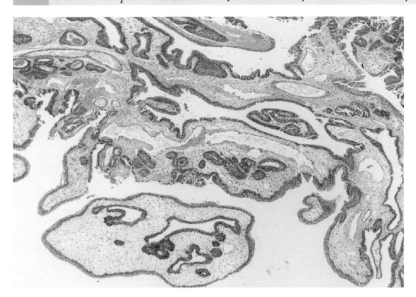

FIGURE 2–17 ▌▌▌ Papillary-polypoid cystitis. The lesion consists of fronds of mucosa with markedly edematous stroma and prominent blood vessels. The overlying urothelium is normal.

Papillary-polypoid and bullous cystitis are reactive conditions most often induced by an indwelling catheter or by the presence of a vesicoenteric fistula. These lesions usually arise in the dome or posterior wall of the bladder. They can be mistaken endoscopically and microscopically for a papillary neoplasm. They are primarily "stromal" reactions, characterized by edema and chronic inflammation in the stroma, resulting in the formation of papillary or polypoid swellings lined by urothelium, which is either normal or hyperplastic (Fig. 2–17). If the edematous mucosal swellings are wider than they are tall, the term *bullous cystitis* is appropriate.

Encrusted cystitis is associated with urinary infection caused by urea-splitting bacteria. The lamina propria is infiltrated by chronic inflammatory cells (which may include giant cells), and the urothelium is denuded. Calcium salts precipitate within fibrinopurulent exudate and amorphous debris, forming encrustations in the lamina propria and on the mucosal surface (Fig. 2–18).

Malakoplakia predominantly affects adult females. Irritative bladder symptoms and hematuria are the most common complaints. Past or current urinary infection, most often with *Escherichia coli*, is very common. Although any portion of the urinary tract may be involved, the bladder is by far the most common site. Cystoscopy reveals soft yellow-brown plaques or nodules (Fig. 2–19). Microscopically, the lamina propria contains sheets of large acidophilic macrophages in a background of other inflammatory cells (Fig. 2–20). Variable numbers of Michaelis-Gutmann bodies are present. These are intracellular or extracellular target-like structures formed by deposition of calcium and iron phosphate on undigested bacterial components; in some instances, special stains are helpful in identifying these structures (Figs. 2–21 and 2–22). Malakoplakia is caused by lysosomal dysfunction; bacteria ingested by macrophages do not undergo the usual sequence of breakdown and lysosomal expulsion.

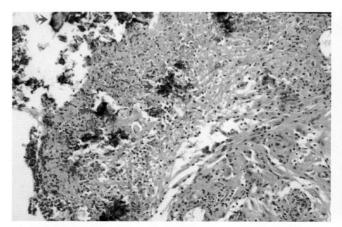

FIGURE 2–18 ▌▌▌ Encrusted cystitis. Deposits of mineral debris are present on the surface and within the lamina propria *(arrows)*.

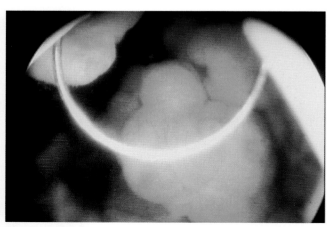

FIGURE 2–19 ▌▌▌ Malakoplakia. Endoscopic photograph of nodular excrescences in the bladder wall in a patient with a long history of urinary infections, complicated by recent gross hematuria. (Courtesy of Howard Goldman, MD, Cleveland, OH.)

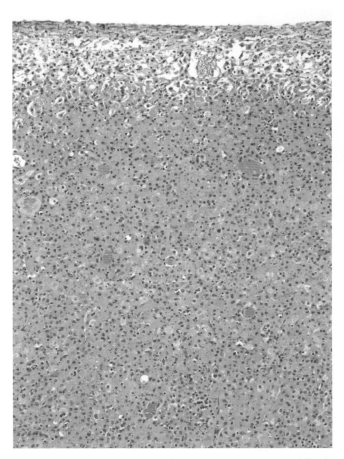

FIGURE 2–20 ▮▮ Malakoplakia. The lamina propria is diffusely infiltrated by von Hansemann histiocytes—macrophages with abundant granular basophilic cytoplasm. Mucosal surface is at top.

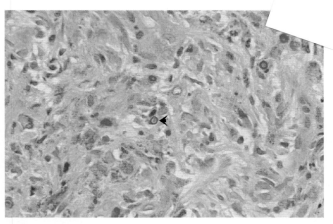

FIGURE 2–22 ▮▮ Malakoplakia. Michaelis-Gutman bodies are highlighted by periodic acid–Schiff (PAS) stain *(arrow)*.

Granulomatous Cystitis

Tuberculous cystitis (non–bacille Calmette-Guérin [BCG] associated) results from spread of tubercle bacilli from an infected kidney. Those at highest risk are women aged 20 to 40 years. The chief complaint is urinary frequency. Urinalysis shows pyuria. In the early phase of disease, cystoscopy shows erythema around the ureteral orifices. Early morning urine culture is the diagnostic test of choice. If the disease progresses untreated, mucosal ulceration, mural fibrosis, and bladder contracture may supervene. Fistulas may form. Microscopically, biopsy specimens may show only surface ulceration with underlying acute and chronic inflammation, edema, and granulation tissue formation. In some cases, classic tubercles with central caseous necrosis surrounded by epithelioid histiocytes, multinucleated giant cells, plasma cells, and lymphocytes may be present. Tubercle bacilli, if present, can be demonstrated by acid-fast stain.

Schistosomiasis is endemic to eastern Africa, the Middle East, and western Asia. The species *Schistosoma hematobium* is capable of living part of its life cycle in humans, having first penetrated the skin of a victim standing in fresh water. The parasites migrate to the urogenital tract, especially the bladder, and mature into adult worms, which lay eggs in the bladder wall. Hematuria is the most common initial complaint, followed by symptoms related to diminution in bladder capacity. The eggs laid by the adult worms cause edema and hyperemia in the lamina propria and urothelial ulceration, forming reddened plaques near the ureteral orifices and on the trigone (Fig. 2–23). A foreign-body granulomatous response with giant cells, and often abundant eosinophils, is initiated by the dead calcified eggs, which may appear endoscopically as "sandy patches" (Fig. 2–24). The relentless inflammation can lead to fibrosis of the bladder, the bladder neck, or the ureteral orifices, complicated by hydronephrosis or voiding difficulty. Epithelial changes develop, including hyperplasia, metaplasia, dysplasia, and carcinoma. Squamous cell carcinoma is the most common associated malignancy, followed by adenocarcinoma.

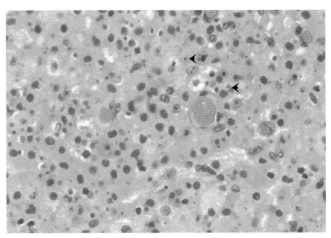

FIGURE 2–21 ▮▮ Malakoplakia. von Hansemann histiocytes and Michaelis-Gutman bodies *(arrows)*.

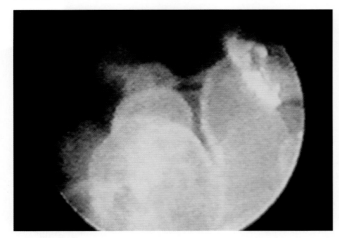

FIGURE 2–23 ▮▮▮▮ Schistosomiasis. Endoscopic photograph of polypoid inflammatory masses in a 9-year-old boy.

Iatrogenic granulomatous cystitis is exemplified by the granulomatous reactions induced by BCG instillation and by surgical procedures in the bladder.

BCG instillation in the management of urothelial carcinoma in situ results in irritative bladder symptoms and sometimes systemic symptoms. The bladder mucosa shows ulceration accompanied by edema, vascular congestion, chronic inflammatory cell infiltrates, and nonnecrotizing granulomas in the lamina propria (Fig. 2–25). Occasionally, acid-fast bacilli are demonstrable in the granulomas, using an acid-fast stain.

Postsurgical granulomas appear grossly as mucosal irregularities with hemorrhage and necrosis. Microscopically, they are "palisading granulomas," with a central zone of necrosis surrounded by palisading epithelioid histiocytes and a peripheral assortment of lymphocytes, eosinophils, histiocytes, giant cells, and plasma cells (Fig. 2–26).

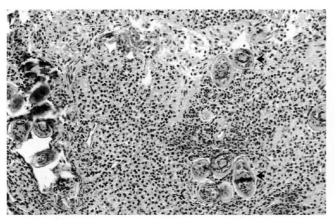

FIGURE 2–24 ▮▮▮▮ Schistosomiasis. Characteristic eggs *(arrows)* are present in association with prominent chronic inflammation. Many of the inflammatory cells are eosinophils.

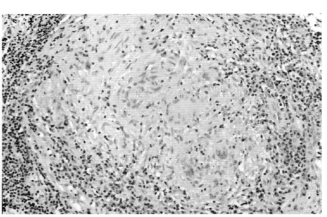

FIGURE 2–25 ▮▮▮▮ Bacille Calmette-Guérin–induced granuloma. A tight cluster of epithelioid histiocytes and multinucleated giant cells is rimmed by lymphocytes. No central necrosis is present in this granuloma.

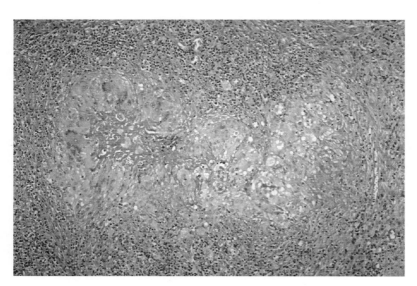

FIGURE 2–26 ▮▮▮▮ Granuloma after transurethral resection, with an elongated serpiginous outline. In the center is acellular debris. Histiocytes are arranged radially around the necrotic material, producing a "palisading" appearance.

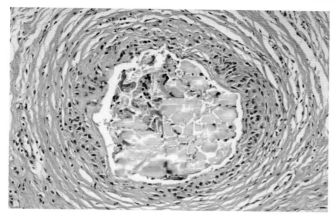

FIGURE 2–27 |■|| Suture granuloma, with residual suture material eliciting an inflammatory response and fibrosis.

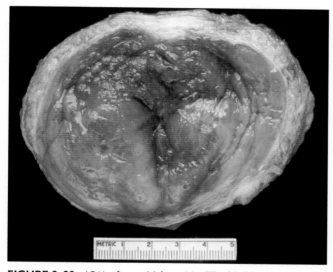

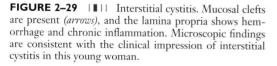

FIGURE 2–28 |■|| Interstitial cystitis. The bladder is small, with mural thickening. Mucosal erosions and erythema are evident.

Suture granuloma of the bladder is a rare complication of hernia repair, sometimes noted many years after surgery (Fig. 2–27). Granulomatous inflammation of the bladder has also been associated rarely with granulomatous disease of childhood, sarcoidosis, Crohn's disease, and rheumatoid arthritis.

MISCELLANEOUS INFLAMMATORY CONDITIONS

Interstitial Cystitis (Hunner's Ulcer)

Interstitial cystitis is an enigmatic disorder affecting predominantly middle-aged and older women, who complain of urgency, frequency, and suprapubic pain with bladder distention. Urine cultures are negative. At cystoscopy, particularly on repeat filling, areas of mucosal bleeding are noted that appear focal (glomerulations) or as linear cracks. In long-standing cases, ulcers and mural scars are evident, usually with diminished bladder capacity (Fig. 2–28).

The microscopic findings vary with the longevity of the process. Mucosal ulceration may or may not be evident. The lamina propria may show a spectrum of findings, ranging from edema and focal hemorrhage to dense infiltrates of lymphocytes and plasma cells (Fig. 2–29). The muscularis propria may appear normal, edematous, or fibrotic. Mast cells are often identifiable at any level of the bladder wall. Attempts to determine their significance have been unsuccessful. Because the histologic findings are so variable and nonspecific, interstitial cystitis is a clinical diagnosis rather than a pathologic diagnosis.

Radiation cystitis is characterized by early and late changes. Histologic findings several weeks after treatment begins include denudation of urothelium and urothelial nuclear atypia, with edema of the lamina propria and telangiectatic changes in blood vessels that may progress over a period of months or years to vascular hyalinization and thrombosis (Figs. 2–30 and 2–31). Atypical stromal cells of the type described in giant cell cystitis are common (Fig. 2–32). Late complications may

FIGURE 2–29 |■|| Interstitial cystitis. Mucosal clefts are present *(arrows)*, and the lamina propria shows hemorrhage and chronic inflammation. Microscopic findings are consistent with the clinical impression of interstitial cystitis in this young woman.

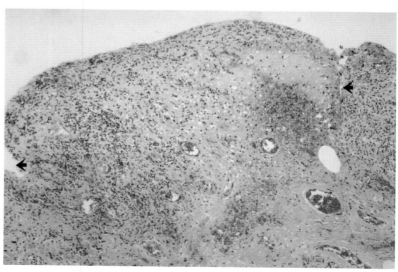

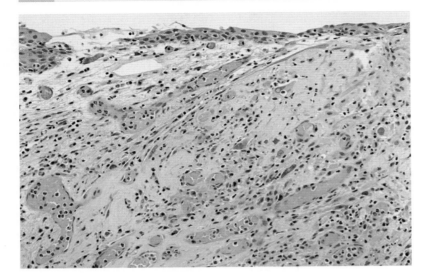

FIGURE 2–30 ▐▐▐ Radiation cystitis, early. The urothelium is thin. The lamina propria is edematous, with chronic inflammation and increased vascularity.

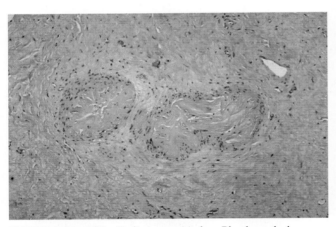

FIGURE 2–31 ▐▐▐ Radiation cystitis, late. Blood vessels show prominent accelerated arteriosclerotic changes.

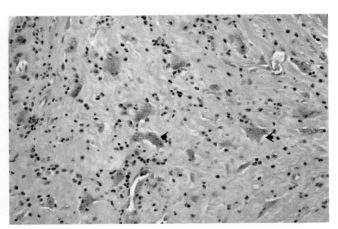

FIGURE 2–32 ▐▐▐ Radiation cystitis. The stroma is fibrotic and contains numerous atypical mesenchymal cells *(arrows)*.

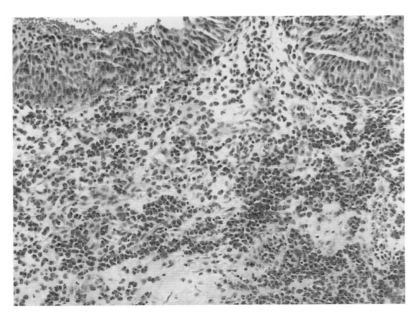

FIGURE 2–33 ▐▐▐ Eosinophilic cystitis. The lamina propria and overlying urothelium are extensively infiltrated by eosinophils. (Case courtesy of Robert Kosick, MD, Baton Rouge, LA.)

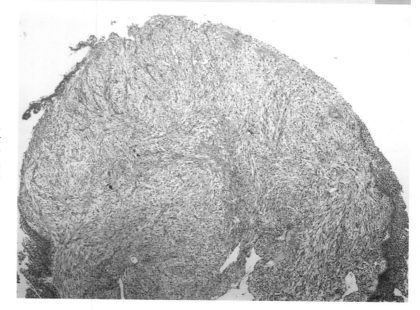

FIGURE 2–34 |▮|| Postoperative spindle cell nodule. This young woman experienced hematuria 3 months after a bladder biopsy showing nonspecific chronic inflammation. Repeat cystoscopy showed this mural nodule, composed of intersecting fascicles of spindle cells in a background of edema and increased vascularity.

include chronic mucosal ulcers, wall fibrosis, bladder contracture, and ureteral stenosis due to fibrosis.

Eosinophilic cystitis denotes bladder inflammation predominated by eosinophils. It is more common in females. One third of affected patients are children. Patients commonly fall into one of two categories: those with a history of allergic disease and those with a history of invasive urothelial carcinoma or transurethral surgery. Patients present with irritative bladder symptoms. Cystoscopy reveals polypoid or bullous lesions, which may raise concern for sarcoma botryoides in a child. Microscopically, the lamina propria is edematous and infiltrated by inflammatory cells, including abundant eosinophils (Fig. 2–33).

Postoperative Spindle Cell Nodule

Postoperative spindle cell nodule is a reactive spindle cell proliferation, which becomes evident within 4 months postoperatively at the site of a previous surgical procedure in the bladder or female genital tract. Endoscopically, it is a friable nodule. Microscopically, it consists of interlacing bundles of bland spindle cells with frequent mitotic figures, often with a background of inflammation, hemorrhage, edema, neovascularity, and myxoid change (Fig. 2–34). Leiomyosarcoma and sarcomatoid carcinoma are included in the microscopic differential. The clinical history is very important. Postoperative spindle cell nodule resolves spontaneously and can be managed conservatively. However, careful endoscopic surveillance is recommended.

Inflammatory Pseudotumor

Inflammatory pseudotumor is grossly and histologically similar to postoperative spindle cell nodule, but a history of surgery is absent. The lesion is most common in women aged 20 to 50 years, and the presenting complaint is hematuria. Grossly, it is usually a solitary broad-based polyp with a mucinous cut surface. It is composed of

spindle cells arranged either haphazardly or in bundles, in a background with a variable degree of vascularity, myxoid change, and inflammation (Fig. 2–35). The process commonly involves the muscularis propria and even perivesical soft tissues. It is often difficult to distinguish from leiomyosarcoma or sarcomatoid carcinoma.

HYPERPLASTIC, REACTIVE, AND METAPLASTIC CHANGES IN UROTHELIUM

Urothelial Hyperplasia

Urothelial hyperplasia may be flat or papillary. In flat urothelial hyperplasia, cytologically normal urothelium more than seven cell layers in thickness is present (Fig. 2–36). This finding is common in settings of chronic bladder inflammation. Papillary urothelial hyperplasia is very rare, consisting of a surface mucosa thrown into undulating folds, without secondary branching of the papillary structures. The papillae are lined by urothelium, which is cytologically normal but usually more than seven cell layers in thickness (Fig. 2–37).

Reactive Changes in Urothelium

Reactive urothelial changes are almost always associated with acute or chronic inflammation in the lamina propria, induced by bacteria, calculi, trauma, chemicals or toxins, and sometimes without an apparent cause (idiopathic). In chronic cystitis, the urothelium commonly shows reactive changes and may be thin, hyperplastic, or denuded. Urothelial cells are crowded and show some loss of polarity, but they are fairly uniform in size and show maturation at the surface. They lack nuclear hyperchromasia, irregularities of the nuclear membrane, and nucleolar prominence (Fig. 2–38). Metaplastic changes are sometimes evident (Fig. 2–39). Patients with reactive changes are not at increased risk for the development of urothelial neoplasia.

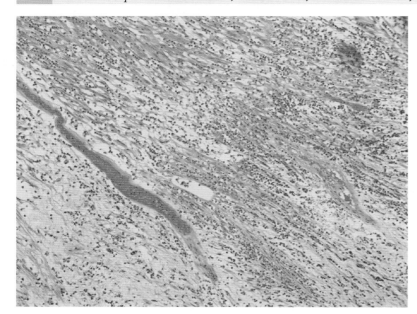

FIGURE 2–35 ▐▌▐▐ Inflammatory pseudotumor. Spindle cells resembling myocytes in cell culture in an inflamed, edematous, and highly vascular stroma. The stroma at lower left shows myxoid change.

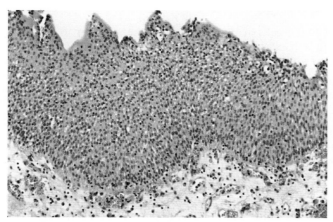

FIGURE 2–36 ▐▌▐▐ Flat urothelial hyperplasia. The urothelium displays normal maturation without papillae, uniform spacing, and no nuclear abnormalities; however, it is substantially thicker than normal.

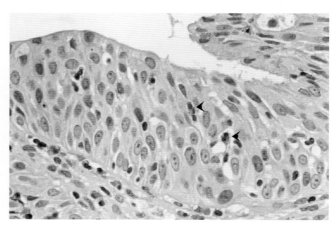

FIGURE 2–38 ▐▌▐▐ Reactive atypia in urothelium. Urothelial cells are crowded and show minimal loss of polarity, but they are relatively uniform in size and show maturation at the surface. Some cells show nuclear enlargement. Intraepithelial eosinophils are present *(arrows)*.

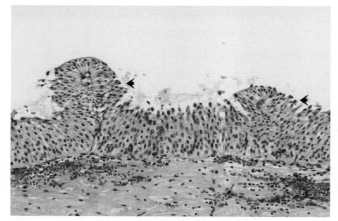

FIGURE 2–37 ▐▌▐▐ Papillary urothelial hyperplasia. Minute papillary excrescences *(arrows)* are present in urothelium that is otherwise normal or only slightly thickened.

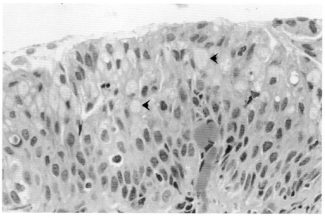

FIGURE 2–39 ▐▌▐▐ Reactive urothelial atypia with mucinous metaplasia. Cell polarity is disturbed, but nuclear size is uniform. In the superficial layers, mucin is present in the cytoplasm of some cells *(arrows)*. Note nuclear hyperchromasia of the basal cells.

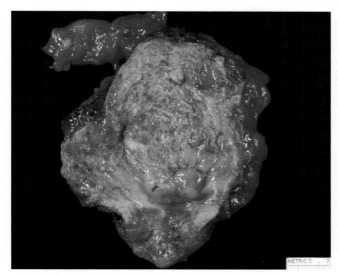

FIGURE 2–40 ▎▊▎▎ Squamous metaplasia of the bladder. The mucosal surface is thickened, leathery, and gray-white.

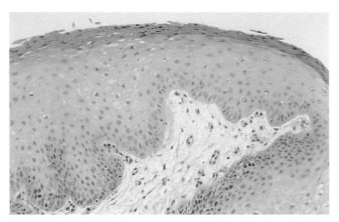

FIGURE 2–41 ▎▊▎▎ Squamous metaplasia of the bladder. Urothelium is replaced by mature squamous epithelium with surface hyperkeratosis and parakeratosis. The epithelium shows no cytologic atypia.

Squamous Metaplasia

Squamous metaplasia is common in patients predisposed to severe chronic cystitis. It appears endoscopically as a gray-white patch, most often anteriorly (Fig. 2–40). The lesions are composed microscopically of layers of squamous epithelium, often with overlying keratin (Fig. 2–41). If marked nuclear atypia is present, one must be concerned about the possibility of in situ or invasive squamous cell carcinoma, which accompanies or follows keratinizing squamous metaplasia in up to 40% of cases. This process is especially prevalent in bladders chronically infected by schistosomiasis.

This term is not used to describe the nonkeratinizing glycogenated squamous epithelium normally present on the trigone and near the bladder neck in the great majority of women.

Nephrogenic Metaplasia

Nephrogenic metaplasia is a reactive mucosal lesion most often encountered in adult males. In most cases, an initiating factor such as trauma, calculus disease, infection, or recent genitourinary surgery can be identified. Nephrogenic metaplasia most often occurs in the bladder but may also occur in the renal pelvis, ureter, or urethra. It may be single or multiple, polypoid, sessile, or papillary. It is usually less than 1 cm in diameter but can be over 4 cm in greatest dimension.

The microscopic architecture may be tubular, cystic, papillary, or polypoid (Figs. 2–42 through 2–45). Secretions are often present within the tubules and cysts. Foci of solid growth pattern are uncommon. The cells lining the luminal and papillary structures generally are uniform and cytologically benign and show virtually no mitotic activity. Clear cells and hobnail cells may be noted focally (Fig. 2–45). In some cases, distinction of this lesion from invasive mucin-producing adenocarcinoma, clear cell adenocarcinoma, or papillary urothelial carcinoma is difficult.

FIGURE 2–42 ▎▊▎▎ Nephrogenic metaplasia, tubular pattern with abundant stromal inflammation. The small, round, hollow acini *(arrows)* are reminiscent of renal tubules.

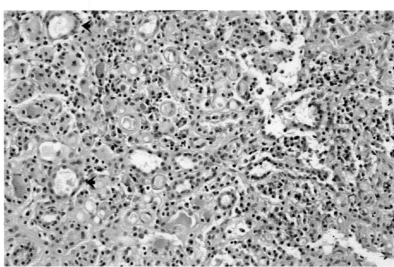

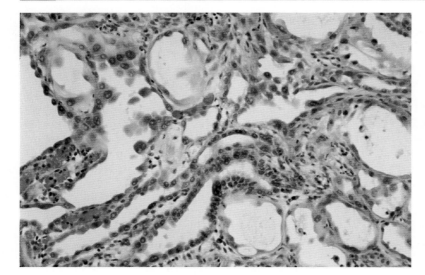

FIGURE 2–43 ▐▐▐▐ Nephrogenic metaplasia, cystic pattern. The lining cells show mild atypia, which is probably reactive/reparative in nature.

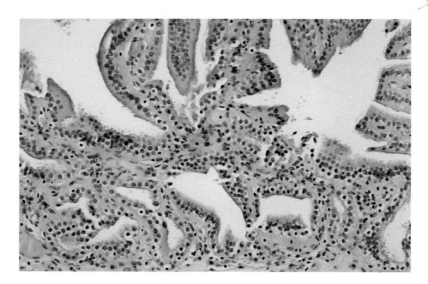

FIGURE 2–44 ▐▐▐▐ Nephrogenic metaplasia, papillary pattern. All structures are lined by a single layer of low columnar or cuboidal cells, in contrast to the multiple layers of cells that typically line structures of papillary urothelial neoplasms.

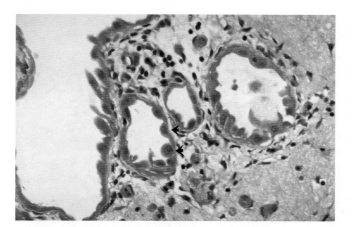

FIGURE 2–45 ▐▐▐▐ Nephrogenic metaplasia. This example illustrates "hobnail cells" *(arrows)*, present in up to 70% of cases.

MISCELLANEOUS BENIGN LESIONS

Ectopic Prostate

Ectopic prostate tissue may present clinically as hematuria in adult males and endoscopically appears as a discrete papillary or polypoid lesion, most commonly on the trigone or near the bladder neck. The lesion is composed of prostatic glands and stroma, covered by urothelium or columnar epithelium.

Fibroepithelial Polyp

A polyp similar to those occasionally noted in the ureter or urethra also occurs in the bladder. It is usually solitary, composed of a fibrovascular core with little or no inflammatory infiltrate, and covered by normal urothelium.

Amyloidosis

Amyloidosis occasionally forms a tumor in the bladder, without evidence of amyloidosis elsewhere, and without evidence of a systemic disease associated with amyloidosis. There is no sex predilection. The presenting complaint is hematuria. Cystoscopy reveals sessile, polypoid, or nodular lesions, which are often ulcerated. Microscopy shows amyloid deposition mainly in the lamina propria and muscularis propria (Fig. 2–46). Amyloidosis of the bladder complicating systemic diseases is less common but may cause more pronounced hematuria. This type of amyloidosis is more subtle endoscopically, appearing as erythema or ulcerated petechiae, without a discernible tumoral mass. The amyloid deposition is mainly in the blood vessels and lamina propria (Fig. 2–47).

Endometriosis

About 1% of women with endometriosis have bladder involvement. Most are in their 30s. Although complaints may include frequency, dysuria, and hematuria, the majority have no bladder symptoms. About half of the patients have a palpable lower abdominal mass. Endoscopically, the mucosa may be normal or ulcerated. Endometriomas appear as blue, red, black, or brown cysts, which may be accompanied by fibrosis or hyperplasia of the muscularis propria (Fig. 2–48). Microscopically, the lesions consist of glandular spaces lined by endometrial epithelium and surrounded by a variable amount of endometrial stroma (Fig. 2–49).

Endocervicosis

This müllerian lesion rarely involves the bladder. Patients are usually in their 30s and 40s, commonly with a history of cesarean section, with irritative bladder symptoms, lower abdominal pain, or hematuria. Lesions are evident

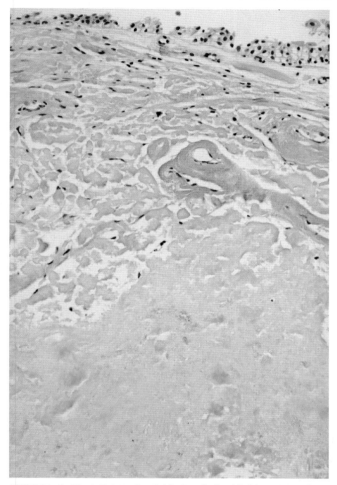

FIGURE 2–46 | ▌ | | Amyloidosis of the bladder. Amorphous eosinophilic deposits of amyloid protein are present in the lamina propria. This pattern of deposition is typical of amyloidosis confined to the bladder.

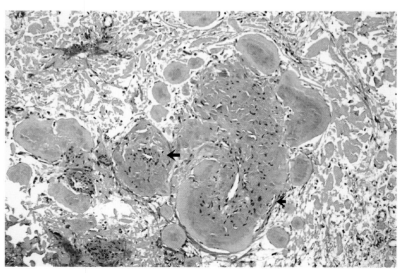

FIGURE 2–47 | ▌ | | Amyloidosis of the bladder, predominantly affecting blood vessels *(arrows)*, with lesser deposits in the lamina propria, a pattern suggestive of systemic amyloidosis.

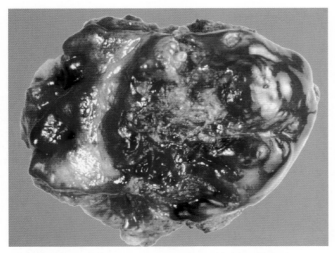

FIGURE 2–48 ▮▮▮ Endometriosis of the bladder. Cystectomy was required to relieve disabling symptoms in this young woman.

as mural nodules at cystoscopy. Microscopically, the nodules are composed of mucin-containing glandular structures of variable shape and size, mainly involving the muscularis propria and lined by a single layer of columnar or flat cuboidal cells (Fig. 2–50). Mucin extravasation with stromal reactive changes may be evident.

Villous Adenoma

Lesions indistinguishable from colonic villous adenoma have been infrequently reported in the bladder and urachus. Villous adenoma is an exophytic papillary tumor, often with a mucinous surface. Microscopically, it is composed of papillary structures lined by atypical columnar epithelium, admixed with goblet cells (Fig. 2–51). Features of invasion, such as a desmoplastic stromal response, are absent. Tumors managed by transurethral resection or open surgical excision have not recurred.

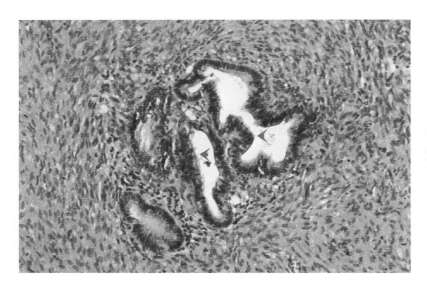

FIGURE 2–49 ▮▮▮ Endometriosis of the bladder. Endometrial glands *(red arrows)* accompanied by small amounts of endometrial stroma *(green arrows)* are present.

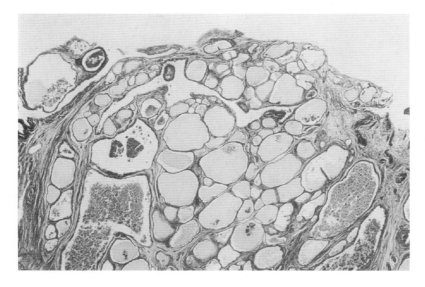

FIGURE 2–50 ▮▮▮ Endocervicosis of the bladder. The lesion consists of crowded, cystically dilated, benign-appearing endocervical-type glands.

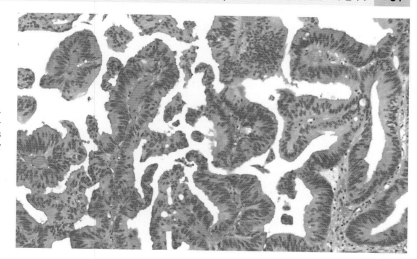

FIGURE 2–51 I▊II Villous adenoma of the bladder. Villoglandular structures lined by enteric-type epithelium with marked cytologic atypia (adenomatous change). The lesion is indistinguishable from similar lesions arising in the gastrointestinal tract.

Urothelial Neoplasms

Dysplasia

The architectural and cytologic abnormalities in dysplasia are less pronounced than in carcinoma in situ. The architectural abnormalities include cell crowding and loss of polarity. Cytologic abnormalities include nuclear enlargement with chromatin coarsening and hyperchromasia, and variation in nuclear shape. Nucleoli are usually small and inconspicuous or, rarely, enlarged. Mitotic figures are usually absent or sparse (Fig. 2–52). Dysplastic features are usually restricted to the basal and intermediate layers of urothelium.

Urothelial dysplasia is a marker for cancer risk, and careful monitoring of patients with dysplasia by endoscopy and urine cytology is prudent. Treatments such as intravesical chemotherapy or BCG are not currently recommended in the management of urothelial dysplasia.

Carcinoma in Situ

Urothelial carcinoma in situ is flat intraepithelial carcinoma. It commonly accompanies papillary or invasive urothelial carcinoma but can present without evidence of either. Most cases of primary carcinoma in situ are encountered in men older than age 50 years, who complain of hematuria, irritative voiding symptoms, and/ or bladder pain of a severity suggestive of interstitial cystitis. Urine cytology is positive for frankly malignant urothelial cells in up to 90% of cases. Cystoscopy may show areas of velvety mucosal erythema; however, the mucosa may appear entirely unremarkable endoscopically, reinforcing the value of urine cytology in diagnosing this entity (Fig. 2–53). Multiple foci of urothelial involvement are commonly present, with involvement of the prostatic urethra and the ureters in many cases.

Urothelial carcinoma in situ (CIS) is characterized by flat disordered proliferation of urothelial cells with

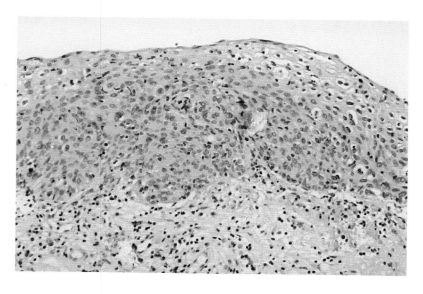

FIGURE 2–52 I▊II Urothelial dysplasia. The lower and middle thirds of the urothelium show cellular crowding with marked loss of polarity, with nuclear enlargement and hyperchromasia. In the upper third, these findings are not evident.

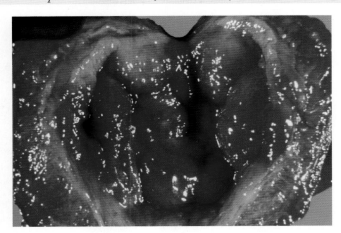

FIGURE 2–53 |▌|| Carcinoma in situ of the bladder. The mucosa is edematous and erythematous. No discrete mucosal lesions are apparent.

marked cytologic abnormalities. The diagnosis of CIS requires the presence of severe cytologic atypia (nuclear anaplasia). The cells of CIS are often dyscohesive and exfoliate freely; much of the surface epithelium may not be present for evaluation in a biopsy specimen (Fig. 2–54). Full-thickness severe cytologic atypia is present, regardless of the thickness of the urothelial layer (Fig. 2–55).

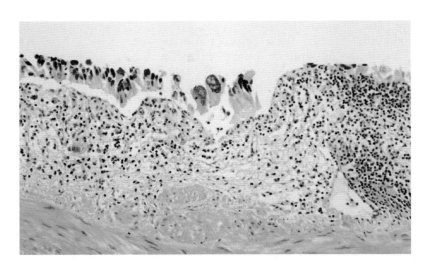

FIGURE 2–54 |▌|| Carcinoma in situ. The urothelium is partially denuded; the residual urothelial cells show marked cytologic atypia.

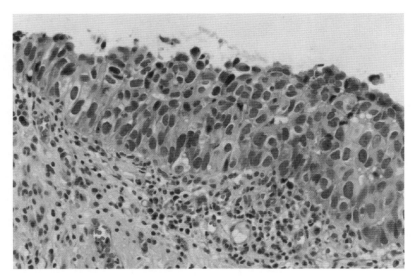

FIGURE 2–55 |▌|| Carcinoma in situ. The urothelial cells show total loss of polarity. There is marked variation in nuclear size and shape. Nuclei are quite hyperchromatic, and some contain prominent nucleoli. The cytologic abnormalities involve the full thickness of the urothelium.

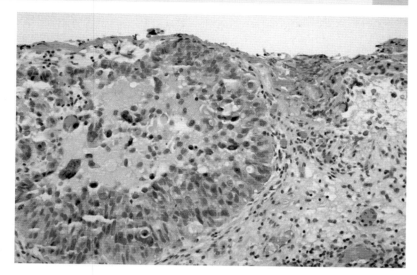

FIGURE 2–56 ❙❚❙❙ Carcinoma in situ, filling a von Brunn's nest. The surface urothelium is almost entirely denuded.

Prominent architectural disorganization of the urothelium is characteristic, with loss of cell polarity and cohesiveness. The tumor cells are large and pleomorphic, with moderate to abundant cytoplasm, although they are sometimes small with a high nucleus to cytoplasmic ratio. The chromatin tends to be coarse and clumped. Nucleoli are usually large and prominent in at least some of the cells and may be multiple. Mitotic figures are often seen in the uppermost urothelium and may be atypical. The adjacent mucosa often contains lesser degrees of cytologic abnormality.

The small cell pattern of CIS is usually associated with an increased number of cell layers. In such cases, the cytoplasm is scant and nuclei are enlarged and hyperchromatic, with coarse unevenly distributed chromatin. Mitotic figures are frequently present, often with abnormal forms. The cells are randomly oriented and disorganized, often with striking cellular dyscohesion, that, in some cases, results in few or no recognizable epithelial cells on the surface, a condition referred to as denuding cystitis. Careful search of all residual mucosa is important in biopsy specimens that have little or no mucosa to exclude the denuding cystitis of CIS.

CIS is often associated with focal discontinuity of the basement membrane. There may be intense chronic inflammation in the superficial lamina propria in some cases, and vascular ectasia and proliferation of small capillaries is frequent. In denuded areas, residual CIS may involve von Brunn's nests (Fig. 2–56). Rarely, CIS exhibits pagetoid growth, characterized by large single cells or small clusters of cells within otherwise normal urothelium, in squamous metaplasia, or within prostatic ducts.

The clinical course of patients with urothelial CIS is variable; up to 83% of patients will develop invasive cancer, and up to 38% of patients will die of bladder cancer.

Papilloma

The World Health Organization criteria for papilloma include the following five main features: (1) small (less than 2 cm in greatest dimension; (2) usually solitary papillary lesion with one or more delicate fibrovascular cores; (3) lined by cytologically and architecturally normal urothelium with orderly maturation; (4) an intact superficial (umbrella) cell layer and no mitotic figures; and (5) occurring in patients usually younger than 50 years of age. The urothelium is usually of normal thickness, although factitious appearance of thickening may be observed owing to tangential cutting at the base of the papilloma (Fig. 2–57). There is little or no variation in nuclear size, shape, or spacing when compared with normal urothelium, and the chromatin texture is finely granular without nucleolar enlargement (Fig. 2–58).

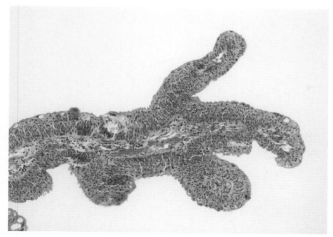

FIGURE 2–57 ❙❚❙❙ Urothelial papilloma. A delicate elongate fibrovascular core lined by cytologically and architecturally normal urothelium.

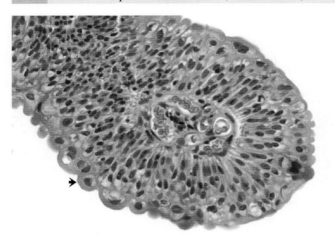

FIGURE 2–58 | ■ | | Urothelial papilloma. The urothelium is of normal thickness, with proper cell polarity and maturation. The surface layer of umbrella cells *(arrow)* is intact.

Papilloma is uncommon, representing less than 3% of papillary urothelial tumors. Such lesions usually occur in patients younger than 50 years of age, but rare cases with otherwise typical features can be seen in patients in their late 50s. An otherwise typical papilloma occurring in an older patient (considerably older than age 50 years) is best considered to be grade 1 urothelial carcinoma.

Urothelial papilloma has a low recurrence rate and very infrequent association with the development of invasive urothelial carcinoma and cancer death; it does not have the capacity to invade or metastasize. However, it is neoplastic, with a small but significant potential for recurrence.

Inverted Urothelial Papilloma

Inverted papilloma accounts for less than 1% of urothelial neoplasms. Median age at presentation is 55 years, but patients as young as 14 years have been reported. Most patients are male. Symptoms include hematuria, irritative voiding symptoms, and, rarely, obstructive voiding symptoms. Lesions may be sessile or pedunculated, are up to 8 cm in diameter, usually have smooth overlying mucosa, and are most often located on or near the trigone. Microscopically, inverted papilloma consists of urothelial cells growing downward into the lamina propria and forming nests, sheets, anastomosing cords, and occasional luminal spaces containing mucin or pink secretions (Fig. 2–59). Cytologic atypia is minimal, and mitotic figures are infrequent (Fig. 2–60). The chief differential consideration is urothelial carcinoma, which can sometimes show an inverted growth pattern. Exophytic growth, mitotic activity, and cytologic atypia favor carcinoma. The recurrence rate of inverted papilloma is less than 1%; however, ongoing clinical surveillance is warranted.

Papillary Urothelial Carcinoma

Carcinoma of the urinary bladder is the fifth most common human cancer. The American Cancer Society predicted 54,300 new cases and 12,400 deaths from bladder cancer in 2001. Urothelial carcinoma affects males 2.7 times as often as females, and the death rate in males is twice that in females. Median age at diagnosis is 65 years, but the lesion has been reported in children and adolescents. Tobacco smoking, exposure to certain chemicals (benzidine, 2-naphthylamine, cyclophosphamide), radiation exposure, and schistosomal bladder infection appear to be significant etiologic factors.

Presenting complaints include hematuria (90%) and/or irritative bladder symptoms (20%); symptoms such as flank pain or lower limb edema are infrequent.

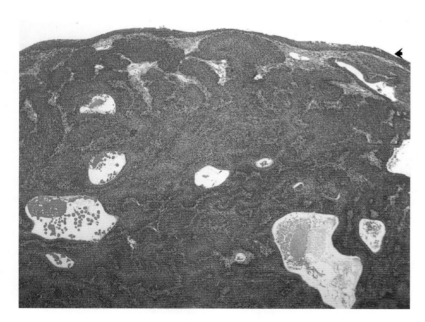

FIGURE 2–59 | ■ | | Inverted urothelial papilloma. Beneath a surface layer of urothelium *(arrow)* are anastomosing trabeculae of urothelial cells. Growth orientation is intramucosal, rather than exophytic.

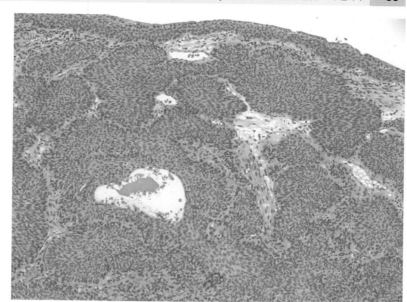

FIGURE 2–60 |▮|| Inverted urothelial papilloma. Islands and trabeculae of cytologically normal urothelial cells bounded by an intact basement membrane and delicate fibrovascular stroma.

Diagnosis is aided by the use of radiologic studies, cystoscopy, and the examination of exfoliated cells in the urine (cytology). Cystoscopy and urine cytology should be considered complementary rather than competitive testing procedures. Urine cytology is not sufficiently sensitive to detect the majority of low-grade urothelial tumors, but these tumors are usually quite readily identified endoscopically. On the other hand, the endoscopic detection of urothelial carcinoma in situ can be very difficult; however, the marked cytologic abnormalities of the cells exfoliated by carcinoma in situ are detected with a high degree of accuracy using urine cytology.

Papillary urothelial carcinoma is an exophytic tumor that may appear solid or composed of numerous papillae when viewed endoscopically (Figs. 2–61 and 2–62). Tumors may be solitary (60%) or multiple (Fig. 2–63). Microscopically, papillary urothelial carcinoma is composed of malignant urothelial cells growing on the surface of papillary fibrovascular cores. The degree of cytologic atypia varies and is used to assign a grade. Areas showing squamous or glandular differentiation are commonly present, particularly in tumors of higher grade. Papillary urothelial carcinoma must be submitted entirely for histologic evaluation in search of an invasive component.

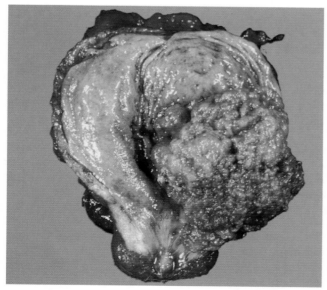

FIGURE 2–61 |▮|| Papillary urothelial carcinoma, grade 2, in a cystectomy specimen.

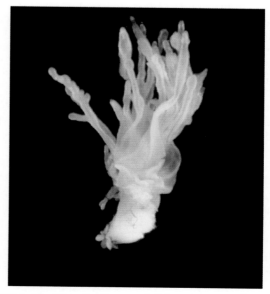

FIGURE 2–62 |▮|| Papillary urothelial carcinoma, grade 1.

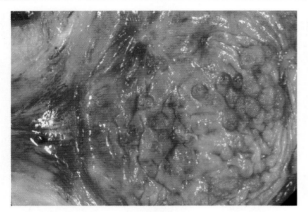

FIGURE 2–63 I▮II Papillary urothelial carcinoma, grade 1, multifocal, in a cystectomy specimen.

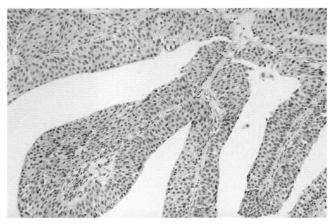

FIGURE 2–64 I▮II Papillary urothelial carcinoma, grade 1. Tumor was large (4 cm), multifocal, and present in a 75-year-old woman. Cell polarity is fairly well preserved, and tumor cells are uniform in size and shape.

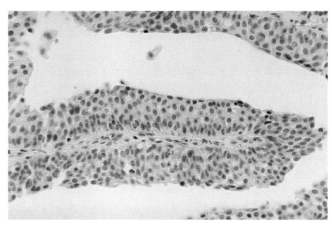

FIGURE 2–65 I▮II Papillary urothelial carcinoma, grade 1. There is minimal loss of cell polarity. Nuclei are quite uniform in size and shape, and nuclear membranes are round. Nuclei lack hyperchromasia and nucleoli. No mitotic figures are evident. Umbrella cells are absent.

Some urothelial carcinomas are nonpapillary; they are invasive from inception. Such cancers are commonly high grade, and they typically produce a prominent desmoplastic stromal reaction. Many of the variants of urothelial carcinoma (nested, giant cell, lymphoepithelioma-like, microcystic, inverted growth pattern, lymphoma-like, sarcomatoid) fall within this category.

Grading Urothelial Neoplasms

The WHO 1973 classification and grading system for bladder tumors has been repeatedly validated and is near-universally used. New grading efforts for bladder tumors were intended to create universal standards of terminology and criteria to allow comparison of results from different centers and promote cooperation. However, the laudable goals of the recent efforts for change have not been attained, and these new schemes appear to have no hope of widespread acceptance. Furthermore, we believe that the WHO 1973 standard, the most widely used system in the world, was not "broken" to begin with and thus did not require substantial repairs or alterations.

Grading of urothelial neoplasms, particularly papillary tumors, may be difficult, owing to intratumoral heterogeneity. Grading is based on the highest level of abnormality noted.

Grade 1 Urothelial Carcinoma

Grade 1 papillary carcinoma consists of an orderly arrangement of normal urothelial cells lining delicate papillae with minimal architectural abnormalities and minimal nuclear atypia (Figs. 2–64 and 2–65). There may be some complexity and fusion of the papillae, but this is usually not prominent. The urothelium is often thickened, with more than seven cell layers, but may be normal. Regardless of thickness, the urothelium displays normal maturation, polarity, and cohesiveness. Nuclei tend to be uniform in shape and spacing, although there may be some enlargement and elongation; the chromatin texture is finely granular, similar to papilloma, without significant nucleolar enlargement. Mitotic figures are rare or absent.

Patients with grade 1 carcinoma are at significant risk of local recurrence, progression, and dying of bladder cancer. Lifelong endoscopic and cytologic surveillance is warranted.

Grade 2 Urothelial Carcinoma

Grade 2 carcinoma retains some of the orderly architectural appearance and maturation of grade 1 carcinoma but displays at least focal moderate variation in orderliness, nuclear appearance, and chromatin texture that should be apparent at low magnification (Figs. 2–66 and 2–67). Cytologic abnormalities are invariably present in grade 2 carcinoma, with moderate nuclear crowding, moderate variation in cell polarity, moderate nuclear hyperchromasia, moderate anisonucleosis, and mild nucleolar enlargement. Mitotic figures are usually present but are limited to the lower half of the urothelium, although this is inconstant. Some tumors may be extremely orderly, reminiscent of grade 1 carcinoma, with only a small focus of obvious disorder or irregularity in cell spacing; these are considered grade 2 cancer, recognizing that grade is based on the highest level

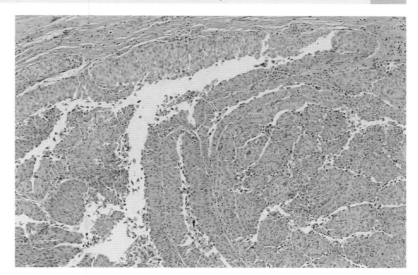

FIGURE 2–66 ❙▮❙❙ Papillary urothelial carcinoma, grade 2. Closely packed papillae are characteristic.

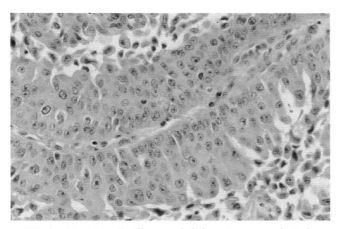

FIGURE 2–67 ❙▮❙❙ Papillary urothelial carcinoma, grade 2. Some preservation of cell polarity is evident. Nuclear membranes are irregular, and conspicuous nucleoli are present. There is moderate diversity in nuclear size and shape.

of abnormality present. Grade 2 carcinomas represent a wide spectrum of tumors that span the morphologic continuum from grade 1 to grade 3.

Most cases of urothelial carcinoma are WHO grade 2, and the outcome is significantly worse than those with lower-grade papillary cancer. The recurrence risk for patients with noninvasive grade 2 cancer is 45% to 67%, with invasion occurring in up to 20% and cancer-specific death in 13% to 20% after surgical treatment. Patients with grade 2 cancer and invasion of the lamina propria are at even greater risk, with recurrence in 67% to 80% of cases, development of muscle-invasive cancer in 21% to 49%, and cancer-specific death in 17% to 51% of those treated surgically.

Grade 3 Urothelial Carcinoma

Grade 3 carcinoma displays the most extreme nuclear abnormalities among papillary urothelial cancers, similar to those seen in CIS (Figs. 2–68 and 2–69). The obvious urothelial disorder and loss of polarity is present at

FIGURE 2–68 ❙▮❙❙ Papillary urothelial carcinoma, grade 3. Complete loss of cell polarity is evident *(black arrow)*. Some of the nuclei are very large, irregular, and hyperchromatic *(blue arrows)*.

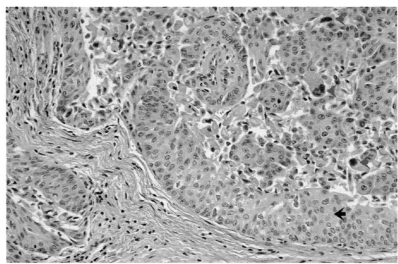

scanning magnification and often includes loss of normal architecture and cell polarity, loss of cell cohesion, and frequent mitotic figures. Cellular anaplasia, characteristic of grade 3 carcinoma, is defined as increased cellularity,

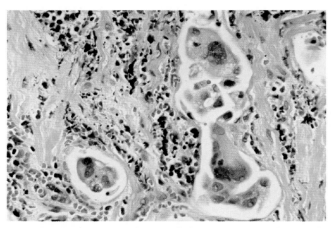

FIGURE 2–69 ▮▮▮ Papillary urothelial carcinoma, grade 3. There is considerable variation in nuclear size and shape. Nuclear membranes are markedly irregular, and nuclei are vacuolated and hyperchromatic. These aggregates of tumor cells are within vascular spaces.

nuclear crowding, disturbance of cellular polarity, absence of differentiation from the base to the mucosal surface, nuclear pleomorphism, irregularity in the size of the cells, variation in nuclear shape and chromatin pattern, increased number of mitotic figures throughout the mucosa, and the occasional presence of neoplastic giant cells.

Recurrence risk for patients with noninvasive grade 3 cancer is 65% to 85%, with invasion occurring in 20% to 52% and cancer-specific death in up to 35% after surgical treatment. Patients with grade 3 cancer and lamina propria invasion experience recurrence in 46% to 71% of cases and develop muscle-invasive cancer in 24% to 48%. Cancer-specific death occurs in 25% to 71% of those treated surgically.

Staging Urothelial Carcinoma

Staging systems for urothelial carcinoma include the Marshall modification of the Jewett-Strong system and the American Joint Commission-Union Internationale Contre le Cancer (AJCC-UICC) systems. The latter is presented in Table 2–1. Stages are defined by depth of invasion, lymph node involvement, and metastatic spread of disease (Figs. 2–70 through 2–73).

TABLE 2–I
TNM STAGING OF BLADDER CARCINOMA

Primary Tumor (T)

TX	Primary tumor cannot be assessed
T0	No evidence of primary tumor
Ta	Noninvasive papillary carcinoma
Tis	Carcinoma *in situ:* "flat tumor"
T1	Tumor invades subepithelial connective tissue
T2	Tumor invades muscle
pT2a	Tumor invades superficial muscle (inner half)
pT2b	Tumor invades deep muscle (outer half)
T3	Tumor invades perivesical tissue
pT3a	microscopically
pT3b	macroscopically (extravesical mass)
T4	Tumor invades any of the following: prostate, uterus, vagina, pelvic wall, abdominal wall
T4a	Tumor invades prostate, uterus, vagina
T4b	Tumor invades pelvic wall, abdominal wall

Regional Lymph Nodes (N)

NX	Regional lymph nodes cannot be assessed
N0	No regional lymph node metastasis
N1	Metastasis in a single lymph node, 2 cm or less in greatest dimension
N2	Metastasis in a single lymph node, more than 2 cm but not more than 5 cm in greatest dimension; or multiple lymph nodes, none more than 5 cm in greatest dimension
N3	Metastasis in a lymph node, more than 5 cm in greatest dimension

Distant Metastasis (M)

MX	Distant metastasis cannot be assessed
M0	No distant metastasis
M1	Distant metastasis

Note: Histopathologic types included are urothelial (transitional cell) carcinoma, squamous cell carcinoma, adenocarcinoma, and undifferentiated carcinoma.

Used with the permission of the American Joint Committee on Cancer (AJCC), Chicago, Illinois. The original source for this material is the *AJCC Cancer Staging Manual, Sixth Edition* (2002) published by Springer-Verlag New York, www.springer-ny.com.

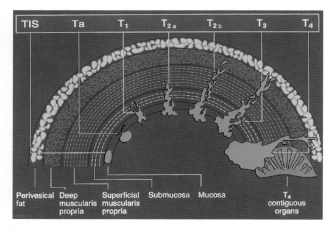

FIGURE 2–70 ▮▮▮ Pictorial representation of staging of urothelial carcinoma according to depth of tumor invasion.

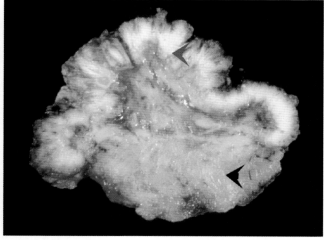

FIGURE 2–71 ▮▮▮ Cross section of surgically excised urothelial carcinoma. Tumor is invasive into lamina propria (*blue arrow*) but does not appear to involve muscularis propria (*black arrow*).

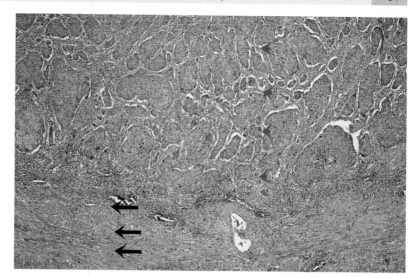

FIGURE 2–72 |■|| Urothelial carcinoma, invasive into lamina propria *(blue arrows)*. Muscularis propria *(black arrows)* appears uninvolved by tumor.

Nonpapillary Variants of Urothelial Carcinoma

Sarcomatoid urothelial carcinoma is characterized by malignant epithelial and sarcomatous components. Tumors containing identifiable sarcomatous components (e.g., bone or cartilage) in addition to carcinoma are designated *carcinosarcoma* by some authorities. These tumors more commonly affect males and patients present with the usual symptoms of urothelial carcinoma. Tumors tend to be large and exophytic, with a polypoid or pedunculated appearance (Fig. 2–74). The carcinoma component may be urothelial, squamous, glandular, or small cell carcinoma. The sarcomatous component may consist of undifferentiated spindle cells, osteosarcoma, chondrosarcoma, or rhabdomyosarcoma (Figs. 2–75 and 2–76). At times, a component of carcinoma may only be detected by extensive tumor sampling or by the use of immunohistochemical stains for keratin markers (Figs. 2–77 and 2–78). All forms of sarcomatoid urothelial carcinoma are associated with poor outcome; only 25% of patients survive 2 years after diagnosis.

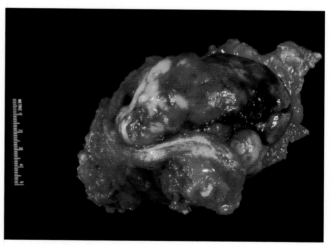

FIGURE 2–74 |■|| Sarcomatoid urothelial carcinoma, surgically excised. Tumor is large, nodular, hemorrhagic, and partially necrotic.

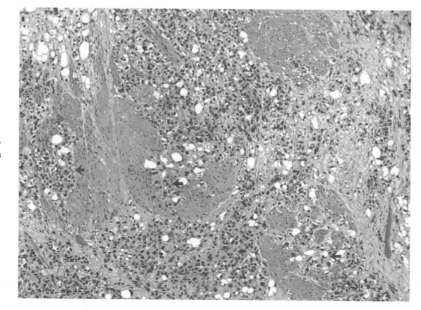

FIGURE 2–73 |■|| Urothelial carcinoma, intersecting and invading thick bundles of muscularis propria *(arrows)*.

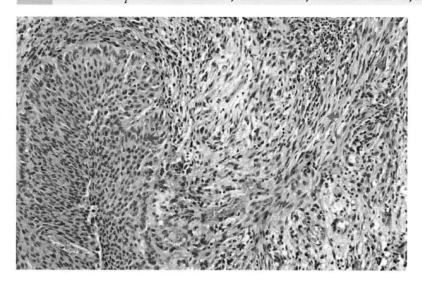

FIGURE 2–75 Sarcomatoid urothelial carcinoma. Part of the tumor is typical urothelial carcinoma *(blue arrow);* the remainder of the tumor shows spindle cell morphology *(red arrows).*

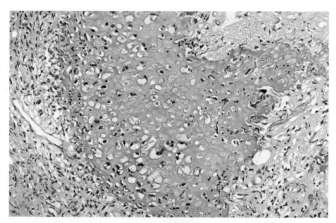

FIGURE 2–76 Sarcomatoid urothelial carcinoma. In a tumor that showed urothelial carcinoma and undifferentiated malignant spindle cells in other areas, this focus of osteosarcoma was present, an example of heterologous differentiation.

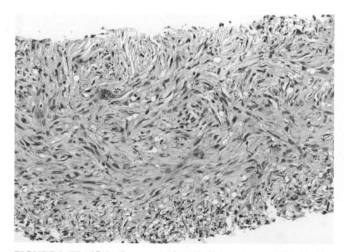

FIGURE 2–77 Sarcomatoid urothelial carcinoma. This bladder tumor is entirely composed of malignant spindle cells.

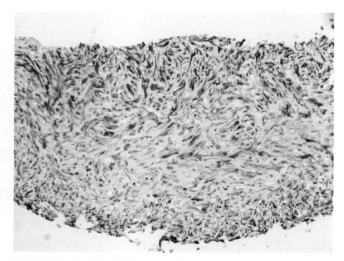

FIGURE 2–78 Sarcomatoid urothelial carcinoma. The spindled tumor cells show immunoreactivity to antibodies against keratin Cam 5.2 *(arrows),* confirming that they are epithelial cells, and that the tumor is carcinoma.

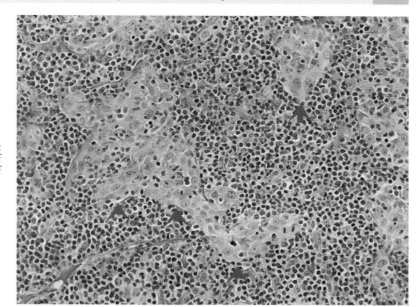

FIGURE 2–79 ▮▮▮ Lymphoepithelioma-like variant of urothelial carcinoma. Discrete or irregular islands of malignant urothelial cells *(arrows)* punctuate sheets of lymphocytes.

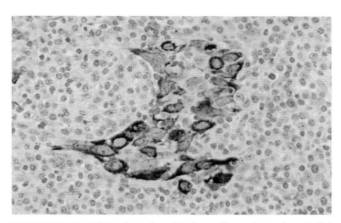

FIGURE 2–80 ▮▮▮ Lymphoepithelioma-like variant of urothelial carcinoma. The epithelial component displays intense immunoreactivity to antibodies against keratin AE1/AE3.

Lymphoepithelioma-like carcinoma is microscopically similar to lymphoepithelioma of the nasopharynx. It most often affects males in their late 60s. It is usually sessile. Microscopically, irregular islands of poorly differentiated cells with large pleomorphic nuclei and large nucleoli are surrounded by abundant lymphoid cells (Fig. 2–79). The inflammatory background may obscure the small component of carcinoma; immunostains for keratin markers may assist by highlighting the carcinoma component (Fig. 2–80). Areas of typical urothelial carcinoma may be present. This variant is often sensitive to chemotherapy.

Other variants of urothelial carcinoma include *nested variant, giant cell variant, lymphoma-like variant and variants with microcystic architecture or inverted growth patterns* (Figs. 2–81 and 2–82). They are predominantly of interest to pathologists because they create unique diagnostic

FIGURE 2–81 ▮▮▮ High-grade urothelial carcinoma with osteoclast-like giant cells *(arrows)*.

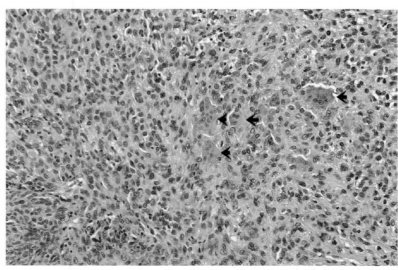

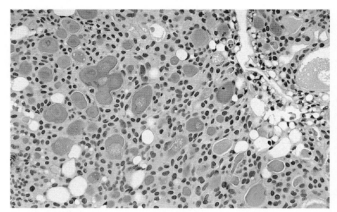

FIGURE 2–82 ▮▮▮ Microcystic variant of urothelial carcinoma. Malignant urothelial cells punctuated by small cystic spaces containing eosinophilic mucin. This variant is difficult to distinguish from nephrogenic metaplasia.

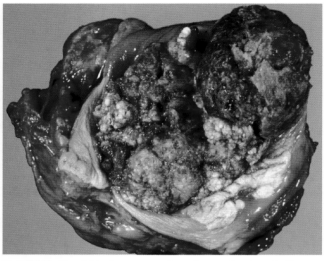

FIGURE 2–83 ▮▮▮ Squamous cell carcinoma, forming a bulky exophytic mass, with gray-white areas reflecting keratin production.

challenges. Their biologic behavior is not significantly different from that of typical urothelial carcinoma.

Squamous Cell Carcinoma

Squamous cell carcinoma (SCC) accounts for about 1 in 20 bladder malignancies in the United States and England and for nearly 3 of 4 bladder malignancies in areas endemic for schistosomiasis. SCC is nearly twice as common in males, and the mean patient age is 65 years. Patients present with hematuria and/or irritative bladder symptoms, and disease stage tends to be high at the time of initial diagnosis. Chronic mucosal inflammation (e.g., chronic urinary retention, calculus disease, schistosomiasis) predisposes to SCC. Keratinizing squamous metaplasia precedes the development of at least half of invasive SCC.

Invasive SCC is usually solid and nodular, with extensive necrosis and accumulated keratin debris on the surface (Fig. 2–83). Some are flat or deeply invasive with surface ulceration. Tumors may occupy much of the bladder lumen. Histologically, the diagnosis of SCC is restricted to tumors composed entirely of SCC. If a component of urothelial carcinoma is present, the lesion is considered urothelial carcinoma with squamous differentiation. The differential diagnosis in cases of bladder SCC includes vascular metastasis or direct extension of SCC from a neighboring site such as the uterine cervix. The degree of differentiation in SCC is variable. In well-differentiated tumors, keratinizing squamous cells with intercellular bridges and fairly uniform nuclei form infiltrating nests and cords (Fig. 2–84). Poorly differentiated tumors show only focal areas of squamous differentiation. The prognostic significance of grading the degree of differentiation is uncertain. Stage at presen-

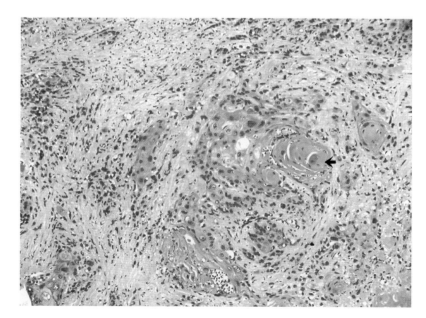

FIGURE 2–84 ▮▮▮ Invasive squamous cell carcinoma. Diagnosis is aided by the presence of keratin pearl formation *(arrow)*.

tation is often high, and this may account for the overall dismal prognosis of bladder SCC (5.3% survival at 10 years in one large series). Death is more commonly the result of local recurrence than of metastatic disease.

ADENOCARCINOMA

Primary adenocarcinoma may arise in the bladder or the urachus.

Nonurachal adenocarcinoma is more common in males than in females, occurs at a mean age of 59 years, and comprises up to 80% of primary bladder adenocarcinoma. Patients present with hematuria or irritative bladder symptoms, and some complain of mucosuria. Up to 40% of patients have metastases when the disease is first detected.

Lesions appear papillary, sessile, or infiltrative with deep central ulceration. Diffuse wall thickening without mucosal ulceration can occur in cases of signet ring cell carcinoma. The diagnosis of adenocarcinoma is restricted to lesions that demonstrate only glandular differentiation. Urothelial carcinoma with a component of adenocarcinoma is not included in this category. There are six subcategories of bladder adenocarcinoma:

1. *Enteric type*—resembling colonic adenocarcinoma (Fig. 2–85)
2. *Mucinous (colloid)*—clusters of tumor cells floating in pools of mucin (Fig. 2–86)
3. *Signet-ring*—tumors composed of diffusely infiltrating signet-ring cells (Fig. 2–87)
4. *Clear cell*—architecturally and cytologically similar to mesonephric adenocarcinoma of the female genital system (Fig. 2–88)
5. *Adenocarcinoma of no specific type*—not resembling one of the above patterns
6. *Mixed*—tumors with two or more of the patterns described above

Entities that may mimic adenocarcinoma include florid cystitis cystica and glandularis, villous adenoma, nephrogenic adenoma, endometriosis, and endocervicosis.

Stage is of considerable prognostic importance in bladder adenocarcinoma. It is assigned using the same criteria one uses to stage urothelial carcinoma. Transmural penetration portends a very poor prognosis in all subtypes. The signet-ring cell type appears to have the worst overall prognosis.

Urachal adenocarcinoma is distinguished from adenocarcinoma arising in bladder mucosa. It must be located in the dome of the bladder, and there must be no cystitis glandularis or intestinal metaplasia in the adjacent bladder mucosa; that is, there should be an abrupt transition from normal urothelium to adenocarcinoma. Furthermore, origin from an adjacent organ must be excluded. Other features favoring urachal origin are tumor extension into the space of Retzius, the presence of urachal remnants, and tumor involvement of detrusor muscle with normal overlying urothelium.

Patients range in age from 15 years to late adulthood; the mean age at diagnosis is 50 years. Males are more commonly affected. Presenting symptoms include

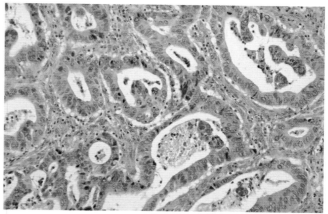

FIGURE 2–85 |▌|| Adenocarcinoma of bladder, enteric type. The tumor resembles typical colonic adenocarcinoma.

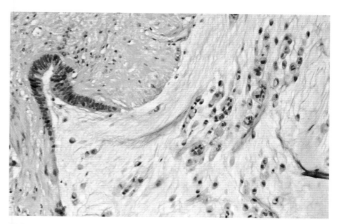

FIGURE 2–86 |▌|| Adenocarcinoma of bladder, mucinous (colloid) type. Malignant cells float in a pool of mucin.

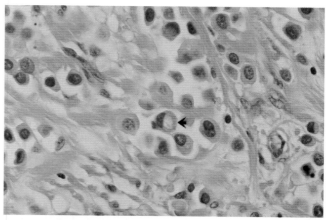

FIGURE 2–87 |▌|| Adenocarcinoma of bladder, signet-ring cell type. *Arrow* indicates a typical signet-ring cell with intracytoplasmic mucin displacing the nucleus to the periphery of the cell.

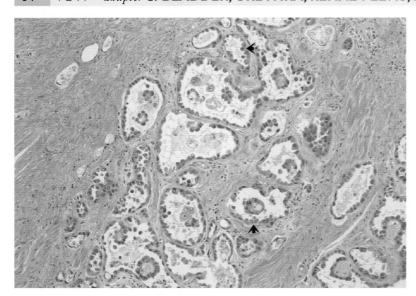

FIGURE 2–88 |█|| Adenocarcinoma of bladder, clear cell type. This example is composed predominantly of tubules lined by cuboidal cells and "hobnail cells" *(arrows)*.

hematuria, mucosuria, umbilical discharge, or irritative voiding symptoms. Cystoscopically, the typical lesion is located in the dome, has a glistening mucinous appearance, and may be covered by normal mucosa, although mucosal ulceration is common (Fig. 2–89). Any of the histologic patterns described for nonurachal adenocarcinoma may be evident microscopically, but mucinous (colloid) carcinoma is most common, followed by enteric-type adenocarcinoma (Fig. 2–90).

The validity of staging urachal adenocarcinoma is uncertain, because virtually all invade muscle from their onset. Survival rates for urachal and nonurachal adenocarcinoma are similar.

Small Cell Carcinoma

Small cell carcinoma accounts for at least 0.5% of bladder malignancies. Males are affected four times as frequently as women, and mean age of patients is 66 years. Hematuria is the common presenting complaint, with irritative or obstructive symptoms in some patients and, occasionally, with symptoms of a paraneoplastic syndrome. In many instances, the tumor is of advanced stage locally, or metastatic, when first discovered.

Endoscopically, small cell carcinoma has no distinctive characteristics. It forms a polypoid or solid sessile mass, up to 10 cm in diameter, often with mucosal ulceration. Microscopically, it consists of sheets of cells that demonstrate either an "oat cell" or an "intermediate cell" appearance. Oat cells have hyperchromatic nuclei with dispersed chromatin and almost no cytoplasm. Nucleoli are inconspicuous or absent. Intermediate cells have larger and less hyperchromatic nuclei and more abundant cytoplasm. Extensive necrosis, abundant mitotic figures, nuclear molding, and DNA encrustation of blood vessels are features seen with both cell types. Associated carcinoma of other types (urothelial, squamous cell, or adenocarcinoma) is present in up to two thirds of cases (Fig. 2–91). Tumor cells show positive immunostaining

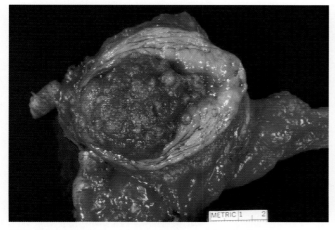

FIGURE 2–89 |█|| Adenocarcinoma originating in the urachus.

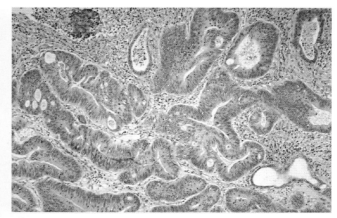

FIGURE 2–90 |█|| Urachal adenocarcinoma. This example resembles typical colonic adenocarcinoma.

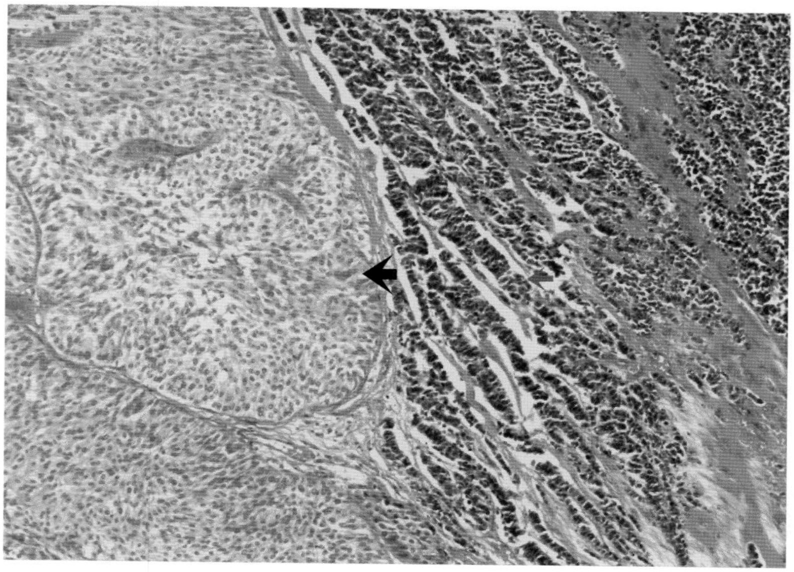

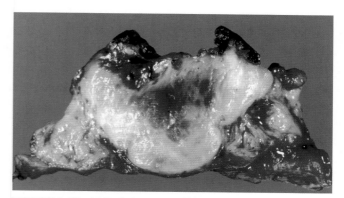

FIGURE 2–91 | ▮ | | Urothelial carcinoma *(black arrow)* admixed with small cell carcinoma *(blue arrow).*

for keratin and neuroendocrine markers in the majority of cases and negative staining for leukocyte common antigen, features helpful in excluding lymphoma. The differential diagnosis also includes small cell carcinoma arising in the prostate. Clinical correlation is required to make these distinctions.

BENIGN SOFT TISSUE NEOPLASMS

Leiomyoma

Nearly 200 cases have been reported, twice as often in women as in men, and rarely in children. Patients present with obstructive voiding symptoms, or less commonly, symptoms of ureteral obstruction. Lesions appear cystoscopically as sessile or pedunculated polyps, usually less than 4 cm in diameter but occasionally much larger. Grossly, leiomyoma is well circumscribed, with a bulging cut surface (Fig. 2–92). Microscopically, it is composed of bundles of spindle cells with pink cytoplasm and cigar-

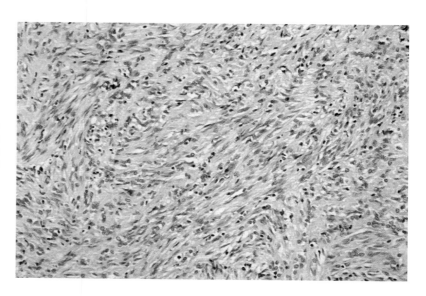

FIGURE 2–92 | ▮ | | Leiomyoma of bladder, surgically excised.

shaped nuclei (Fig. 2–93). Necrosis, mitotic figures, nuclear atypia, and an infiltrative interface with surrounding tissue are absent in leiomyoma; their presence raises concern for low-grade leiomyosarcoma.

FIGURE 2–93 | ▮ | | Leiomyoma of bladder. The tumor consists of swirling fascicles of benign smooth muscle cells without cytologic atypia, necrosis, or mitotic figures. The patient was alive and free of disease after 11 years.

Hemangioma

Bladder hemangioma occurs more often in males and most often in patients younger than 30 years of age, many of whom also have cutaneous hemangiomas. Hematuria is the most common complaint, but irritative or obstructive symptoms may predominate. Endoscopy reveals purple mural nodules, which may mimic endometriosis, sarcoma, or melanoma. Most hemangiomas are less than 2 cm in diameter, but lesions up to 10 cm rarely occur. The extent of mural involvement varies. Microscopically, hemangioma is composed of blood-filled vascular channels of variable size and shape, lined by benign endothelial cells that lack mitotic activity. Cavernous hemangioma is most common.

Neurofibroma

Neurofibroma of the bladder occasionally occurs in patients with von Recklinghausen's disease. There is a slight male preponderance, and age at presentation ranges from infancy to late adulthood. Symptoms include hematuria and irritative or obstructive voiding complaints. Multiplicity and recurrence are common. At cystoscopy, solitary or multiple sessile or pedunculated submucosal polyps are observed, up to several centimeters in diameter. Microscopically, neurofibroma is composed of elongated spindle cells with thin wavy nuclei in a collagenized fibrillar matrix.

Granular Cell Tumor

Granular cell tumor is a rare cause of hematuria in adults. It is usually a solitary yellow-white submucosal nodule, up to 12 cm in diameter. Microscopically, it is composed of polygonal cells with abundant pink cytoplasm, which appears coarsely granular. It is believed to be of Schwann cell origin; the cytoplasm typically shows positive immunostaining for S-100 protein.

BLADDER SARCOMAS

Rhabdomyosarcoma

Most patients with rhabdomyosarcoma are younger than 5 years old, and a slight majority are male. Hematuria or symptoms of bladder outlet obstruction are common. At cystoscopy, the classic finding is a pale gray multinodular polypoid mass centered around the bladder neck and trigone, sometimes resembling a cluster of grapes (sarcoma botryoides) (Figs. 2–94 and 2–95) Microscopically, the common finding is a small round blue cell tumor, that is, small round blue cells with minimal cytoplasm in a loose myxoid stroma. These cells congregate beneath the urothelium to form a cambium layer (Fig. 2–96). In some cases, the diagnosis is assisted by the presence of rhabdoid cells or strap cells with cross striations (Fig. 2–97). In the majority of cases, confirmation of the diagnosis requires immunohistochemical, cyto-

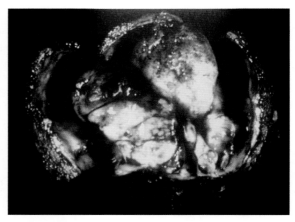

FIGURE 2–94 | ▮ | | Rhabdomyosarcoma of bladder.

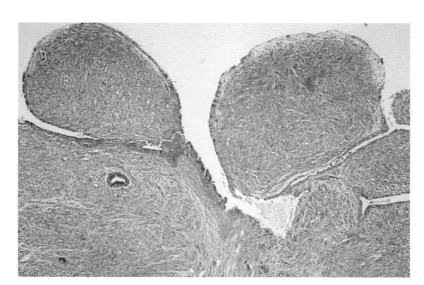

FIGURE 2–95 | ▮ | | Rhabdomyosarcoma of bladder. Polypoid masses of tumor are characteristic of a botryoides growth pattern.

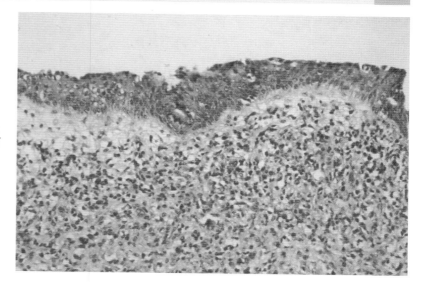

FIGURE 2–96 |▮|| Rhabdomyosarcoma of bladder. Intact urothelium with underlying cambium layer of malignant spindle cells.

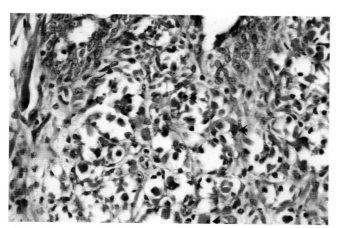

FIGURE 2–97 |▮|| Rhabdomyosarcoma of bladder. Diagnostic malignant rhabdomyoblasts *(arrows)* are present.

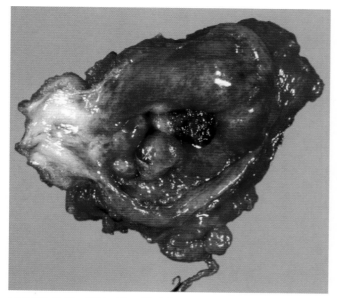

FIGURE 2–98 |▮|| Myxoid leiomyosarcoma of bladder. The bladder lumen contains a hemorrhagic and necrotic mass.

genetic, or ultrastructural studies to differentiate the lesion from several other small round blue cell tumors that afflict children.

Leiomyosarcoma

The majority of patients are middle-aged adults, although some are younger than 21 years old at the time of diagnosis. Patients complain of hematuria or obstructive voiding symptoms. Leiomyosarcoma appears lobulated or mushroom-shaped at cystoscopy (Fig. 2–98). Most tumors are between 2 and 5 cm in diameter, but some are much larger. Microscopically, leiomyosarcoma is composed of interlacing bundles of spindle cells with cigar-shaped nuclei and pink cytoplasm (Fig. 2–99). In contrast to leiomyoma, nuclear pleomorphism, mitotic figures, and necrosis are frequently present. Any level of mitotic activity in a smooth muscle neoplasm of the bladder, especially if an infiltrative interface is noted between the tumor and surrounding tissue, raises concern for leiomyosarcoma. Other lesions that may be difficult to differentiate from leiomyosarcoma are inflammatory pseudotumor, postoperative spindle cell nodule, and sarcomatoid urothelial carcinoma.

Other Sarcomas

Other rare sarcomas of the bladder include malignant fibrous histiocytoma (Fig. 2–100), osteogenic sarcoma, fibrosarcoma, angiosarcoma (Fig. 2–101), hemangiopericytoma, and liposarcoma. Sarcomatoid urothelial carcinoma can contain components indistinguishable from pure sarcoma and must be included in the differential diagnosis of bladder sarcoma.

HEMATOPOIETIC MALIGNANCIES

Lymphoma

Involvement of the bladder by systemic lymphoma is relatively common and usually asymptomatic, but primary involvement of the bladder in the absence of systemic lymphoma accounts for only 0.2% of extranodal lymphoma cases. The majority of patients are women in their

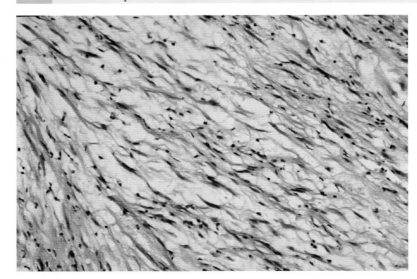

FIGURE 2–99 | ❚ | | Myxoid leiomyosarcoma of bladder. Malignant spindle cells arranged in fascicles with a prominent myxoid stroma.

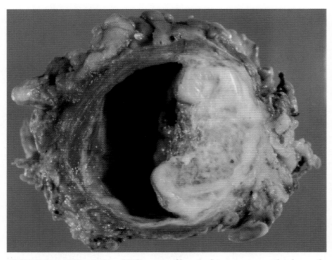

FIGURE 2–100 | ❚ | | Malignant fibrous histiocytoma (high-grade sarcoma). This whole mount of the bladder reveals a large fleshy mural mass on one side partially filling the lumen.

60s or 70s, who complain of hematuria, dysuria, or irritative symptoms. The infiltrates of malignant lymphoid cells may involve the bladder diffusely, without forming a discrete mass, or may form one or more sessile or polypoid nodules. Generally, the mucosa appears intact at cystoscopy. Biopsy specimens show diffuse infiltration of normal structures by lymphoid cells (Fig. 2–102). The differential diagnosis includes small cell carcinoma and lymphoepithelioma-like carcinoma. The use of immunohistochemical stains for lymphoid, neuroendocrine, and cytokeratin markers aids in establishing the correct diagnosis and subclassifying the type of lymphoma. Mucosa-associated lymphoid tissue (MALT)-type lymphoma, diffuse large cell lymphoma, and small lymphocytic lymphoma are most commonly encountered. Primary Hodgkin's lymphoma involving the bladder has been reported in three instances.

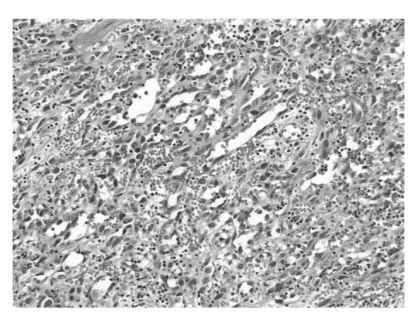

FIGURE 2–101 | ❚ | | Angiosarcoma of bladder, with typical vascular channels lined by malignant endothelial cells.

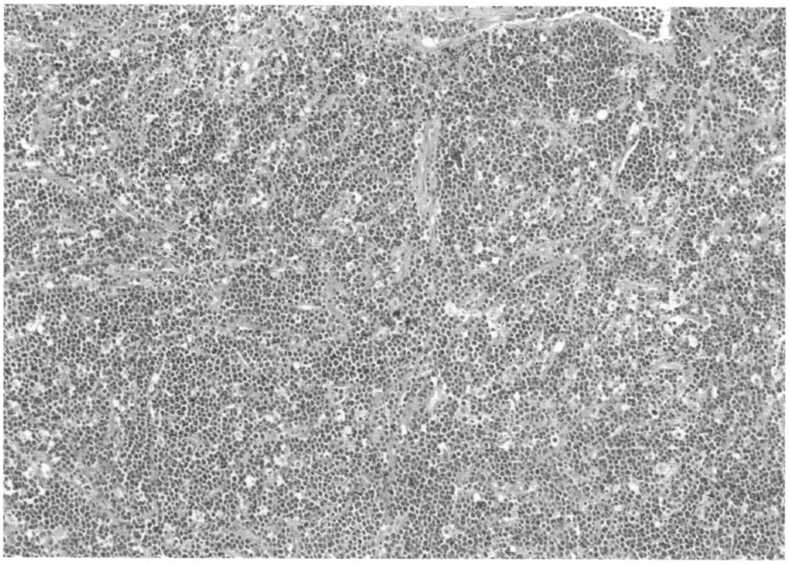

FIGURE 2–102 Lymphoma of bladder. The lamina propria is densely infiltrated by malignant lymphoid cells (small lymphocytic lymphoma).

Plasmacytoma

Bladder involvement by malignant plasma cells may be a component of systemic disease (multiple myeloma) or may be limited to the bladder (plasmacytoma). Patients are adults with hematuria. Tumor infiltrates form sessile or pedunculated mural nodules, with intact overlying mucosa. Microscopically, the infiltrates are composed of sheets of atypical plasma cells. Cases of solitary plasmacytoma have been treated successfully with radiation therapy without subsequent development of multiple myeloma.

Leukemia

Bladder involvement by leukemia is reported in up to 26% of patients dying of leukemia. Symptoms are generally insufficient to prompt investigation. The infiltrates of leukemic cells, although evident microscopically, only rarely form visible mural mass lesions.

MISCELLANEOUS BLADDER NEOPLASMS

Melanoma

Most patients with primary bladder melanoma are in their 50s or 60s and present either with hematuria or with symptoms related to metastases. The bladder lesions range in size up to 8 cm in diameter. At cystoscopy, they have a fungating or polypoid appearance, usually with dark pigmentation evident (Fig. 2–103). Microscopically, they are composed of aggregates of polygonal or spindle-shaped cells, some of which may contain pigment (Fig. 2–104). Diagnosis is supported by positive immunostaining for S-100 protein and HMB45. Melanoma metastatic to the bladder is much more common than primary bladder melanoma. Clinical correlation is required to ascertain whether the bladder lesion is primary or metastatic.

Pheochromocytoma (Paraganglioma)

This tumor occurs in adolescents and adults, with approximately equal frequency in males and females. Hematuria is common, and about half of patients ex-

perience symptoms caused by release of catecholamines from the tumor, particularly when the bladder is full or during voiding. Tachycardia, fainting, dizziness, or headaches are reported. Cystoscopy reveals an intramural nodule varying in size up to 15 cm, often with mucosal ulcerations. Paraganglioma is lobulated, circumscribed, pink, or yellow-brown. It is composed of nests of cells (zellballen) with bland round to oval nuclei of variable size and abundant pink or clear cytoplasm (Fig. 2–105). The cell nests are surrounded by a network of small vessels. Mitotic activity and necrosis are limited or absent. Immunostains for keratin markers are negative, whereas various neuroendocrine markers are positive. Sustentacular cells around the zellballen show positive

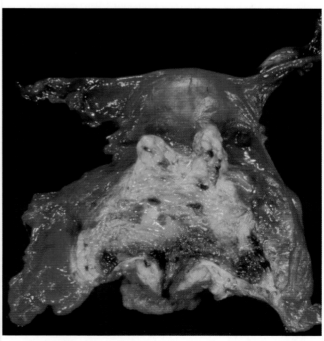

FIGURE 2–103 Primary melanoma of the urethra and bladder neck. Part of the tumor displays jet-black pigmentation.

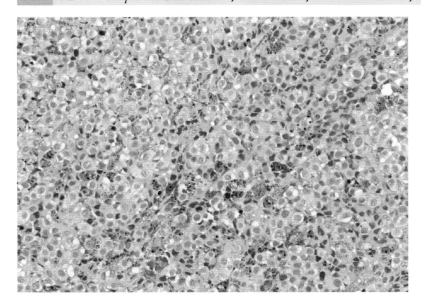

FIGURE 2–104 ▮▮▮ Melanoma of bladder, composed of a mixture of pigmented and nonpigmented malignant melanocytes.

immunostaining for S-100 protein. Up to 15% of bladder paragangliomas are malignant.

Cancer Metastatic to the Bladder

About 13% of bladder cancers originate outside the bladder and involve the bladder by direct extension from an adjacent site such as colon, prostate, or uterine cervix (72%), metastasis from a distant site (17%), or infiltration by systemic hematopoietic disease (11%). Metastases account for 2.3% of bladder cancers. Melanoma is the most common primary site, followed in order by carcinoma of the stomach, breast, kidney, and lung. Although the majority of metastases to the bladder are not clinically evident during life, bladder symptoms occasionally are the first indication of malignancy originating in a distant organ.

URETHRA

NON-NEOPLASTIC DISORDERS

Congenital Urethral Polyp

This rare lesion is found only in males, most of whom present between the ages of 6 and 9 years with obstructive or irritative voiding symptoms, hematuria, or urethral bleeding. Most lesions are located in the prostatic urethra near the verumontanum, but some arise in the distal urethra. The polyp is composed of a stalk containing blood vessels, loose fibrous tissue, and sometimes smooth muscle, covered by urothelium, which may show reactive or reparative features or ulceration (Fig. 2–106).

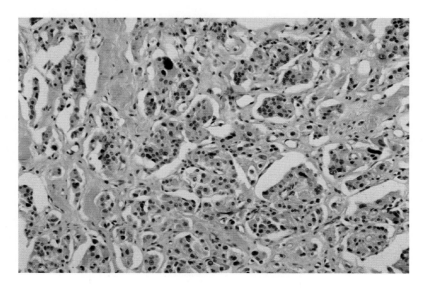

FIGURE 2–105 ▮▮▮ Pheochromocytoma (paraganglioma) of bladder. Tumor cells are typically arranged in discrete nests ("zellballen").

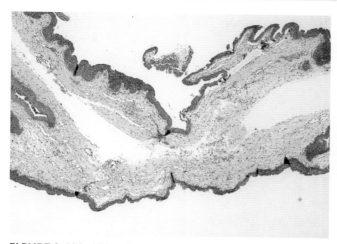

FIGURE 2–106 | ▌ | | Congenital urethral polyp. The patient was a 7-year-old boy with urethral bleeding. A long thin polyp was noted arising in the prostatic urethra and protruding into the bulbous urethra. It consists of a fibrovascular core lined by normal urothelium.

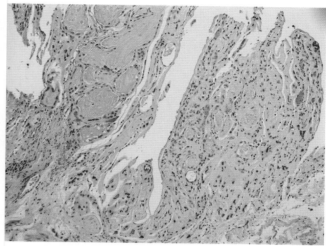

FIGURE 2–108 | ▌ | | Nephrogenic metaplasia, tubular and cystic types, noted incidentally in the urothelium lining a surgically excised urethral diverticulum.

Prostatic-type Urethral Polyp

Discovery of this lesion may be incidental or may be prompted by hematuria or hematospermia, most commonly in men younger than 30 years old. It forms short papillary fronds in the urethral mucosa, of variable extent, usually in the prostatic urethra but sometimes at the bladder neck or even in the distal urethra. Microscopically, it consists of papillary or polypoid fronds lined by cuboidal or columnar epithelial cells that are indistinguishable from those lining normal prostatic acini (Fig. 2–107). Appropriate immunostains help to confirm that the cells are of prostatic origin. In older men, careful attention to cytologic details is important to exclude adenocarcinoma, which can present with similar symptoms and endoscopic findings.

Urethral Diverticulum

This is a saccular outpouching of urethral mucosa, most commonly affecting females. Although it may be of congenital origin, the vast majority are probably acquired as a result of infection and inflammation superimposed on obstruction and dilatation of paraurethral glands. Urethral pain, drainage of urine or purulent material, or irritative voiding symptoms draw attention to the lesion, which may be palpable. Microscopically, there is acute and chronic inflammation in the soft tissues surrounding the diverticulum. The diverticulum is lined by urothelium; however, the development of squamous, glandular, or nephrogenic metaplasia is quite common (Fig. 2–108). Reported complications include stone formation and carcinoma, which

FIGURE 2–107 | ▌ | | Prostatic urethral polyp. This polypoid structure was noted in the prostatic urethra of an adult male. It is composed of prostatic acini and lacks any urothelial lining. In this instance, part of the polyp is replaced by prostatic adenocarcinoma *(arrows)*.

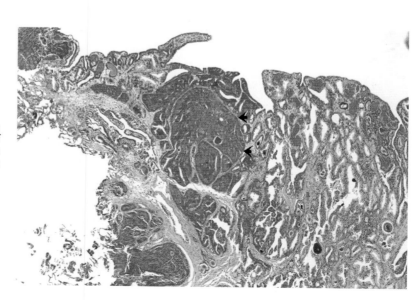

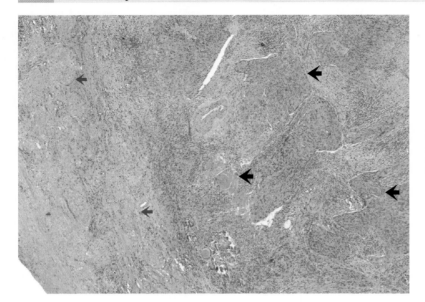

FIGURE 2–109 |▌|| Squamous cell carcinoma *(black arrows)* discovered unexpectedly in a surgically excised urethral diverticulum. The thickened and fibrotic wall of the diverticulum is at far left *(blue arrows).*

may be urothelial, squamous, conventional adenocarcinoma, or clear cell adenocarcinoma (Fig. 2–109).

Urethral Caruncle

This lesion is noted only in females, most of whom are postmenopausal. The etiology is uncertain, but mucosal prolapse and/or obstructive/inflammatory changes in paraurethral glands and stroma may be involved. The lesion may be asymptomatic or may cause pain or bloody spotting. Grossly, caruncle is a red or pink, polypoid or pedunculated lesion immediately adjacent to the urethral meatus. Microscopically, there are variable components of proliferative epithelium, neovascularity, and inflammatory infiltrate (Fig. 2–110). Reactive atypical stromal cells and glandular elements derived from preexisting paraurethral glands are sometimes present. Caruncles have no association with neoplasia.

Urethral Meatal Cyst

Urethral meatal cyst is a median raphe cyst arising at the urethral meatus (Figs. 2–111 and 2–112). The gross and microscopic findings in median raphe cyst are described in Chapter 6.

Nephrogenic Metaplasia

Metaplastic changes in the urethral epithelium may be of squamous, intestinal, or nephrogenic type, similar to changes encountered in the bladder and upper tracts, and with similar etiology and symptomatology. Nephrogenic metaplasia in the prostatic urethra may appear endoscopically as a papillary or sessile erythematous lesion. In females, the lesion is usually encountered incidentally during examination of an excised urethral diverticulum. The microscopic features are as described in the section on bladder pathology.

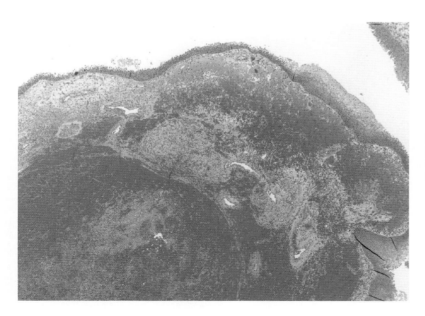

FIGURE 2–110 |▌|| Urethral caruncle. The lesion is polypoid, with marked edema, hemorrhage, and chronic inflammation in the stroma. The overlying epithelium is partly squamous and partly urothelial.

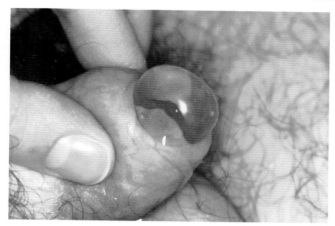

FIGURE 2–111 | ▮ | | Urethral meatal cyst. (Courtesy of Allan Decter, MD, Winnipeg, Manitoba.)

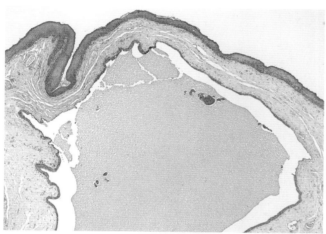

FIGURE 2–112 | ▮ | | Urethral meatal cyst. The cyst is lined by pseudostratified columnar epithelium and contains mucoproteinaceous material.

Amyloidosis

The urethra is the portion of the urinary tract least commonly involved by amyloidosis. Amyloid deposition in the urethra may be "tumoral," without evidence of systemic illness, or nontumoral and associated with systemic disease. Either form can cause hematuria; the tumoral type may obstruct urination. Any portion of the urethra may be involved. Tumoral deposits appear as plaques or mucosal nodules, sometimes with surface ulceration, and mimic neoplasia when viewed endoscopically. The tumoral lesions show amyloid deposits diffusely in lamina propria and underlying soft tissue; amyloid deposits occurring in a setting of systemic illness are usually concentrated around blood vessels. Appropriate special stains assist in making the correct diagnosis.

Malakoplakia

Urethral involvement by this disorder is rare. Women are affected much more often than men. Patients complain of irritative or obstructive voiding symptoms. Cystoscopy

reveals a nodular, polypoid or plaquelike mass. The histologic features of this lesion were described previously in the section on bladder disorders.

Condyloma Acuminatum

This lesion is caused by human papillomavirus and is sexually transmitted. It is estimated to account for up to 30% of male urethral tumors. Symptoms include urethral bleeding or deviation of the urinary stream. Lesions appear endoscopically as solitary or multiple white papillomatous mucosal excrescences. Microscopically, condyloma consists of flat or papillary hyperplastic squamous epithelium, with nuclear features collectively called koilocytic atypia—eccentrically placed hyperchromatic nuclei with irregular nuclear outlines and cytoplasmic retraction artifact that produces a perinuclear halo effect.

Malignancies of the Urethra

The urethra is composed of tissues similar to those found in the renal pelvis, ureter, and bladder. Not surprisingly, malignancies such as urothelial carcinoma, squamous cell carcinoma (Fig. 2–113), various types of adenocarcinoma (Figs. 2–114 and 2–115), and melanoma (Fig. 2–116) arise in the urethra and are not unique to this site. They are not discussed in detail in this section.

Other Urethral Lesions

Some urethral lesions are managed without a need to submit tissue for pathologic evaluation. Urethritis, posterior urethral valves (Fig. 2–117), urethral strictures, and certain congenital disorders such as megalourethra fall into this category.

RENAL PELVIS AND URETER

CONGENITAL MALFORMATIONS

The renal pelvis and ureter are conduits composed of interlacing fascicles of spirally oriented smooth muscle and lined by urothelial mucosa. Their function is dependent on the presence of intrinsically normal musculature and proper spatial orientation with respect to the bladder. Surgical correction of malformations involves the excision of an intrinsically defective segment of the collecting system (as in congenital uretero-pelvic

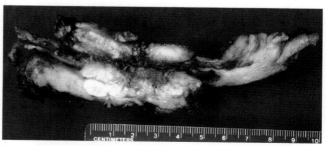

FIGURE 2–113 | ▮ | | Squamous cell carcinoma of the urethra. Patient was a 27-year-old man. (*Red arrow* indicates tumor extension into periurethral soft tissues.) (Courtesy of Wei Yang, MD, Cleveland, Ohio.)

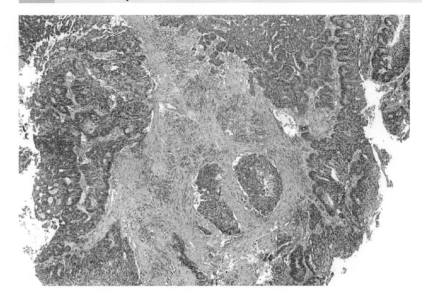

FIGURE 2–114 ▎▉▎▎ Adenocarcinoma of urethra. This tumor originated in the urethra of a 68-year-old woman.

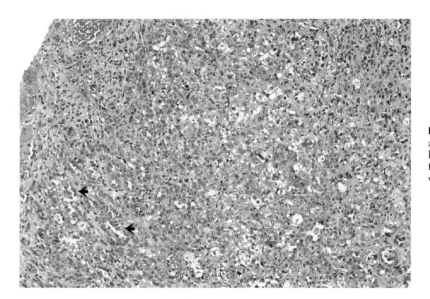

FIGURE 2–115 ▎▉▎▎ Clear cell adenocarcinoma that arose in the urethra of a 63-year-old woman. At lower left *(black arrows)* the tumor forms luminal structures focally lined by hobnail cells. Small aggregates of cells with clear cytoplasm are also present *(red arrows)*.

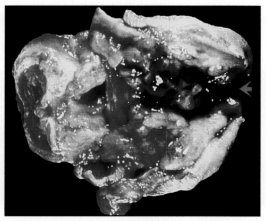

FIGURE 2–116 ▎▉▎▎ Melanoma arising in the distal urethra (distal penectomy specimen). The tumor is darkly pigmented and hemorrhagic *(red arrow)*.

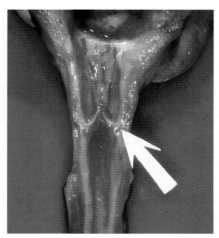

FIGURE 2–117 ▎▉▎▎ Posterior urethral valves *(arrow)*.

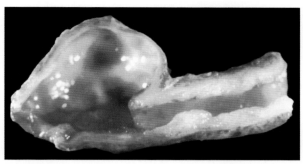

FIGURE 2–118 |▮|| Ureterocele, evident at left as a cystic dilatation of the distal ureter.

junction obstruction [see Fig. 1–19], ureterocele [Fig. 2–118], ureteral diverticulum [Fig. 2–119], and primary megaureter), or the reestablishment of proper anatomy (as in correction of ureteral reflux, ureteral ectopia, or paraureteral diverticulum). Evaluation of an excised segment of the drainage system usually centers on the status of the musculature; the overlying mucosa is generally normal.

Congenital Ureteropelvic Junction Obstruction

The microscopic findings in this condition are variable. The muscle layers are normal, attenuated, disorganized, or predominantly longitudinal. In a minority of cases, the obstruction is extrinsic to the collecting system and caused by impingement of polar vessels associated with renal malrotation.

Ureterocele

Ureterocele may show absence of musculature, muscular atrophy, or muscular hypertrophy.

Primary Megaureter

Primary megaureter includes two separate pathologic entities. In the great majority of cases, the proximal ureteral muscle is hypertrophic and the thin distal ureteral segment shows mural fibrosis, muscular hypoplasia, predominance of circular muscle fibers, or fibromuscular thickening of the wall. In 20% of cases, the thin distal segment appears intrinsically normal and the proximal dilated segment shows marked diminution or absence of musculature. Marked diminution of ureteral muscle with absence of fascicle formation is also noted in conditions known as *ureteral dysplasia.* These malformed ureters are associated with renal dysplasia in about two thirds of cases.

Vesicoureteric Reflux

Reflux of urine from the bladder into the ureter is primarily an anatomic problem related to shortness of the intravesical portion of the distal ureter. Distal ureteral segments excised during correction of reflux may show diminution in the number of longitudinal muscle fibers. The fact that establishment of an adequate intravesical tunnel corrects the vast majority of reflux conditions suggests that there is no significant intrinsic ureteral abnormality in these cases. Similarly, the abnormalities involved in ureteral ectopia are anatomic rather than intrinsic.

Paraureteral Diverticulum

This is a congenital or acquired defect in bladder wall musculature in the region of the intravesical portion of the ureter. Lack of anatomic support of the distal ureter predisposes to reflux. The ureter in such cases is either intrinsically normal or dysplastic (with associated renal dysplasia).

NON-NEOPLASTIC CONDITIONS

Ureteritis Cystica and Pyelitis Cystica

These are reactive conditions that are sometimes noted in association with inflammation or neoplasia and rarely may be grossly evident as cystic lesions in the mucosa of the ureter or renal pelvis (Fig. 2–120). Their microscopic features are similar to those of cystitis cystica, previously described.

Squamous Metaplasia

When squamous metaplasia occurs in the renal pelvis or ureter, it is usually a response to a chronic irritant, such

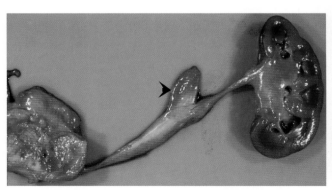

FIGURE 2–119 |▮|| Ureteral diverticulum *(arrow).*

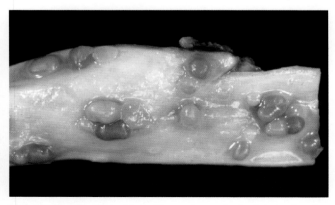

FIGURE 2–120 |▮|| Ureteritis cystica and glandularis, forming numerous small nodules in the ureteral mucosa.

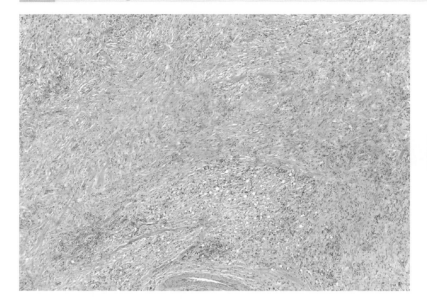

FIGURE 2–121 ▮▮▮ Retroperitoneal fibrosis at low magnification. The plaque consists of fibrous tissue diffusely infiltrated by inflammatory cells.

as a calculus or indwelling catheter, and is more often keratinizing than nonkeratinizing. Exfoliation of keratinous debris and squamous cells can result in the formation of a *cholesteatoma*, a white mass lesion that mimics a neoplasm. Keratinizing squamous metaplasia is also associated with increased risk of squamous cell carcinoma and urothelial carcinoma.

Nephrogenic Metaplasia

Nephrogenic metaplasia rarely occurs in the ureter. Its microscopic appearance is similar to that of its counterpart in the bladder.

Malakoplakia

Malakoplakia is encountered in the renal pelvis and ureter, but far less commonly than in the bladder. Its pathogenesis was discussed in the section on bladder pathology. It forms soft yellow-brown nodular masses or plaques. The microscopic findings are as described previously.

Retroperitoneal Fibrosis

This is a fibrosing inflammatory condition that exerts its adverse effects on the abdominal portion of the ureters. Its etiology is usually indeterminate, although some cases are related to a diversity of factors, such as aneurysms, vasculitis, inflammatory bowel disease, use of ergot compounds, and neoplasms. It mainly affects men 40 to 60 years of age. Symptoms in the early phase of the disease are usually constitutional, often with pain in the lower flanks and back. As the disease progresses, symptoms of uremia supervene. Radiologic studies show medial deviation of the ureters, with varying degrees of hydronephrosis. Grossly, retroperitoneal fibrosis is a pale gray irregular plaque that encases the ureters and blood vessels. Microscopically, the plaque is composed of a variable mixture of fibrous tissue with a polymorphous assortment of chronic inflammatory cells (Figs. 2–121 and 2–122).

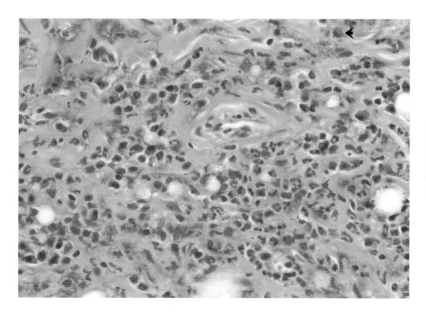

FIGURE 2–122 ▮▮▮ Retroperitoneal fibrosis at high magnification. In a background of fibrous tissue is a polymorphous assortment of acute and chronic inflammatory cells: neutrophils *(blue arrow)*, mature lymphocytes *(green arrow)*, plasma cells *(red arrow)*, macrophages *(yellow arrow)*, and eosinophils *(black arrow)*.

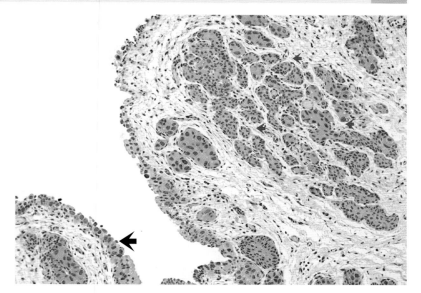

FIGURE 2–123 |▌| | In situ *(black arrow)* and invasive *(blue arrows)* urothelial carcinoma of the proximal ureter. Carcinoma cells were identified in urine from this collecting system several times, but ureteroscopy and retrograde pyelograms showed no lesion. Nephroureterectomy was performed entirely on the basis of positive urine cytology.

NEOPLASMS OF URETER AND RENAL PELVIS

Neoplasms occur with approximately equal frequency in the ureter and renal pelvis. The spectrum of neoplasia in these sites is similar to that encountered in the bladder, but with only one tenth the frequency. The vast majority are epithelial, and 80% are malignant.

BENIGN EPITHELIAL NEOPLASMS

Urothelial Papilloma

This uncommon noninvasive papillary tumor is usually asymptomatic and is found incidentally. Its microscopic features are as described previously.

Inverted Papilloma

Inverted papilloma is more common in the ureter than in the renal pelvis. It occurs most often in men in their 60s and may present with hematuria or may be found incidentally during radiologic studies of the upper tracts. Its gross and microscopic appearance has been described previously.

CARCINOMA

Urothelial Carcinoma in Situ

Urothelial carcinoma in situ of the ureter and renal pelvis has been shown to have the same predisposition to the development of urothelial carcinoma as its counterpart in the urinary bladder. It is found in the mucosa adjacent to invasive urothelial cancers in these sites in 95% of cases (Fig. 2–123). Mucosa involved by carcinoma in situ may appear normal or erythematous. The microscopic findings were described previously.

Urothelial Carcinoma

Urothelial carcinoma arising in the upper tracts has been noted to be associated with tobacco use, Balkan nephropathy, and exposure to industrial carcinogens, thorium-containing contrast materials, and excess phenacetin usage. Patients present with hematuria and/or flank pain.

The calyces and renal pelvis are involved by urothelial carcinoma twice as often as the ureters, and the distal ureter is more often involved than the proximal ureter. Tumors are often multifocal, and about half of affected patients have a prior history of urothelial carcinoma or experience the development of a subsequent urothelial carcinoma elsewhere in the urinary tract. The occurrence of subsequent tumors in the ureteral stump after standard nephrectomy in 15% of cases has resulted in the adoption of nephroureterectomy as the standard surgical procedure for these tumors.

Urothelial carcinoma is typically exophytic and papillary (Figs. 2–124 and 2–125) or solid and infiltrative with a scirrhous, desmoplastic response (Fig. 2–126).

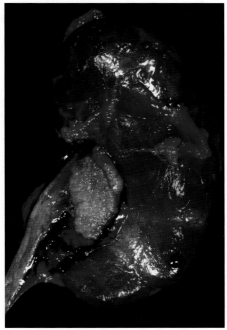

FIGURE 2–124 |▌| | Urothelial carcinoma, almost entirely filling the renal pelvis.

Infiltrative tumors of the pelvis or calyces can diffusely invade renal parenchyma as well as hilar or perirenal fat; this occurrence is especially likely in high-grade and sarcomatoid cancers (Figs. 2–127 and 2–128). The microscopic findings are identical to those described in the section on bladder neoplasms.

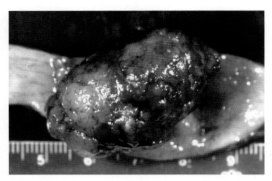

FIGURE 2–125 |▮|| Urothelial carcinoma forming a polypoid ureteral mass.

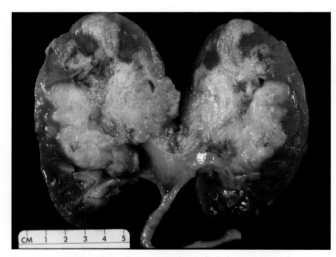

FIGURE 2–126 |▮|| Sarcomatoid urothelial carcinoma forming a polypoid mass in the renal pelvis and diffusely infiltrating renal parenchyma.

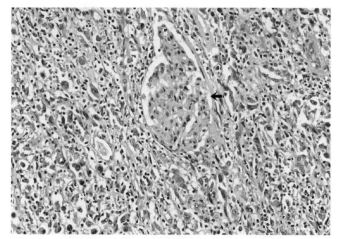

FIGURE 2–127 |▮|| High-grade urothelial carcinoma composed of spindle and pleomorphic cells (sarcomatoid carcinoma) infiltrating renal parenchyma. A residual glomerulus is present centrally *(arrow)*.

Prognosis is related to tumor grade, tumor stage, and tumor multiplicity. Grading is the same as for bladder urothelial neoplasms.

A widely used staging system is given in Table 2–2.

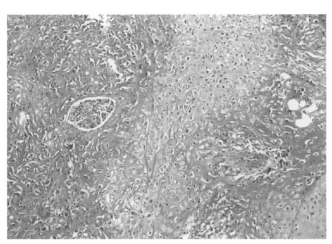

FIGURE 2–128 |▮|| Sarcomatoid urothelial carcinoma infiltrating renal parenchyma. Part of the tumor was osteosarcoma with a large cartilaginous component. Tumor originated as a high-grade papillary urothelial carcinoma in the renal pelvis.

TABLE 2–2

TNM STAGING OF CARCINOMA OF RENAL PELVIS AND URETER

Primary Tumor (T)

TX	Primary tumor cannot be assessed
T0	No evidence of primary tumor
Ta	Noninvasive papillary carcinoma
Tis	Carcinoma *in situ*
T1	Tumor invades subepithelial connective tissue
T2	Tumor invades muscularis
T3	(For renal pelvis only) Tumor invades beyond muscularis into peripelvic fat or the renal parenchyma
T3	(For ureter only) Tumor invades beyond muscularis into periureteric fat
T4	Tumor invades adjacent organs, or through the kidney into the perinephric fat

Regional Lymph Nodes (N)

NX	Regional lymph nodes cannot be assessed
N0	No regional lymph node metastasis
N1	Metastasis in a single lymph node, 2 cm or less in greatest dimension
N2	Metastasis in a single lymph node, more than 2 cm but not more than 5 cm in greatest dimension; or multiple lymph nodes, none more than 5 cm in greatest dimension
N3	Metastasis in a lymph node, more than 5 cm in greatest dimension

Note: Laterality does not affect the N classification

Distant Metastasis (M)

MX	Distant metastasis cannot be assessed
M0	No distant metastasis
M1	Distant metastasis

Note: Histopathologic types included are urothelial (transitional cell) carcinoma, squamous cell carcinoma, adenocarcinoma, and undifferentiated carcinoma.

Used with the permission of the American Joint Committee on Cancer (AJCC), Chicago, Illinois. The original source for this material is the *AJCC Cancer Staging Manual, Sixth Edition* (2002) published by Springer-Verlag New York, www.springer-ny.com.

Squamous Cell Carcinoma

This tumor is rare in the ureter but accounts for about 10% of renal pelvic neoplasms. There is commonly a history of chronic infection and calculus disease. It is an aggressive tumor, which tends to infiltrate the renal parenchyma, and stage at the time of diagnosis is often advanced, leading to a very poor prognosis (Fig. 2–129). Few patients survive 5 years. The gross and microscopic findings are similar to those noted in the bladder.

Adenocarcinoma

Primary adenocarcinoma of the renal pelvis or ureter is rare. It usually arises in a background of chronic infection and calculus disease. Papillary architecture or abundant mucin production is frequently noted. Advanced stage at the time of diagnosis is common, and prognosis is poor.

Metastases to the Ureter

Vascular metastases of cancer to the ureter most commonly originate from breast or colon primaries. Direct extension from adjacent malignancy arising in the bladder, prostate, or uterine cervix is a more common mode of involvement than vascular spread.

SOFT TISSUE TUMORS

Fibroepithelial Polyp

This lesion occurs more often in the upper tracts than in the bladder. It affects patients of all ages, although most are middle aged, and the majority are males. In children, it is the most common benign ureteral polyp. Patients present with hematuria and renal colic. The lesion consists of one or more polypoid projections, is lined by smooth shiny mucosa, and is localized to a single site. Microscopically, it has an edematous, noninflamed fibrovascular core, and its surface is covered by normal or ulcerated urothelium (Fig. 2–130).

Smooth Muscle Neoplasms

Leiomyoma and *leiomyosarcoma* are encountered in the ureter and renal pelvis less frequently than in the bladder. They present as hematuria or flank pain and form polypoid or infiltrative masses that mimic urothelial carcinoma grossly. Their microscopic features are discussed in the section on bladder pathology.

Miscellaneous Neoplasms

Other rare neoplasms that have been reported to arise in the ureter or renal pelvis are hemangioma, osteogenic sarcoma, malignant schwannoma, malignant melanoma, sarcomatoid carcinoma, and pure choriocarcinoma. Ureteral obstruction due to mural infiltration by lymphoma has been reported.

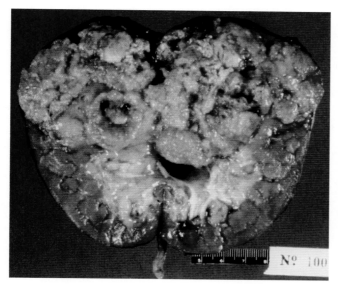

FIGURE 2–129 |▮|| Squamous cell carcinoma of the renal pelvis, extensively obliterating renal parenchyma.

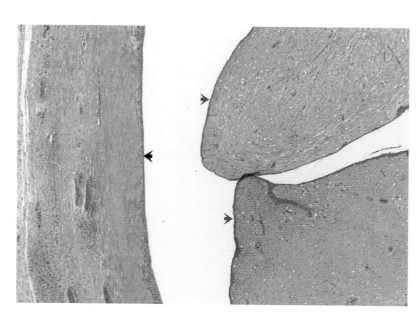

FIGURE 2–130 |▮|| Fibroepithelial polyp of the ureter. Ureteral wall is at left (*black arrow*). The polyp (*blue arrows*) consists of a fibrovascular core lined by thin urothelium, some of which appears to show squamous metaplasia.

Chapter 3

PROSTATE, SEMINAL VESICLES, AND PROSTATIC URETHRA

NORMAL HISTOLOGY OF THE PROSTATE, SEMINAL VESICLES, AND COWPER'S GLANDS

The prostate is composed of tubules and acinar structures supported by fibromuscular stroma. The acini have smooth, rounded contours. The lining epithelium forms arches, ridges, and papillary infoldings. The epithelium lining prostatic ducts and acini is composed of three principal cell types: secretory cells, basal cells, and neuroendocrine cells. The secretory luminal cells are cuboidal to columnar, with pale to clear cytoplasm, and produce prostate-specific antigen (PSA), prostatic acid phosphatase (PAP), acidic mucin, and other secretory products (Figs. 3–1 and 3–2). Melanin-like or lipofuscin-like pigment is sometimes seen in prostatic epithelial cells or in the stroma (Fig. 3–3). It probably represents cellular degeneration and has no apparent significance. The basal cells possess the highest proliferative activity of the pro-

static epithelium, albeit low, and are thought to contain a subset of stem cells that repopulate the secretory cell layer. Basal cells are selectively labeled with antibodies to high-molecular-weight keratins such as clone 34βE12, a property that is exploited immunohistochemically in separating benign acinar processes such as atrophy (which retains a basal cell layer) from adenocarcinoma (which lacks a basal cell layer) (Fig. 3–4). The neuroendocrine cells are the least common cell type of the prostatic epithelium and are usually not identified in routine hematoxylin and eosin–stained sections except for rare cells with large eosinophilic granules (Fig. 3–5). Although their function is unknown, neuroendocrine cells probably have an endocrine-paracrine regulatory role in growth and development.

The seminal vesicles are paired accessory sex glands situated adjacent to the posterolateral aspect of the prostate. Their excretory ducts merge with the ampullary portions of the vasa deferentia to form the ejaculatory ducts, which enter the prostatic urethra at the

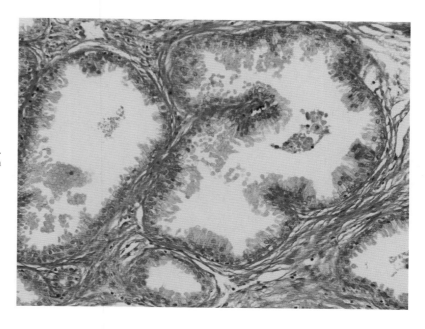

FIGURE 3–1 ▮▮▮ Benign prostatic epithelium. Although there is cell proliferation, spacing is uniform and nuclei are small without nucleolomegaly.

Several images in this chapter are courtesy of Mayo Clinic Foundation, Rochester, MN.

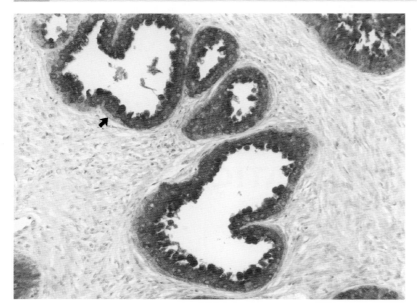

FIGURE 3–2 ▏▊▏▏ Benign prostatic epithelium. The secretory cells show strong cytoplasmic immunoreactivity to antibodies against prostate-specific antigen. The basal cells show no immunostaining *(arrow)*.

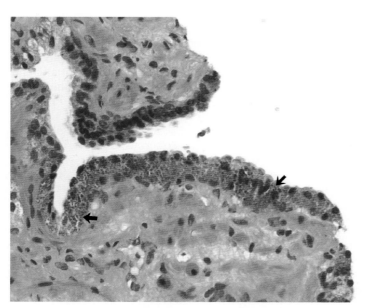

FIGURE 3–3 ▏▊▏▏ Melanin-like pigment in benign prostatic epithelium *(arrows)*.

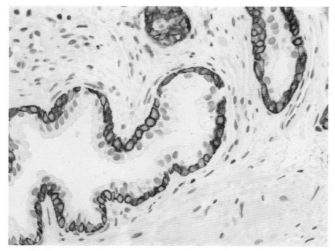

FIGURE 3–4 ▏▊▏▏ Benign prostatic epithelium. The basal cells show strong immunoreactivity to antibodies against keratin 34βE12. The overlying secretory cells show no immunostaining.

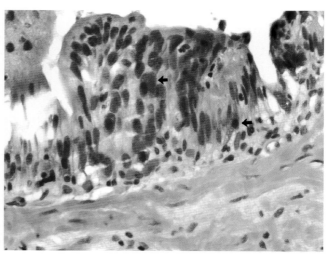

FIGURE 3–5 ▏▊▏▏ Neuroendocrine cells with dark red cytoplasmic granules *(arrows)*.

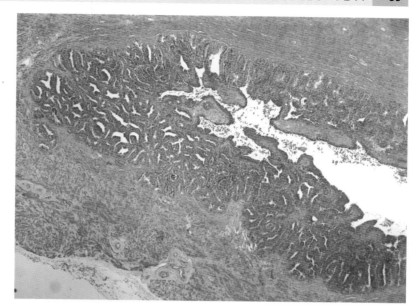

FIGURE 3–6 ⏐▮⏐⏐ Low-power view of normal seminal vesicle. A thick muscular wall surrounds complex tubulopapillary structures bordering a large central lumen.

verumontanum. Microscopically, the seminal vesicle is composed of complex papillary structures and small tubules arranged in lobular units around large central ducts (Fig. 3–6). The wall of the seminal vesicle consists of thick smooth muscle. The luminal structures are lined by basal cells and cuboidal to columnar secretory cells. The secretory cells often contain bright golden granules of lipofuscin and commonly exhibit marked cytologic atypia: hyperchromasia, multinucleation, and pronounced nucleomegaly (Fig. 3–7). In contrast to prostatic epithelium, seminal vesicle secretory cells do not show immunoreactivity to antibodies against PSA.

Although Cowper's glands are not part of the prostate, they are occasionally sampled inadvertently at the time of prostate needle biopsy, and they may create diagnostic uncertainty. They are small, paired bulbomembranous urethral glands composed of circumscribed lobules of closely packed uniform acini lined by cytologically benign cells with abundant apical mucinous cytoplasm (Fig. 3–8). Nuclei are inconspicuous. The secretory cells of Cowper's glands show no immunoreactivity to antibodies against PSA (Fig. 3–9).

INFLAMMATION

Patchy mild acute and chronic inflammation is present in most adult prostates and probably is a normal finding (Fig. 3–10). When the inflammation is severe, extensive, or clinically apparent, the term *prostatitis* is warranted.

FIGURE 3–7 ⏐▮⏐⏐ Seminal vesicle epithelium. Many cells contain bright golden lipofuscin granules *(arrow)*. Cell nuclei are hyperchromatic and vary considerably in size but lack nucleoli and mitotic figures.

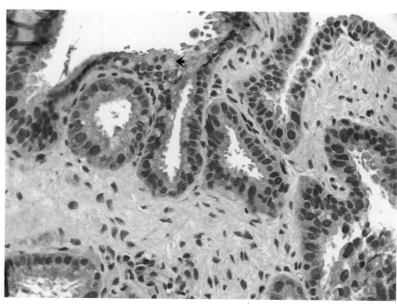

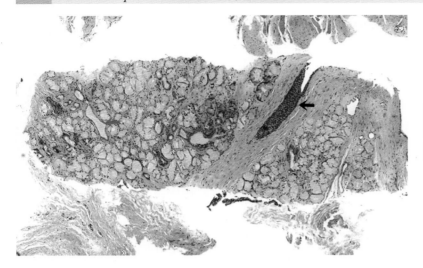

FIGURE 3–8 ▐▌▐▐ Cowper's gland. Circumscribed lobules of closely packed uniform acini lined by cytologically benign mucin-producing cells surround a central duct *(red arrow)*. Urethral urothelium is included in the biopsy core *(black arrow)*.

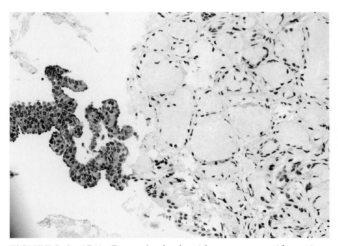

FIGURE 3–9 ▐▌▐▐ Cowper's gland, with prostate-specific antigen immunostain. The epithelial cells of Cowper's gland acini show no staining; a detached and unoriented strip of prostatic epithelium at left shows strong positive immunostaining.

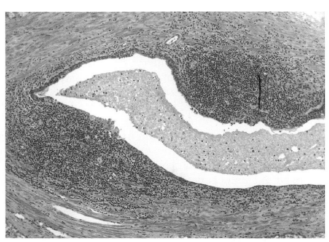

FIGURE 3–10 ▐▌▐▐ Nonspecific chronic inflammation. A large prostatic duct is surrounded by mature lymphocytes and a few macrophages. This type of chronic inflammation is very commonly observed in adult prostates.

There is a wide spectrum of prostatitides, many of which are rare and poorly understood.

ACUTE BACTERIAL PROSTATITIS

Patients with acute bacterial prostatitis present with sudden onset of fever, chills, irritative voiding symptoms, and pain in the lower back, rectum, and perineum. The prostate is swollen, firm, tender, and warm. Microscopically, there are sheets of neutrophils surrounding prostatic glands, often with marked tissue destruction and cellular debris (Fig. 3–11). The stroma is edematous and hemorrhagic, and microabscesses may be present. Diagnosis is based on culture of urine and expressed prostatic secretions; biopsy is contraindicated owing to the potential for sepsis. Most cases of acute prostatitis are caused by bacteria responsible for other

urinary tract infections, including *Escherichia coli* (80% of infections), other Enterobacteriaceae, *Pseudomonas, Serratia, Klebsiella* (10% to 15%), and *enterococci* (5% to 10%). Abscess is a rare complication, usually occurring in immunocompromised patients such as those with the acquired immunodeficiency syndrome (AIDS).

CHRONIC PROSTATITIS

Chronic abacterial prostatitis is more common than bacterial prostatitis and rarely follows infection elsewhere in the urinary tract. Patients often complain of painful ejaculation. Cultures of urine and expressed prostatic secretions are negative. The etiologic agent is unknown, but *Chlamydia, Ureaplasma,* and *Trichomonas* have been proposed. This form of prostatitis has a prolonged indolent course with relapses and remissions. Chronic bacterial

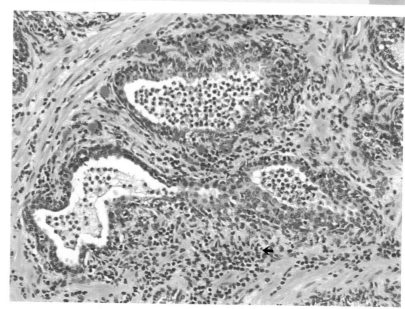

FIGURE 3–11 ▮▮ ▮▮ Acute prostatic inflammation. Neutrophils are present in the stroma *(black arrow)*, in prostatic epithelium *(red arrow)*, and within the lumens of the prostatic ducts *(blue arrow)*.

prostatitis is a common cause of relapsing urinary tract infection and is usually caused by *E. coli.* Clinical diagnosis is difficult, often requiring multiple urine cultures obtained after prostatic massage.

GRANULOMATOUS PROSTATITIS

Granulomatous prostatitis is a group of morphologically distinct forms of chronic prostatitis, the pathogenesis of which often cannot be determined. It accounts for about 1% of benign inflammatory conditions of the prostate. Causes include infection, tissue disruption after biopsy, bacille Calmette-Guérin (BCG) therapy, and others. The majority of patients have a prior history of urinary tract infection. The prostate is hard, fixed, and nodular, and cancer is usually suspected clinically. Urinalysis often shows pyuria and hematuria. Granulomatous prostatitis is probably caused by blockage of prostatic ducts and stasis of secretions, regardless of its etiology. The epithelium is destroyed, and cellular debris, bacterial toxins, and prostatic secretions escape into the stroma, eliciting an intense localized inflammatory response.

Idiopathic Granulomatous Prostatitis

Idiopathic (nonspecific) granulomatous prostatitis accounts for the majority of cases of granulomatous prostatitis (69%). The granulomas are usually noncaseating and associated with parenchymal loss and marked fibrosis (Figs. 3–12 and 3–13). Classification of eosinophilic and noneosinophilic types is probably of no clinical value.

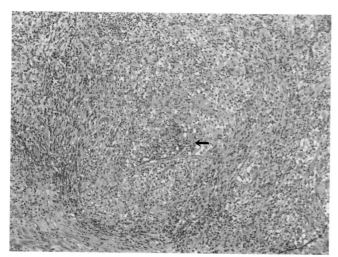

FIGURE 3–12 ▮▮ ▮▮ Nonspecific granulomatous prostatitis. The remnants of a prostatic duct, filled with inflammatory exudate, are present centrally *(arrow)*, surrounded by non-necrotizing granulomatous inflammation.

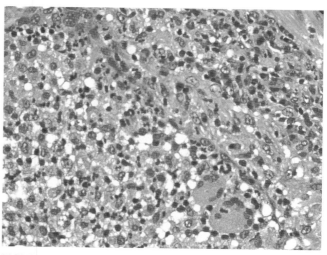

FIGURE 3–13 ▮▮ ▮▮ Nonspecific granulomatous prostatitis. There is a polymorphous assortment of inflammatory cells, including macrophages, plasma cells, lymphocytes, multinucleated giant cells, and occasional eosinophils.

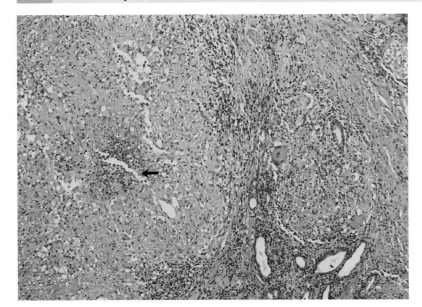

FIGURE 3–14 | ■ | | Granulomatous prostatitis in a patient who underwent cystoprostatectomy for bladder cancer after therapy with bacille Calmette-Guérin. At left is a granuloma with central necrosis *(black arrow);* at right is a non-necrotizing granuloma *(red arrow).* Special stains for acid-fast bacilli were negative.

Infectious Granulomatous Prostatitis

This is an unusual form of granulomatous prostatitis and may be caused by bacteria, fungi, parasites, and viruses. *Mycobacterium tuberculosis* infection of the prostate only occurs after pulmonary infection with miliary dissemination. Small, 1- to 2-mm caseating granulomas coalesce within the prostatic parenchyma, forming yellow nodules and streaks. Brucellosis may mimic tuberculosis clinically and pathologically. Mycotic infections of the prostate are rare and invariably follow fungemia. Most of the deep mycoses induce necrotizing and non-necrotizing granulomas and fibrosis. *Candida albicans* is usually only associated with acute inflammation. Granulomas caused by *Schistosoma hematobium* are frequently found in the prostate as well as the bladder and seminal vesicles in endemic areas. The organisms lodge in vesicular and pelvic venous plexuses as the final habitat. The adult female schistosome migrates into the submucosa of the urinary bladder and prostatic stroma where it lays eggs that induce granuloma formation and fibrosis.

Bacille Calmette-Guérin–Induced Granulomatous Prostatitis

This occurs in virtually all patients treated with intravesicular BCG immunotherapy for urothelial malignancy. The granulomas are characteristically discrete, with or without necrosis, and often contain numerous acid-fast bacilli (Fig. 3–14). No therapy is required.

MALAKOPLAKIA

Malakoplakia is a granulomatous disease associated with defective intracellular lysosomal digestion of bacteria. It occasionally occurs in the prostate, presenting as a diffuse indurated mass clinically suggestive of prostatic carcinoma. *E. coli* is commonly isolated from urine cultures. Microscopically, the prostate is effaced by sheets of

macrophages admixed with lymphocytes and plasma cells. Intracellular and extracellular Michaelis-Gutmann bodies are identified, appearing as sharply demarcated spherical structures with concentric "owl's eyes" measuring 5 to 10 μm in diameter. Periodic acid–Schiff stain is useful in identifying nonmineralized forms, and von Kossa stain can be used for mineralized forms (Fig. 3–15).

XANTHOMA AND XANTHOGRANULOMATOUS PROSTATITIS

Xanthoma is a rare form of idiopathic granulomatous prostatitis that consists of a localized collection of cholesterol-laden histiocytes; it may also be seen in patients with hyperlipidemia (Fig. 3–16).

Postsurgical Granulomatous Prostatitis

This can be identified years after transurethral resection owing to cauterization and surgical disruption of tissues. The granulomas are characteristically circumscribed and rimmed by palisading histiocytes with central fibrinoid necrosis (Fig. 3–17). Multinucleated giant cells are frequently present. Treatment is unnecessary.

OTHER FORMS OF GRANULOMATOUS PROSTATITIS

Other rare causes include sarcoidosis, rheumatoid nodule, polyarteritis nodosa, Wegener's granulomatosis, allergic (eosinophilic) prostatitis, Teflon-induced prostatitis, silicone-induced prostatitis, and giant cell arteritis (Fig. 3–17).

METAPLASIA

SQUAMOUS METAPLASIA

Squamous metaplasia may result from any of a variety of insults to the prostate, including acute inflammation,

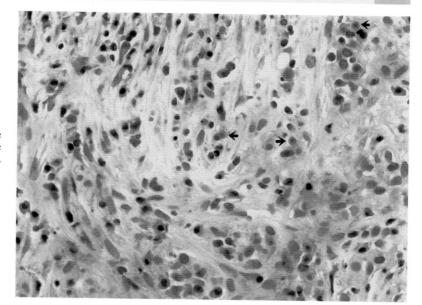

FIGURE 3–15 ▍▊▍▍ Malakoplakia in a prostate needle biopsy. Numerous Michaelis-Gutmann bodies are present *(arrows)*, as well as macrophages, plasma cells, and lymphocytes.

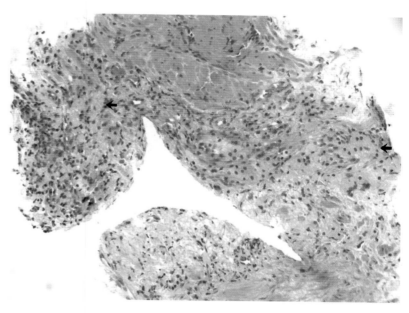

FIGURE 3–16 ▍▊▍▍ Xanthoma in a prostate needle biopsy, consisting of a large aggregate of foamy macrophages *(arrows)*. The findings in xanthoma may raise concern for Gleason pattern 4 adenocarcinoma.

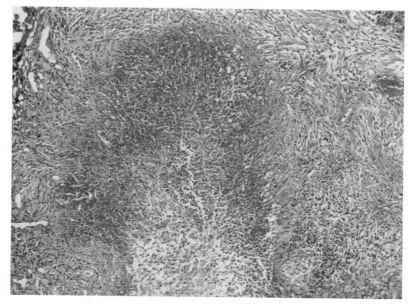

FIGURE 3–17 ▍▊▍▍ Necrotizing granuloma in a prostate chip obtained after transurethral resection. Histiocytes and fibroblasts are aligned at right angles to the area of central necrosis ("palisading granuloma"). This patient had Wegener's granulomatosis. Similar findings are often seen in prostates previously sampled or resected endoscopically.

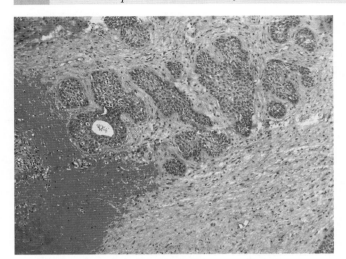

FIGURE 3–18 ▮▮▮ Squamous metaplasia of the epithelium of ducts and acini adjacent to a prostate infarct. The hemorrhage seen at left typically accompanies recent infarcts.

infarction, radiation therapy, and androgen deprivation therapy. The changes may be focal or diffuse, appearing as intraductal syncytial aggregates of flattened cells with abundant eosinophilic cytoplasm or cohesive aggregates of glycogen-rich clear cells with shrunken hyperchromatic nuclei (Fig. 3–18). Squamous metaplasia commonly involves the prostatic urethra in patients with an indwelling catheter.

MUCINOUS METAPLASIA

Mucinous metaplasia refers to clusters of tall columnar cells or goblet cells that are infrequently observed in the prostatic acinar epithelium. This finding is invariably microscopic and can also be seen in the urothelium of large periurethral prostatic ducts, foci of urothelial metaplasia, atrophy, nodular hyperplasia, basal cell hyperplasia, and postatrophic hyperplasia (Fig. 3–19).

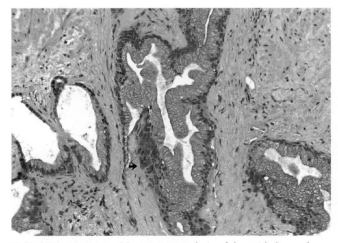

FIGURE 3–19 ▮▮▮ Mucinous metaplasia of the epithelium of prostatic ducts and acini, characterized by the presence of numerous tall, columnar, mucin-producing cells. In this image, numerous neuroendocrine cells with red granular cytoplasm are seen *(arrow)*.

NEPHROGENIC METAPLASIA

Nephrogenic metaplasia most often occurs in adult patients in the urinary bladder, renal pelvis, ureter, and urethra; prostatic urethral involvement is rare, and extension into the prostatic parenchyma may create diagnostic confusion with adenocarcinoma. It usually follows instrumentation, urethral catheterization, infection, or calculi.

Nephrogenic metaplasia appears as an exophytic papillary mass of cystic and solid tubules protruding from the urethral mucosa. The tubules may extend into the underlying prostate as a proliferation of small round to oval tubules, sometimes filled with colloid-like material. The lining consists of flattened or simple cuboidal cells, often with a distinctive hobnail appearance. (See Figures 2–42 and 2–45 in Chapter 2.)

HYPERPLASIA

NODULAR HYPERPLASIA (BENIGN PROSTATIC HYPERPLASIA)

Enlargement of the prostate, also known as nodular hyperplasia or benign prostatic hyperplasia (BPH), consists of overgrowth of the epithelium and fibromuscular tissue of the transition zone and periurethral area. Development of nodular hyperplasia includes three pathologic changes: nodule formation, diffuse enlargement of the transition zone and periurethral tissue, and enlargement of nodules. In men younger than 70 years of age, diffuse enlargement predominates; in older men, epithelial proliferation and expansile growth of existing nodules predominate, probably as the result of androgenic and other hormonal stimulation. The proportion of epithelium to stroma increases as obstructive symptoms become more severe.

Grossly, nodular hyperplasia consists of variably sized nodules that are soft or firm, rubbery, and yellow-gray and bulge from the cut surface on transection (Fig. 3–20). Degenerative changes include calcification and infarction. Nodular hyperplasia usually involves the transition zone, but occasionally nodules arise from the periurethral tissue at the bladder neck. Protrusion of bladder neck nodules into the bladder lumen is referred to as median lobe hyperplasia (Fig. 3–21).

Microscopically, nodular hyperplasia is composed of varying proportions of epithelium and stroma (fibrous connective tissue and smooth muscle) (Figs. 3–22 and 3–23). The most common are adenomyofibromatous nodules that contain all elements. The epithelial lining of the verumontanum may become abundant and proliferative (some refer to this as verumontanum mucosal gland hyperplasia), but criteria for separating normal and hyperplastic mucosa are not well defined (Fig. 3–24).

Vascular insufficiency probably accounts for infarction of hyperplastic nodules, seen in up to 20% of resected cases. The center of the nodule undergoes hemorrhagic necrosis, often with reactive changes in the residual epithelium at the periphery, including squamous metaplasia and transitional cell metaplasia (Fig. 3–25).

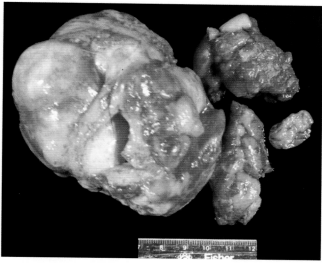

FIGURE 3–20 | ▌ | | Nodules of benign hyperplastic prostate tissue enucleated at open prostatectomy.

FIGURE 3–23 | ▌ | | Benign prostatic hyperplasia, predominantly stromal. Low-power view of the same case shown in Figure 3–22. In this area, there was marked stromal hyperplasia and very few glands.

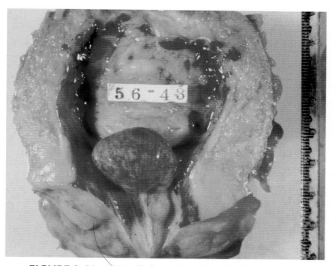

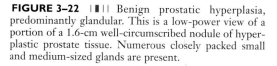

FIGURE 3–21 | ▌ | | Enlarged "median lobe" of prostate.

Nodular hyperplasia is not a precursor of cancer, but there are a number of similarities. Both display a parallel increase in prevalence with patient age according to autopsy studies, although cancer lags by 15 to 20 years. Both require androgens for growth and development, and both may respond to androgen deprivation treatment. Most cancers arise in patients with concomitant nodular hyperplasia, and cancer is found incidentally in a significant number (10%) of transurethral prostatectomy specimens.

ATROPHY AND POSTATROPHIC HYPERPLASIA (POSTINFLAMMATORY HYPERPLASIA; PARTIAL ATROPHY; POSTSCLEROTIC HYPERPLASIA)

Atrophy is a near-constant microscopic finding in the prostate, consisting of small distorted glands with flattened epithelium, hyperchromatic nuclei, and stromal

FIGURE 3–22 | ▌ | | Benign prostatic hyperplasia, predominantly glandular. This is a low-power view of a portion of a 1.6-cm well-circumscribed nodule of hyperplastic prostate tissue. Numerous closely packed small and medium-sized glands are present.

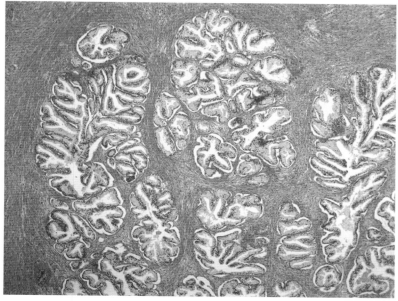

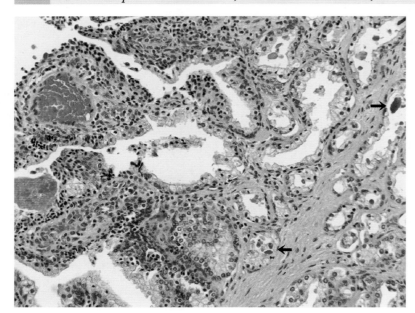

FIGURE 3–24 ▮▮▮▮ Normal verumontanum. Note the tubulopapillary architecture, relative paucity of stroma, and red-brown luminal secretions *(arrows)*.

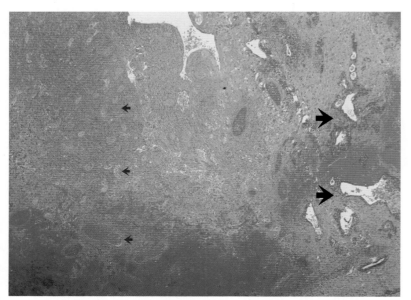

FIGURE 3–25 ▮▮▮▮ Prostate infarct. Only the ghostly outlines of infarcted ducts and acini are seen in some areas *(blue arrows)*. Viable acini and ducts are present on the right *(black arrows)*. There is extensive stromal hemorrhage.

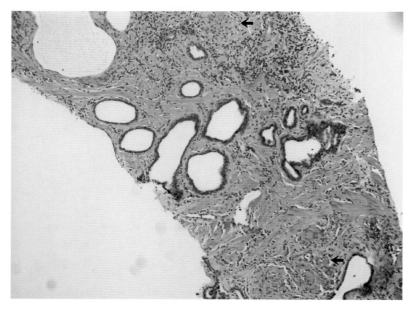

FIGURE 3–26 ▮▮▮▮ Atrophy. Some glands are small, and some appear dilated. The secretory cells appear shrunken and hyperchromatic. The surrounding stroma is fibrotic. Nonspecific granulomatous inflammation is also present *(arrows)*.

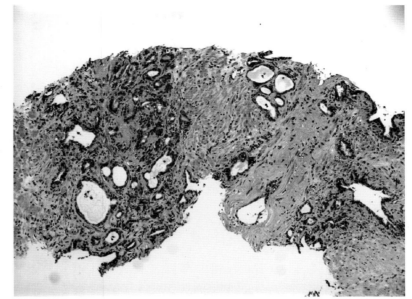

FIGURE 3–27 |▮|| Postatrophic hyperplasia. Lobules of closely packed small atrophic acini appear centered around large central ducts. The light purple stroma is markedly sclerotic.

fibrosis (Fig. 3–26). The prevalence and extent increase with advancing age, particularly in men older than age 40 years. Atrophy may be confused with adenocarcinoma because of prominent acinar architectural distortion, but it lacks significant nuclear and nucleolar enlargement. The nucleus-to-cytoplasmic ratio may be high because of scant cytoplasm, and nuclei are hyperchromatic.

Postatrophic hyperplasia (PAH) is at the extreme end of the morphologic continuum of acinar atrophy that most closely mimics adenocarcinoma. PAH consists of a microscopic lobular cluster of 5 to 15 small acini with distorted contours reminiscent of atrophy. One or more larger dilated acini are usually present within these round to oval clusters, and the small acini appear to bud off of the dilated acinus, imparting a lobular appearance

to the lesion (Fig. 3–27). The small acini are lined by a layer of cuboidal secretory cells with mildly enlarged nuclei with an increased nucleus-to-cytoplasmic ratio when compared with adjacent benign epithelial cells (Fig. 3–28).

BASAL CELL HYPERPLASIA

Basal cell hyperplasia (BCH) consists of a proliferation of basal cells two or more cells in thickness at the periphery of prostatic acini. It sometimes appears as small nests of cells surrounded by compressed stroma, often associated with chronic inflammation (Fig. 3–29). The nests may be solid or cystically dilated, and occasionally are punctuated by irregular round luminal spaces, creating a cribriform

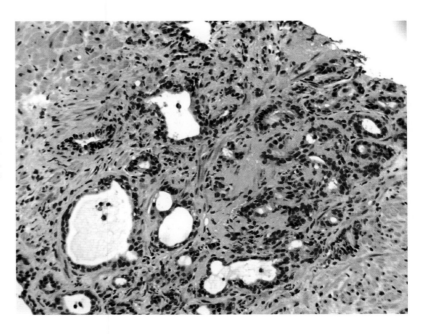

FIGURE 3–28 |▮|| Postatrophic hyperplasia. The acini are closely packed and irregular in shape and size, and acinar lining cells have hyperchromatic nuclei and minimal cytoplasm. Malignancy is excluded by absence of nucleomegaly and nucleolomegaly.

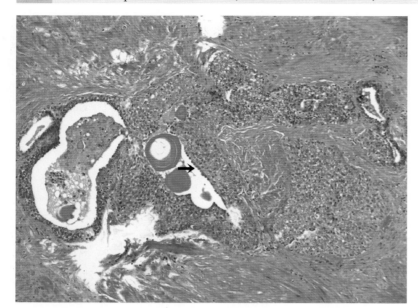

FIGURE 3–29 |▐| | Basal cell hyperplasia. Nearly all the cells lining these ducts are basal cells. The *arrow* indicates an attenuated layer of secretory cells adjacent to the lumen.

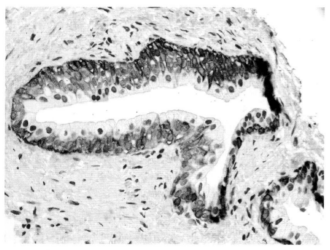

FIGURE 3–30 |▐| | Basal cell hyperplasia. Two or more layers of basal cells are highlighted by immunostaining with antibodies against keratin 34βE12.

pattern. BCH frequently involves only part of an acinus and sometimes protrudes into the lumen, retaining the overlying secretory cell layer; less commonly, there is symmetric duplication of the basal cell layer at the periphery of the acinus. Nucleoli are usually inconspicuous except in atypical BCH (see later). BCH displays intense cytoplasmic immunoreactivity in virtually all of the cells with high-molecular-weight keratin 34βE12 and other basal cell–specific markers (Fig. 3–30). Clear cell change is common in BCH, often with a cribriform pattern; this is referred to as cribriform hyperplasia or clear cell cribriform hyperplasia (Fig. 3–31).

Basal Cell Adenoma

Basal cell adenoma is a form of florid BCH characterized by one or more large circumscribed nodules of acini with BCH in a background of nodular hyperplasia. The nodules contain uniformly spaced aggregates of hyperplastic basal cells that form small solid nests or cystically

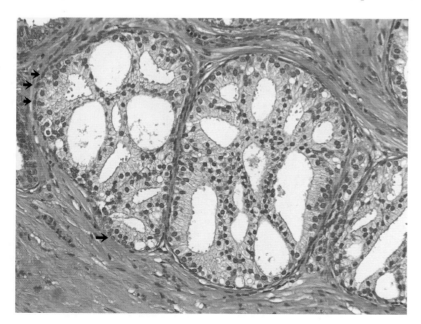

FIGURE 3–31 |▐| | Clear cell cribriform hyperplasia. *Arrows* indicate the presence of basal cells, excluding adenocarcinoma. The absence of nucleomegaly and nucleolomegaly in the secretory cells excludes high-grade prostatic intraepithelial neoplasia.

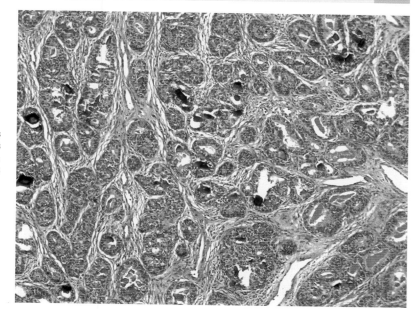

FIGURE 3–32 ▎▊▎▎ Basal cell adenoma. Numerous closely spaced acini are present, all lined by several layers of basal cells. Many acini contain calcified secretions. Several other similar aggregates were observed in this specimen obtained by transurethral resection.

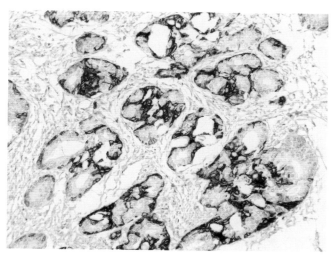

FIGURE 3–33 ▎▊▎▎ Basal cell adenoma, immunostained with antibodies against keratin 34βE12, illustrating the abundance of basal cells (same case as shown in Fig. 3–32).

dilated acini. Prominent calcific debris is often present within acinar lumens (Figs. 3–32 and 3–33).

Atypical Basal Cell Hyperplasia

Atypical BCH refers to BCH with large prominent nucleoli. The nucleoli are round to oval and lightly eosinophilic (Fig. 3–34). There is chronic inflammation in the majority of cases, suggesting that nucleolomegaly is a reflection of reactive atypia. A morphologic spectrum of nucleolar size is observed in basal cell proliferations, and only those with more than 10% of cells exhibiting prominent nucleoli are considered atypical. This lesion is significant because of the potential for misdiagnosis as adenocarcinoma.

ATYPICAL ADENOMATOUS HYPERPLASIA (ATYPICAL HYPERPLASIA; ATYPICAL ADENOSIS)

Atypical adenomatous hyperplasia (AAH) is a localized proliferation of small acini within the prostate arising in

FIGURE 3–34 ▎▊▎▎ Atypical basal cell hyperplasia. The two small acini indicated by *black arrows* contain numerous basal cells whose nuclei are larger than those of normal basal cells. Many nuclei have conspicuous nucleoli *(yellow arrow)*. The nuclear and nucleolar enlargement are less than that observed in high-grade prostatic intraepithelial neoplasia or adenocarcinoma.

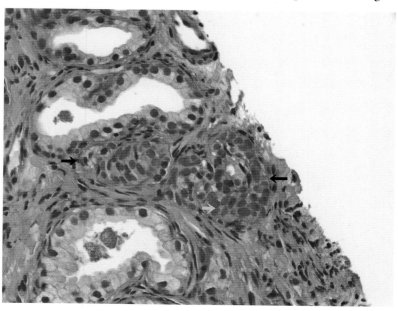

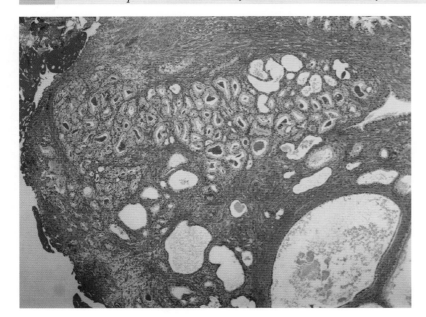

FIGURE 3–35 ▮▮▮ Atypical adenomatous hyperplasia. A well-circumscribed aggregate of closely packed acini is present in a background of hyperplasia. The findings raise concern for low-grade adenocarcinoma.

intimate association with nodular hyperplasia (Fig. 3–35). AAH varies in incidence from 19.6% (transurethral resection specimens) to 24% (autopsy series in 20- to 40-year-old men). The mean size of AAH is 0.03 cm³, but mass-forming AAH measuring up to 21.1 cm³ has been documented.

AAH is distinguished from well-differentiated carcinoma by the presence of inconspicuous nucleoli, partially intact but fragmented basal cell layer, and infrequent crystalloids (Fig. 3–36). All measures of nucleolar size allow separation of AAH from adenocarcinoma, including mean nucleolar diameter, largest nucleolar diameter, and percentage of nucleoli greater than 1 μm in diameter. The majority of Gleason pattern 1 cancers are now thought to represent foci of AAH.

AAH may be linked to a subset of prostate cancers that arise in the transition zone, but the evidence is circumstantial: increased incidence in association with carcinoma (15% in 100 prostates without carcinoma at autopsy and 31% in 100 prostates with cancer at autopsy), topographic relationship with small-acinar carcinoma, age peak incidence that precedes that of carcinoma, increased nuclear area and diameter, a proliferative cell index that is similar to that of small-acinar carcinoma but significantly higher than that of normal and hyperplastic prostatic epithelium, and rare cases with genetic instability.

SCLEROSING ADENOSIS

Sclerosing adenosis of the prostate consists of a benign solitary circumscribed proliferation of small acini set in a dense spindle cell stroma (Fig. 3–37). It is present in about 2% of specimens obtained by transurethral resection of the prostate. The unique immunophenotype of

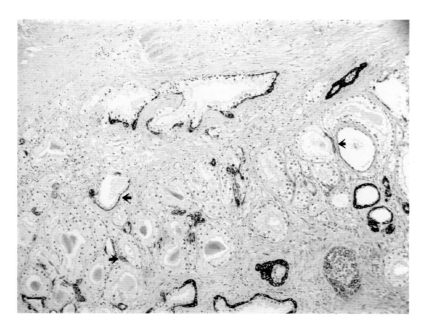

FIGURE 3–36 ▮▮▮ Atypical adenomatous hyperplasia. Some of the crowded acini have partial basal cell layers, as shown by keratin 34βE12 immunostaining *(arrows)*. Nucleomegaly and nucleolomegaly were absent.

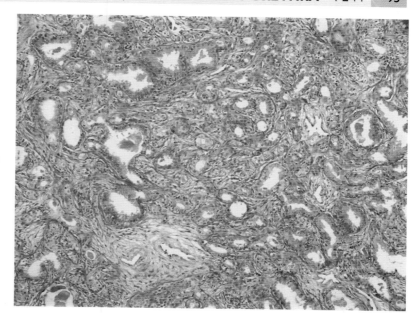

FIGURE 3–37 | ▌| | Sclerosing adenosis with crowded, small, benign acini set in a cellular stroma.

sclerosing adenosis is a valuable diagnostic clue that distinguishes it from adenocarcinoma. The basal cells show immunoreactivity for S-100 protein and muscle specific actin, unlike normal prostatic epithelium or carcinoma (Fig. 3–38); consequently, sclerosing adenosis is considered a form of metaplasia. The basal cell layer is intact or fragmented and discontinuous in sclerosing adenosis, as demonstrated by immunohistochemical stains for high-molecular-weight keratin 34βE12, compared with absence of staining in carcinoma (Fig. 3–39). PSA and PAP are present within secretory luminal cells.

STROMAL HYPERPLASIA WITH ATYPICAL CELLS

Stromal hyperplasia with atypia consists of stromal nodules in the transition zone with increased cellularity and nuclear atypia. These may appear as solid stromal nodules (often erroneously referred to as atypical leiomyoma) or with atypical degenerative smooth muscle cells interspersed with benign glands. Stromal nuclei are large, hyperchromatic, and rarely multinucleated or vacuolated, with inconspicuous nucleoli (Fig. 3–40). There are no mitotic figures and no necrosis. Stromal hyperplasia with atypia has no malignant potential, and the atypical cells are considered degenerative.

PROSTATIC CYSTS

Cysts are unusual in the prostate (Fig. 3–41). Giant multilocular prostatic cystadenoma is a large tumor composed of acini and cysts lined by prostatic-type epithelium set in a hypocellular fibrous stroma. This rare tumor arises in men between ages 28 and 80 years

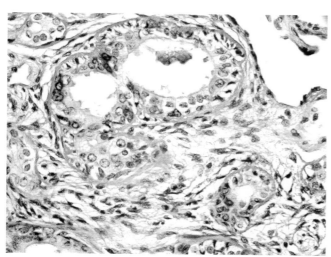

FIGURE 3–38 | ▌| | Sclerosing adenosis, immunostained with antibodies against S-100 protein. Many of the basal cells show immunoreactivity, a finding not observed in other small acinar proliferations of the prostate.

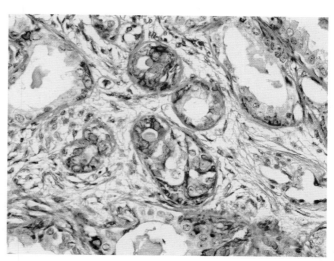

FIGURE 3–39 | ▌| | Sclerosing adenosis, immunostained with antibodies against keratin 34βE12. Positive immunostaining is evident in basal cells.

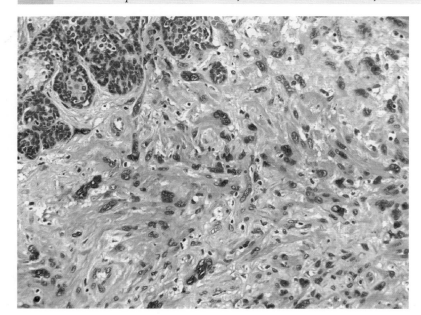

FIGURE 3–40 ❙▎❙❙ Stromal hyperplasia with atypia. Stromal nuclei are large and hyperchromatic. Many show multinucleation or vacuolization. Nucleoli are inconspicuous, and mitotic figures and necrosis are absent.

as a large midline prostatic or extraprostatic mass causing urinary obstruction. The epithelial lining displays PSA immunoreactivity. Surgical excision is usually curative, although the cyst may recur if excision is incomplete. Other benign cysts include seminal vesicle cyst, ejaculatory duct cyst, and müllerian duct cyst. Location is often useful, recognizing that seminal vesicle cyst is typically lateral whereas müllerian duct cyst is midline. Phyllodes tumor is described under soft tissue tumors below. Echinococcal cyst is usually associated with prominent inflammation, and organisms are often demonstrable.

PROSTATIC INTRAEPITHELIAL NEOPLASIA

High-grade prostatic intraepithelial neoplasia (PIN) is now accepted as the most likely preinvasive stage of adenocarcinoma, a decade after its first formal description. PIN is characterized by cellular proliferations within preexisting ducts and acini with cytologic changes mimicking cancer, including nuclear and nucleolar enlargement. It coexists with cancer in more than 85% of cases but retains an intact or fragmented basal cell layer, unlike

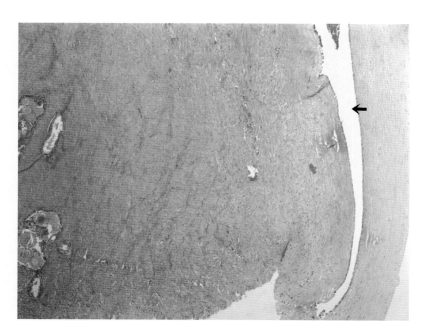

FIGURE 3–41 ❙▎❙❙ Prostatic cyst. This 1.5-cm cyst *(arrow)*, lined by small inconspicuous cuboidal cells, was found incidentally in a radical prostatectomy specimen.

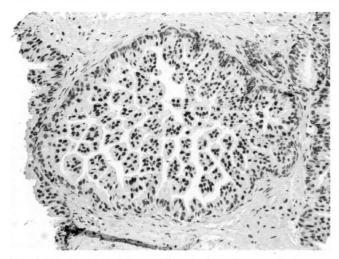

FIGURE 3–42 |█|| Micropapillary high-grade prostatic intraepithelial neoplasia immunostained with antibodies against keratin 34βE12. A basal cell layer is present in this acinus, although it appears discontinuous in some areas.

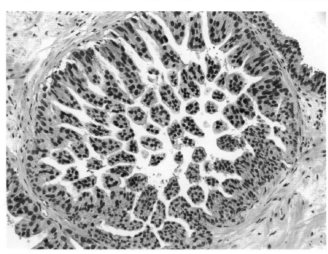

FIGURE 3–44 |█|| High-grade prostatic intraepithelial neoplasia, micropapillary type.

cancer, which lacks a basal cell layer. The only method of detection is biopsy; PIN does not significantly elevate total and free serum PSA concentration and cannot be detected by ultrasonography.

The incidence of PIN varies according to the population of men under study and increases with patient age. The lowest likelihood is in men participating in PSA screening and early detection studies, with an incidence of PIN in biopsy specimens ranging from 0.7% to 20%. Prostate biopsies performed in routine urologic practice show PIN in 4.4% to 25% of cases; the incidence in transurethral prostatic resections varies from 2.8% to 33%. Select antikeratin antibodies such as 34βE12 (high-molecular-weight keratin) may be used to stain tissue sections for the presence of basal cells, recognizing that PIN retains an intact or fragmented basal cell layer whereas cancer does not (Fig. 3–42).

DIAGNOSTIC CRITERIA

Prostatic intraepithelial neoplasia (PIN) refers to the putative precancerous end of the continuum of cellular proliferations within the lining of prostatic ducts, ductules, and acini. There are two grades of PIN (low grade and high grade), although the term *PIN* is usually used to indicate high-grade PIN. The high level of interobserver variability with low-grade PIN limits its clinical utility, and many pathologists do not report this finding except in research studies, including us. Interobserver agreement for high-grade PIN is "good to excellent."

There are four main patterns of high-grade PIN: tufting, micropapillary, cribriform, and flat (Figs. 3–43 through 3–46). The tufting pattern is the most common, present in 97% of cases, although most cases have

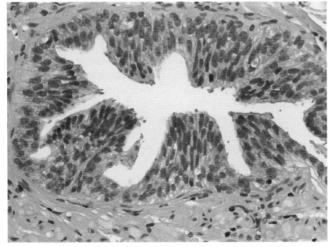

FIGURE 3–43 |█|| High-grade prostatic intraepithelial neoplasia, tufting type. The majority of the secretory cells have prominent nucleoli, and many have two nucleoli.

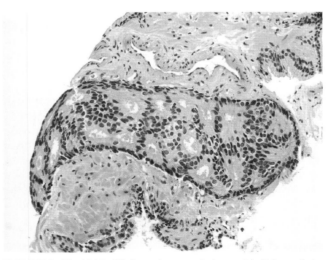

FIGURE 3–45 |█|| High-grade prostatic intraepithelial neoplasia, cribriform type.

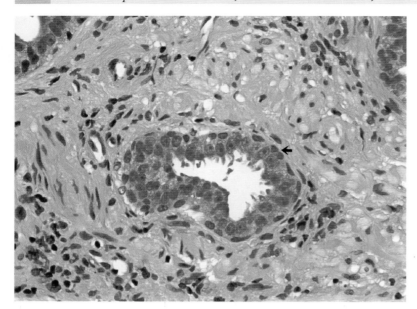

FIGURE 3–46 | ▮ | | High-grade prostatic intraepithelial neoplasia, flat type. Basal cells *(arrow)* are easily identified in this acinus.

multiple patterns. There are no known clinically important differences between the architectural patterns of high-grade PIN, and their recognition appears to be only of diagnostic utility.

There is inversion of the normal orientation of epithelial proliferation with PIN; most proliferation normally occurs in the basal cell compartment, whereas in PIN the greatest proliferation occurs on the luminal surface, similar to preinvasive lesions in the colon (tubular adenoma) and other sites.

PIN spreads through prostatic ducts in multiple different patterns, similar to prostatic carcinoma. In the first pattern, neoplastic cells replace the normal luminal secretory epithelium, with preservation of the basal cell layer and basement membrane. This pattern often has a cribriform or near-solid appearance. In the second pattern, there is direct invasion through the ductal or acinar wall, with disruption of the basal cell layer. In the third pattern, neoplastic cells invaginate between the basal cell layer and columnar secretory cell layer ("pagetoid spread"), a very rare finding.

Early stromal invasion, the earliest evidence of carcinoma, occurs at sites of acinar outpouching and basal cell disruption in acini with high-grade PIN. Such microinvasion is present in about 2% of high-power microscopic fields of PIN and is seen with equal frequency with all architectural patterns.

PIN is associated with progressive abnormalities of phenotype and genotype that are intermediate between normal prostatic epithelium and cancer, indicating impairment of cell differentiation and regulatory control with advancing stages of prostatic carcinogenesis. A model of prostatic carcinogenesis has been proposed based on the morphologic continuum of PIN and the multistep theory of carcinogenesis, and animal models appear to confirm this model.

CLINICAL SIGNIFICANCE

PIN has a high predictive value as a marker for adenocarcinoma, and its identification warrants repeat biopsy for concurrent or subsequent invasive carcinoma. Adenocarcinoma was identified in 36% of subsequent biopsies from cases with PIN, compared with 13% in the control group. The likelihood of finding cancer increased as the time interval from first biopsy increased (32% incidence of cancer within 1 year compared with 38% incidence in follow-up biopsies obtained after more than 1 year). High-grade PIN, patient age, and serum PSA concentration were jointly highly significant predictors of cancer, with PIN providing the highest risk ratio (14.9). These data underscore the strong association of PIN and adenocarcinoma and indicate that vigorous diagnostic follow-up is needed.

There is a marked decrease in the prevalence and extent of high-grade PIN in cases after combination androgen deprivation therapy when compared with untreated cases. The prevalence and extent of PIN are also decreased after radiation therapy.

ADENOCARCINOMA

Prostate cancer is the most common cancer of men in the United States and is second only to lung cancer as a cause of cancer death. For all men, the overall lifetime probability of developing clinical evidence of prostate cancer is greater than 1 in 6. Despite an 80% prevalence at autopsy by age 80 years, the clinical incidence is much lower, indicating that most men die with prostate carcinoma rather than of prostate carcinoma.

GROSS PATHOLOGY OF PROSTATIC ADENOCARCINOMA

Gross identification of prostatic adenocarcinoma is often difficult in radical prostatectomy specimens, and definitive diagnosis requires microscopic examination. Adenocarcinoma tends to be multifocal, with a predilection for the peripheral zone. Grossly apparent tumor foci are at least 5 mm in greatest dimension and appear yellow-white with a firm consistency owing to stromal

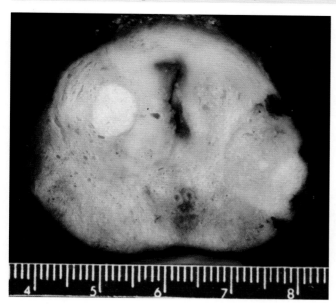

FIGURE 3–47 ❚❚❚❚ Adenocarcinoma, forming a yellow-white circumscribed nodule in this radical prostatectomy specimen. In most cases, adenocarcinoma is not readily identified by gross inspection.

desmoplasia (Fig. 3–47). Some tumors appear as yellow granular masses that stand in contrast to the normal spongy prostatic parenchyma.

MICROSCOPIC FEATURES OF PROSTATIC ADENOCARCINOMA

Most prostatic adenocarcinomas are composed of acini arranged in one or more patterns. The diagnosis relies on a combination of architectural and cytologic findings. The light microscopic features are usually sufficient for diagnosis, but rare cases may benefit from immunohisto-chemical studies.

Architecture

Architectural features are assessed at low- to medium-power magnification and include variation in acinar spacing, size, and shape. The arrangement of the acini is diagnostically useful and is the basis of Gleason grade. Malignant acini usually have an irregular haphazard arrangement, randomly scattered in the stroma in clusters or single acini, usually with variation in spacing except in the lowest Gleason grades. The acini in suspicious foci are usually small or medium sized, with irregular contours that stand in contrast to the smooth round to elongate contours of benign and hyperplastic acini. Comparison with the adjacent benign prostatic acini is always of value. Variation in acinar size is a particularly useful criterion, particularly when there are small irregular abortive acini with primitive lumens at the periphery of a focus of well-differentiated carcinoma.

Stroma

The stroma in cancer frequently contains young collagen that appears lightly eosinophilic, although desmoplasia may be prominent. There is sometimes splitting or dis-tortion of muscle fibers in the stroma, but this is an inconstant and unreliable feature by itself.

Cytology

The cytologic features of adenocarcinoma include nuclear and nucleolar enlargement, and these are present in the majority of malignant cells. The identification of two or more nucleoli is virtually diagnostic of malignancy, particularly when the nucleoli are eccentrically located in the nucleus; we find this criterion useful, but employ it sparingly. Artifacts often obscure the nuclei and nucleoli, and overstaining of nuclei by hematoxylin creates one of the most common and difficult problems encountered in interpretation of suspicious foci. Differences in fixation and handling of biopsy specimens influence nuclear size and chromasia, so comparison with cells from the same specimen is important and serves as an internal control.

Luminal Mucin

Acidic sulfated and nonsulfated mucin is often seen in acini of adenocarcinoma, appearing as amorphous or delicate threadlike faintly basophilic secretions in routine sections (Fig. 3–48). Acidic mucin is not specific for carcinoma.

Crystalloids

Crystalloids are sharp needle-like eosinophilic structures that are often present in the lumens of well differentiated and moderately differentiated carcinoma (Fig. 3–49). They result from abnormal protein and mineral metabolism within benign and malignant acini and are probably related to the hard eosinophilic proteinaceous secretions commonly found in the lumens of malignant acini. Crystalloids are not pathognomonic for malignancy; they are also seen occasionally in benign glands, hyperplastic glands, and atypical adenomatous hyperplasia (Fig. 3–50). The presence of crystalloids in metastatic adenocarcinoma of unknown site of origin is strong presumptive evidence of prostatic origin, although it is an uncommon finding and is not conclusive.

Collagenous Micronodules

Collagenous micronodules are a specific but infrequent and incidental finding in prostatic adenocarcinoma, consisting of microscopic nodular masses of paucicellular eosinophilic fibrillar stroma that impinge on acinar lumens (Fig. 3–51).

Perineural Invasion

Perineural invasion is common in adenocarcinoma and may be the only evidence of malignancy in biopsy specimens. This finding is strong presumptive evidence of malignancy but may rarely occur with benign acini. Complete circumferential growth, intraneural invasion, and ganglionic invasion are found only with cancer (Fig. 3–52). This is probably not a useful predictive factor.

Vascular/Lymphatic Invasion

Microvascular invasion is a strong indicator of malignancy, and its presence correlates with histologic grade, although it is sometimes difficult to distinguish from fixation-associated retraction artifact of acini (Fig. 3–53).

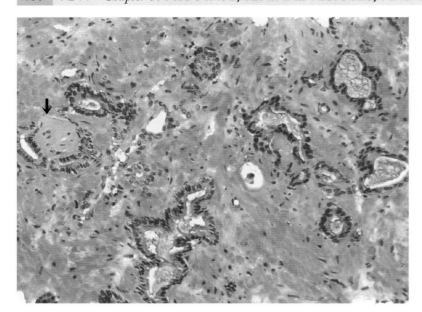

FIGURE 3–48 ▌█▌▌ Adenocarcinoma. Wispy blue mucin is present in most of the malignant acini. A nerve at left *(arrow)* is almost completely encircled by cancer.

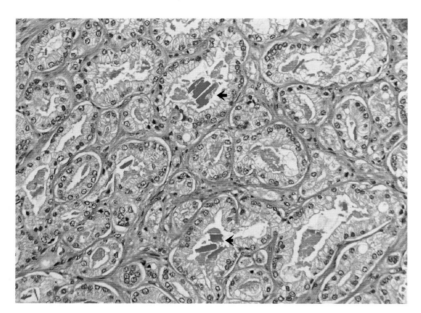

FIGURE 3–49 ▌█▌▌ Adenocarcinoma. Dark red crystalloids with sharp contours *(arrows)* are present in many of the glands in this low-grade cancer.

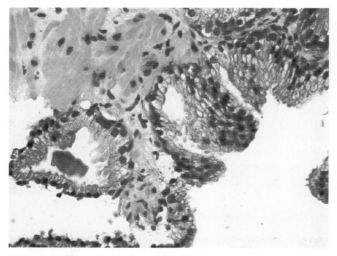

FIGURE 3–50 ▌█▌▌ A sharp crystalloid is seen in a benign acinus at left, illustrating that crystalloids are not pathognomonic for cancer.

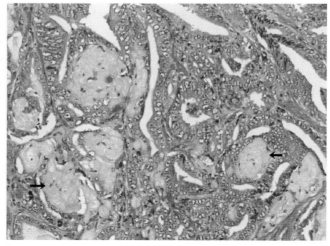

FIGURE 3–51 ▌█▌▌ Collagenous micronodules. These paucicellular eosinophilic fibrillar stromal nodules *(arrows)* are seen only in adenocarcinoma.

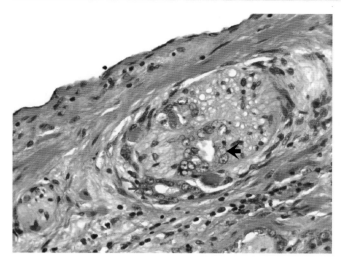

FIGURE 3–52 |▊|| Nerve with intraneural *(black arrow)* and perineural *(blue arrow)* adenocarcinoma.

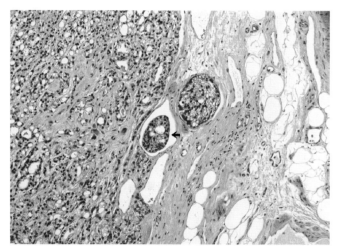

FIGURE 3–53 |▊|| Angiolymphatic invasion by adenocarcinoma *(arrow).*

IMMUNOHISTOCHEMISTRY OF PROSTATIC ADENOCARCINOMA

Immunohistochemical studies are utilized commonly in prostate cancer for diagnosis.

Basal Cell–Specific Anti–Keratin 34βE12 (Keratin 903; High-Molecular-Weight Keratin)

Basal cell–specific anti–keratin 34βE12 stains virtually all of the normal basal cells of the prostate; there is no staining in the secretory and stromal cells. Basal cell layer disruption is present in the majority of cases of high-grade PIN, more commonly in glands adjacent to invasive carcinoma than in distant glands. Basal cells are absent in adenocarcinoma. Prostate cancer cells do not react with this antibody (Fig. 3–54).

Prostate-Specific Antigen

Immunohistochemical staining for PSA is useful in identifying poorly differentiated prostate cancer in close proximity to the bladder and the rectum; it can also verify prostatic origin of metastatic carcinoma (Figs. 3–55 and 3–56). The intensity of PSA immunoreactivity often varies from field to field within a tumor, and the correlation of staining intensity with tumor differentiation is inconsistent. PSA expression is generally greater in low-grade tumors than in high-grade tumors, but there is significant heterogeneity from cell to cell. Up to 1.6% of poorly differentiated cancers will be negative for both PSA and PAP. Extraprostatic expression of PSA has been reported in a number of tissues and tumors, including periurethral gland adenocarcinoma in women, rectal carcinoid, and extramammary Paget's disease.

Prostatic Acid Phosphatase

PAP is a valuable immunohistochemical marker for identifying prostate cancer when used in combination with stains for PSA. There is more intense and uniform staining of tumor cells and the glandular epithelium of

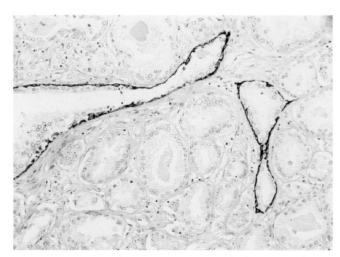

FIGURE 3–54 |▊|| Immunostain using antibodies against keratin 34βE12. Two benign ducts are lined by positive-staining basal cells; a layer of secretory cells lies above them. The malignant acini are devoid of basal cells.

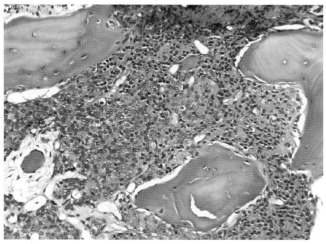

FIGURE 3–55 |▊|| Bone biopsy, showing poorly differentiated malignant cells filling the space between bone trabeculae. In such cases, immunohistochemical stain may help determine the type of malignancy, and site of origin (see Fig. 3–56).

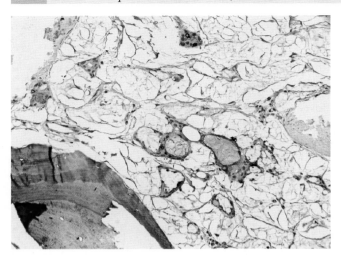

FIGURE 3–56 ▌▐▌▐▌ Bone biopsy showing marrow involvement by acinar structures that show positive immunostaining for prostate-specific antigen. Findings are consistent with metastatic prostatic adenocarcinoma.

well-differentiated adenocarcinoma, whereas less intense and more variable staining is seen in moderately and poorly differentiated adenocarcinoma.

CANCER GRADE

Grade is one of the strongest predictors of biologic behavior in prostate cancer, including invasiveness and metastatic potential, but is not sufficiently reliable when used alone for predicting pathologic stage or patient outcome for individual patients. The Gleason score, recommended for routine use in all pretherapy specimens by the College of American Pathologists, is a scalar measurement that combines discrete primary and secondary groups (patterns or grades) into a total of nine discrete groups (scores 2 to 10). The primary grade is the most common or predominant grade; the secondary grade is the next most common but should comprise at least 5% of the tumor. It is often hard to apply this rule when the amount of cancer in the specimen is small; in such cases, there may be no secondary pattern and the primary grade is simply doubled. Significant histologic changes in adenocarcinoma occur as a result of radiation and androgen deprivation therapy that make grading difficult and of questionable value. Interobserver and intraobserver variability has been reported with the Gleason grading system and other grading systems. Gleason noted exact reproducibility of score in 50% of needle biopsies and ± one score in 85%, similar to the findings of others.

Gleason pattern 1 adenocarcinoma is uncommon and difficult to diagnose, particularly in biopsy specimens. It consists of a circumscribed mass of simple monotonously replicated round acini that are uniform in size, shape, and spacing (Fig. 3–57). Nuclear and nucleolar enlargement is moderate but allows separation from its closest mimic, atypical adenomatous hyperplasia. Crystalloids are observed in more than half of cases.

Gleason pattern 2 is very similar to pattern 1 except for the lack of circumscription of the focus, indicating the ability of the cancer to spread through the stroma. Slightly greater variation in acinar size and shape is observed, but the acinar contours are chiefly round and smoothly sculpted. Acinar packing is somewhat more variable than pattern 1, and separation is usually less than one acinar diameter (Fig. 3–58).

Gleason pattern 3 is the most common pattern of prostatic adenocarcinoma and encompasses a wide and diverse group of lesions. The hallmark of pattern 3 adenocarcinoma is prominent variation in size, shape, and spacing of acini (Fig. 3–59). Despite this variation, the acini remain discrete and separate, unlike the fused acini of pattern 4. Acini are haphazardly arranged in the stroma, sometimes with prominent stromal fibrosis.

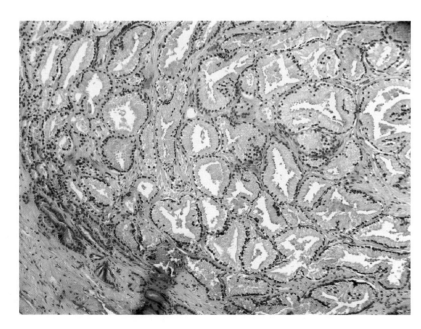

FIGURE 3–57 ▌▐▌▐▌ Adenocarcinoma, Gleason grade 1. The focus of cancer has a well-circumscribed border with the adjacent stroma, and the glands show minimal variation in size and shape. Prominent nucleoli were seen in most cells at high power.

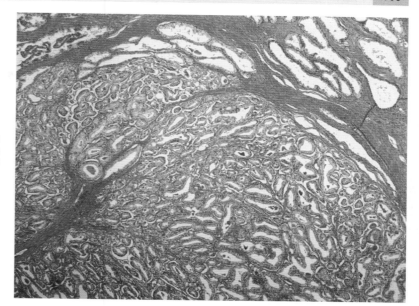

FIGURE 3–58 | ▌| | Adenocarcinoma, Gleason grade 2. The border of the tumor is well circumscribed. The individual glands vary in shape and size more than is observed in grade 1 cancer.

Gleason pattern 4 characteristically shows fusion of acini, with ragged infiltrating cords and nests at the edges (Fig. 3–60). Unlike the simple entwined acinar tubules of pattern 3, this pattern consists of an anastomosing network or spongework of epithelium. In some cases, the fused and irregularly infiltrating glands and cell nest are composed of cells with abundant clear cytoplasm, superficially resembling renal cell carcinoma at low power; this pattern is sometimes described as "hypernephroid" (Fig. 3–61). Pattern 4 adenocarcinoma is considered poorly differentiated and is more malignant than pattern 3.

Gleason pattern 5 adenocarcinoma is characterized by fused sheets and masses of haphazardly arranged acini in the stroma, often displacing or overrunning adjacent tissues (Fig. 3–62). In biopsy specimens, these cases raise the serious concern for anaplastic carcinoma or sarcoma. Cases with scattered acinar lumens indicative of glan-

dular differentiation are included within this pattern. Comedocarcinoma is an important subtype of this pattern, consisting of luminal necrosis within an otherwise cribriform pattern (Fig. 3–63). Pattern 5 also includes rare histologic variants such as signet-ring cell carcinoma and small cell undifferentiated carcinoma.

Needle core biopsy underestimates tumor grade in up to 45% of cases and overestimates grade in up to 32%. Exact correlation is present in about one third of biopsy specimens, and agreement within one Gleason unit occurs in another one third. Grading errors are common in biopsy specimens with small amounts of tumor and low-grade tumor and are probably caused by tissue sampling variation, tumor heterogeneity, and undergrading of needle biopsy specimens. Gleason grading should be used for all needle biopsies, even those with small amounts of tumor.

On average, there are 2.7 (range 1 to 5) different

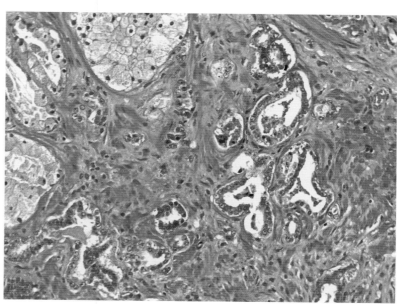

FIGURE 3–59 | ▌| | Adenocarcinoma, Gleason grade 3. Glands are irregular in shape and size and are randomly distributed in the stroma. Each gland is discrete and separate.

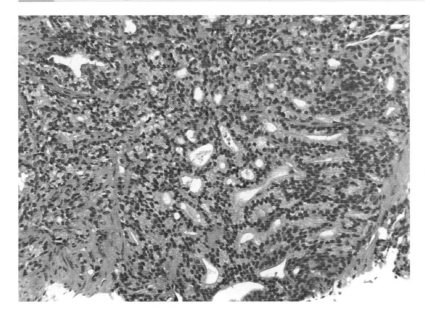

FIGURE 3–60 ▐▌▐▐ Adenocarcinoma, Gleason grade 4. Numerous very small acini without apparent separation from one another by stroma ("gland fusion"). Some glands are so crowded and compressed that their lumens are not readily discerned.

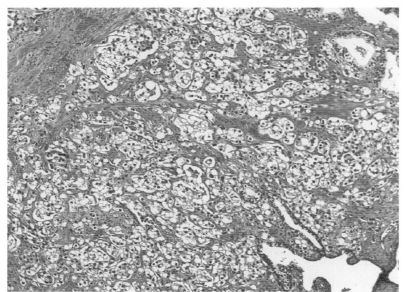

FIGURE 3–61 ▐▌▐▐ Adenocarcinoma, Gleason grade 4. The tumor shows gland fusion and diffuse stromal infiltration by cell nests and individual tumor cells. The majority of the cells have abundant clear cytoplasm, reminiscent of renal cell carcinoma, a feature sometimes described as "hypernephroid."

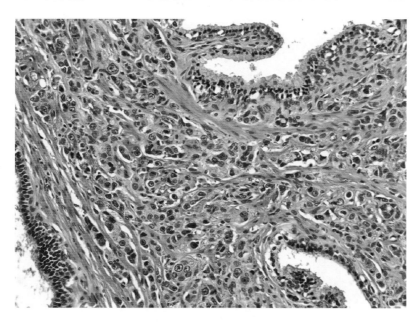

FIGURE 3–62 ▐▌▐▐ Adenocarcinoma, Gleason grade 5. The stroma between several benign glands is diffusely infiltrated by sheets of carcinoma cells. No gland formation is apparent.

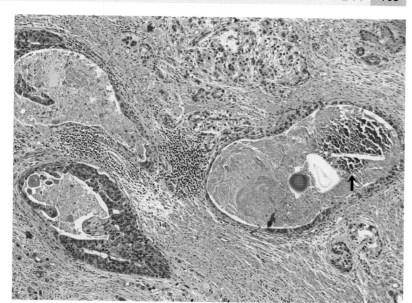

FIGURE 3–63 |▮|| Adenocarcinoma, Gleason grade 5 (ductal carcinoma with central necrosis). Several large ductal spaces are involved by solid and cribriform carcinoma. Necrotic debris, focally calcified *(arrow)*, is present in the center of the ducts.

Gleason primary patterns (grades) in prostate cancer treated by radical prostatectomy. More than 50% of cancers contain at least three different grades. The number of grades increases with greater cancer volume, the most common finding being high-grade cancer within the center of a larger well-differentiated or moderately differentiated cancer occurring in some 53% of cases. Grade is an invariable component of most clinical nomograms in prostate cancer.

HISTOLOGIC VARIANTS OF PROSTATIC ADENOCARCINOMA

The biologic behavior of histologic variants of adenocarcinoma may differ from typical acinar adenocarcinoma, and proper clinical management depends on accurate diagnosis and separation from tumors arising in other sites.

Ductal Carcinoma (Adenocarcinoma with Endometrioid Features; Endometrioid Carcinoma)

Ductal carcinoma accounts for about 0.8% of prostatic adenocarcinomas. It typically arises as a polypoid or papillary mass within the prostatic urethra and large periurethral prostatic ducts and may histologically resemble endometrial adenocarcinoma of the female uterus (Figs. 3–64 and 3–65). Most refer to this tumor as adenocarcinoma with endometrioid features or simply ductal carcinoma. The term *endometrial* should not be used in describing prostate specimens. Most cancers with papillary or cribriform pattern are located in the peripheral zone at a great distance from the urethra, indicating that the histologic findings are not specific. Ductal carcinoma invariably displays intense cytoplasmic immunoreactivity for PAP and PSA. Focal carcinoembryonic

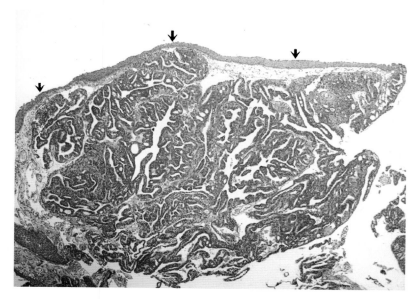

FIGURE 3–64 |▮|| Ductal (endometrioid) adenocarcinoma. A layer of transitional-type epithelium overlying the tumor nodule *(arrows)* is consistent with protrusion of tumor into the lumen of the prostatic urethra. Tumor architecture is predominantly papillary.

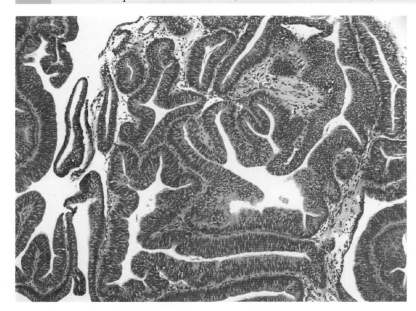

FIGURE 3–65 ▮▮▮ Ductal (endometrioid) adenocarcinoma. The tumor shows papillary architecture, with complex branching and infolding. The tumor cells are tall, columnar, and pseudostratified. There is a strong resemblance to endometrial adenocarcinoma.

antigen (CEA) immunoreactivity is occasionally present. The prognosis of ductal carcinoma appears to be the same as for typical acinar adenocarcinoma.

Mucinous Carcinoma (Colloid Carcinoma)

Pure mucinous carcinoma of the prostate is rare, although typical acinar adenocarcinoma often produces mucin focally, particularly after high-dose estrogen therapy. The clinical presentation of mucinous carcinoma is similar to that of typical acinar carcinoma, and there are no apparent differences in patient age, stage at presentation, cancer volume, serum PSA concentration, or pattern of metastases. This tumor may not respond well to endocrine therapy or radiation therapy and is highly aggressive. Focal mucinous differentiation is observed in at least one third of cases of prostatic carcinoma, but the accepted diagnosis of mucinous carcinoma

arbitrarily requires that at least 25% of the tumor consists of pools of extracellular mucin. Three patterns of mucinous carcinoma have been described: acinar carcinoma with luminal distention, cribriform carcinoma with luminal distention, and "colloid carcinoma" with cell nests embedded in mucinous lakes (Fig. 3–66). In some cases, the nuclei are low grade, with uniform finely granular chromatin and inconspicuous nucleoli, but their presence within mucin pools is diagnostic of malignancy.

Adenocarcinoma with Vacuolated Cytoplasm (Foamy Gland Carcinoma)

In rare cases, the cells of adenocarcinoma contain abundant cytoplasm packed with minute vacuoles, giving them a "foamy" or "xanthomatous" appearance. The nuclei in most instances are small, and there may be little or no nucleolar prominence, making the diagnosis challenging,

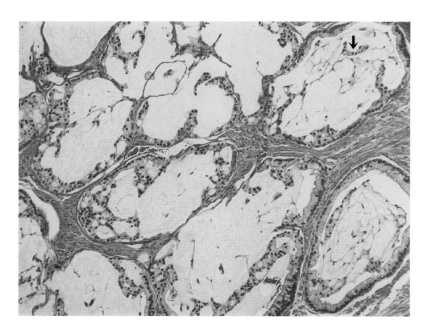

FIGURE 3–66 ▮▮▮ Mucinous adenocarcinoma. The majority of the tumor consists of mucin. Tumor cells border the mucin lakes and focally appear to "float" on a mucin lake *(arrow)*. If more than 25% of a tumor shows this morphology, the name is applicable.

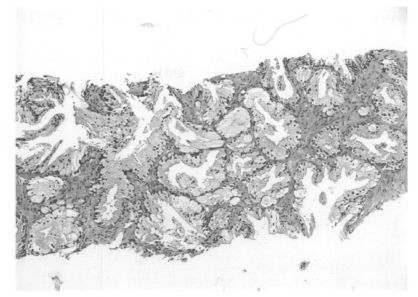

FIGURE 3–67 ❘▮❘❘ Foamy gland carcinoma, low power. At this power, the most striking and unusual finding is the great abundance of cytoplasm in the tumor cells.

particularly in needle biopsies (Figs. 3–67 and 3–68). Adenocarcinoma with foamy gland morphology is often associated with more readily recognized high-grade adenocarcinoma (Gleason pattern 4).

Signet-Ring Cell Carcinoma

Signet-ring cell carcinoma of the prostate is rare. The clinical presentation is similar to that of typical acinar adenocarcinoma except that all are high stage. The prognosis is poor. The diagnosis of signet-ring cell carcinoma arbitrarily requires that 25% or more of the tumor is composed of signet-ring cells. Most often, it is a minor component of Gleason pattern 5 carcinoma. Tumor cells show distinctive nuclear displacement by clear cytoplasm (Fig. 3–69). Signet-ring cells are present in 2.5% of cases of acinar adenocarcinoma but rarely in sufficient numbers to be considered signet-ring cell carcinoma.

Carcinoma with Neuroendocrine Differentiation

Virtually all prostatic adenocarcinomas contain at least a small number of neuroendocrine cells, but special studies such as histochemistry and immunohistochemistry are usually necessary to identify them. The clinical features of adenocarcinoma with neuroendocrine differentiation are similar to typical acinar adenocarcinoma. Neuroendocrine differentiation in adenocarcinoma has no impact on prognosis, so there is no role for immunohistochemical stains for neuroendocrine markers in routine practice (Fig. 3–70).

Neuroendocrine Carcinoma (Small Cell Carcinoma and Carcinoid)

Most cases of neuroendocrine carcinoma have typical local signs and symptoms of prostatic adenocarcinoma, although paraneoplastic syndromes are frequent in these

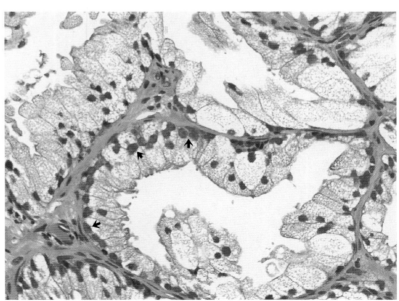

FIGURE 3–68 ❘▮❘❘ Foamy gland carcinoma, high power. The cytoplasm of tumor cells is abundant and remarkably vacuolated. Cell nuclei in this variant of adenocarcinoma are often small and may not have prominent nucleoli. Only a few of the nuclei in this case have prominent nucleoli *(arrows)*.

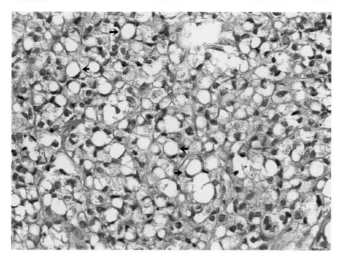

FIGURE 3–69 ▮▮▮ Signet-ring cell carcinoma. The tumor is composed of sheets of cells with large cytoplasmic vacuoles that compress the cell nuclei to the periphery, creating a "signet ring" appearance *(arrows).*

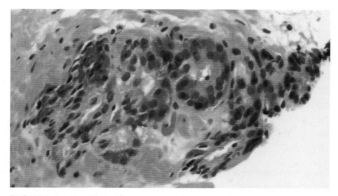

FIGURE 3–70 ▮▮▮ Carcinoma with neuroendocrine differentiation, indicated by the presence of abundant dark red cytoplasmic granules in many of the tumor cells.

patients. Small cell carcinoma is aggressive and rapidly fatal. Neuroendocrine carcinoma of the prostate varies histopathologically from carcinoid-like pattern (low-grade neuroendocrine carcinoma) to small cell undifferentiated (oat cell) carcinoma (high-grade neuroendocrine carcinoma) (Fig. 3–71). Typical acinar adenocarcinoma is present, at least focally, in about half of cases, and transition patterns may be seen. A wide variety of secretory products may be detected within the malignant cells, including serotonin, calcitonin, adrenocorticotropic hormone, human chorionic gonadotropin, thyroid-stimulating hormone, bombesin, calcitonin gene-related peptide, and inhibin.

Squamous Cell and Adenosquamous Carcinoma

Squamous cell carcinoma is very rare in the prostate. Adenosquamous carcinoma refers to the combination of squamous cell carcinoma and typical acinar carcinoma and is also rare (Fig. 3–72). Presenting signs and symptoms are similar to those of typical prostatic adenocarcinoma, although there is often a history of hormonal therapy or radiation therapy. Squamous cell carcinoma of the prostate may also arise in patients with *Schistosoma hematobium* infection. Serum PSA and PAP concentration is usually normal, even with metastases, and bone metastases are typically osteolytic rather than osteoblastic. The prognosis is poor, and these tumors are unresponsive to androgen deprivation therapy. Squamous cell carcinoma of the prostate is histopathologically similar to its counterpart in other organs, consisting of irregular nests and cords of malignant cells with keratinization and squamous differentiation, rarely with squamous pearls. Keratinizing squamous cell carcinoma of the prostate usually arises in the periurethral ducts and is very rare; otherwise, the site of origin of squamous cell carcinoma is unknown.

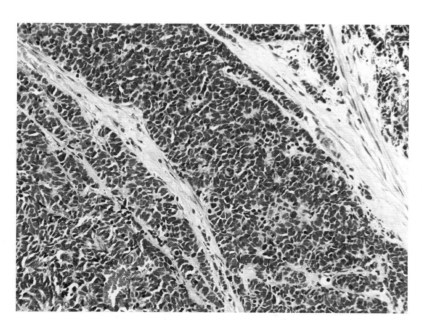

FIGURE 3–71 ▮▮▮ Small cell carcinoma of prostate. Tumor cells have minimal cytoplasm and hyperchromatic nuclei with absent or inconspicuous nucleoli and nuclear molding.

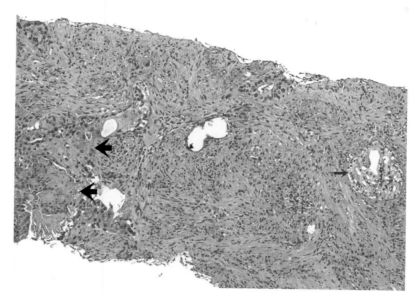

FIGURE 3–72 I∎II Adenosquamous carcinoma. In this prostate needle biopsy, the *black arrows* indicate a focus of keratinizing squamous cell carcinoma; the *blue arrow* indicates a focus of cribriform adenocarcinoma.

Sarcomatoid Carcinoma (Carcinosarcoma; Metaplastic Carcinoma)

Sarcomatoid carcinoma is considered by many to be synonymous with carcinosarcoma. Authors who separate these tumors define sarcomatoid carcinoma as an epithelial tumor showing spindle cell (mesenchymal) differentiation and carcinosarcoma as adenocarcinoma intimately admixed with heterologous malignant soft tissue elements (Figs. 3–73 and 3–74). Regardless of terminology, these tumors are rare and aggressive. Patients tend to be older men who present with symptoms of urinary outlet obstruction, similar to those of typical adenocarcinoma. Serum PSA concentration may be normal at the time of diagnosis. About half of patients have a prior history of typical acinar adenocarcinoma treated by radiation therapy or androgen deprivation therapy. Treatment is variable and has no apparent influence on the poor prognosis. Metastases may consist of carcinoma and/or sarcoma, so careful search of the primary tumor is useful to identify a component of carcinoma. Coexistent adenocarcinoma is almost always high grade (Fig. 3–75). The most common soft tissue elements are osteosarcoma, with or without cartilaginous differentiation, and leiomyosarcoma.

Adenoid Cystic Carcinoma/Basal Cell Carcinoma

Adenoid cystic carcinoma/basal cell carcinoma is very rare, consisting of basal cell nests of varying size infiltrating the stroma. The malignant potential is uncertain owing to the small number of reported cases and limited follow-up, but some cases are malignant with extraprostatic extension and distant metastases. At present, adenoid basal cell tumor is probably best considered a tumor of low malignant potential. There are two

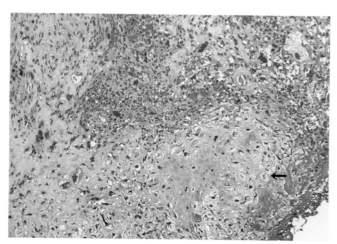

FIGURE 3–73 I∎II Carcinosarcoma (sarcomatoid carcinoma). The cancer in this specimen obtained by transurethral resection had several morphologic variations, including ductal carcinoma with necrosis, areas resembling small cell carcinoma, and several areas that resembled chondrosarcoma *(arrow)*.

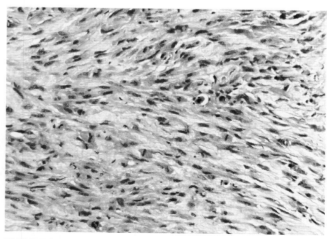

FIGURE 3–74 I∎II Sarcomatoid carcinoma. This spindle cell prostate cancer resembles high-grade sarcoma. Tumor cells showed strong diffuse immunoreactivity to antibodies against pan-keratin, confirming that it is carcinoma.

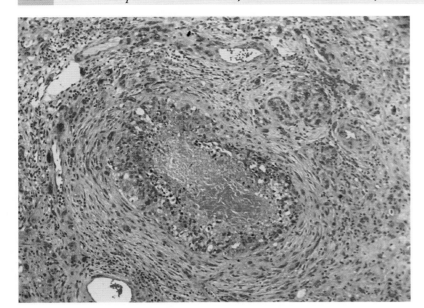

FIGURE 3–75 ▮▮▮ Sarcomatoid carcinoma (same case as illustrated in Figure 3–73). A focus of ductal carcinoma with central necrosis (Gleason grade 5) is present in a background of poorly differentiated spindle and pleomorphic malignant cells.

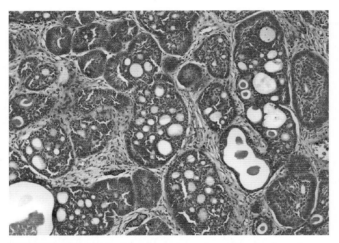

FIGURE 3–76 ▮▮▮ Adenoid cystic carcinoma/basal cell carcinoma. This image demonstrates the adenoid cystic pattern: nests of tumor cells, punctuated by rounded fenestrations containing mucinous material.

architectural patterns of adenoid cystic carcinoma/basal cell carcinoma: adenoid cystic and basaloid. The adenoid cystic pattern consists of irregular clusters of crowded basal cells punctuated by rounded fenestrations, many of which contain mucinous material resembling salivary gland adenoid cystic carcinoma (Fig. 3–76). The basaloid pattern consists of variably sized rounded basaloid cell nests with prominent peripheral palisading. These patterns frequently coexist.

Atrophic Pattern of Adenocarcinoma

Cancer acini with dilated lumens and flattened lining cells with modest-sized nucleoli are referred to as "atrophic" cancer. This is an unusual pattern that is easily mistaken for atrophy (Fig. 3–77). Useful diagnostic features include the presence of adjacent typical acinar adenocarcinoma and identification of enlarged prominent nucleoli in at least some of the cells in the "atrophic" focus, but caution is warranted in rendering this difficult diagnosis on needle biopsies with only a small amount of cancer.

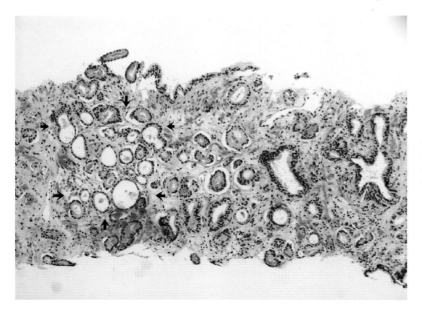

FIGURE 3–77 ▮▮▮ Atrophic carcinoma. The clustered acini with dilated lumens and flattened epithelium outlined by *arrows* resemble atrophic glands. Inspection at higher magnification confirmed that most of the lining cells have prominent nucleoli.

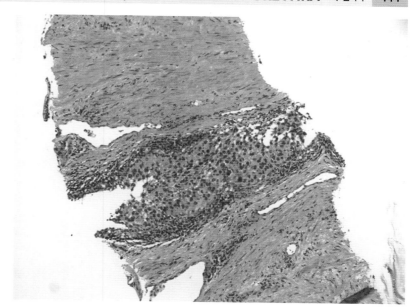

FIGURE 3–78 |▋|| Urothelial carcinoma with squamous differentiation filling a prostatic duct in a specimen obtained by needle biopsy performed before the discovery of this patient's poorly differentiated urothelial carcinoma of the bladder.

UROTHELIAL CARCINOMA INVOLVING THE PROSTATE AND PROSTATIC URETHRA

Urothelial carcinoma of the prostate usually represents synchronous or metachronous spread from carcinoma in the bladder and urethra. It involves the prostate and urethra in about 40% of radical cystoprostatectomy specimens for bladder carcinoma. Patients usually present with symptoms of hematuria, urinary obstruction, or prostatitis. Serum PSA and PAP concentrations are not elevated. Diagnostic criteria are identical to those for urothelial cancer of the bladder and urethra (Figs. 3–78 and 3–79).

TREATMENT CHANGES IN ADENOCARCINOMA

Treatment changes in the benign and cancerous prostate create diagnostic challenges in pathologic interpretation, particularly in needle biopsy specimens and evaluation of possible extraprostatic metastases. It is critical that the clinician provide the pertinent history of androgen deprivation or radiation therapy to assist the pathologist in rendering the correct diagnosis.

Androgen Deprivation Therapy

There are a variety of agents that are used for androgen deprivation, and the histopathologic effects of most are similar. Hormonal treatment alters the benign and cancerous prostatic epithelium, causing acinar atrophy, apoptosis (programmed cell death), cytoplasmic clearing, nuclear and nucleolar shrinkage, and chromatin condensation. Squamous metaplasia and glycogenic acanthosis are common findings after orchiectomy and diethylstilbestrol but are uncommon after contemporary forms of treatment. Tumor cell nuclei are frequently small and

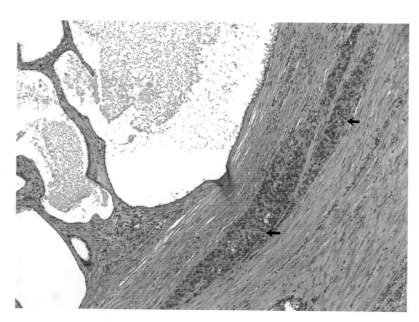

FIGURE 3–79 |▋|| Urothelial carcinoma of bladder, infiltrating prostatic stroma *(arrows)*. This is the cystoprostatectomy specimen from the patient illustrated in Figure 3–78.

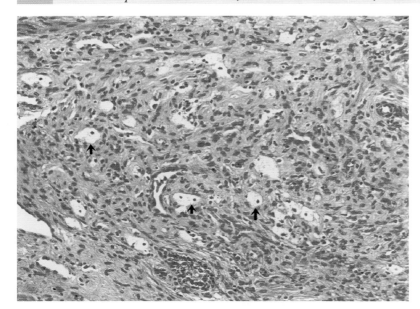

FIGURE 3–80 ▮▮▮ Adenocarcinoma after total androgen ablation therapy. Residual carcinoma cells with small hyperchromatic nuclei and cytoplasmic clearing are indicated by *arrows.*

hyperchromatic, obscuring the nucleoli and creating a "nucleolus-poor" appearance in many areas (Fig. 3–80). PSA and PAP are retained in tumor cells after 3 months of therapy but decline with longer duration of therapy; keratin 34βE12 remains negative, regardless of duration, indicating an absent basal cell layer.

The volume of prostate cancer is reduced by more than 40% after treatment, and there is a 20% to 25% decline in positive margins at radical prostatectomy. Pathologic stage is similar in untreated and treated prostatic adenocarcinoma, according to retrospective reports of radical prostatectomies, although there is a trend toward lower stage in treated cases. Occasional cases after therapy display the "vanishing cancer phenomenon" in which no residual cancer was found in the radical prostatectomy specimen.

Radiation Therapy

Histologic changes of radiation injury in benign and hyperplastic epithelium include acinar atrophy and distortion, marked cytologic abnormalities of the epithelium, basal cell hyperplasia, stromal fibrosis, decreased ratio of acini to stroma, and vascular changes (Fig. 3–81). PIN after radiation therapy retains characteristic features of untreated PIN, but the prevalence and extent decline. For about 12 months after completion of external-beam irradiation, needle biopsy is of limited value, owing to ongoing tumor cell death. After this period, however, biopsy is a good method for assessing local tumor control, with a low level of sampling variation that is minimized by obtaining multiple specimens. The changes after three-dimensional conformal therapy are

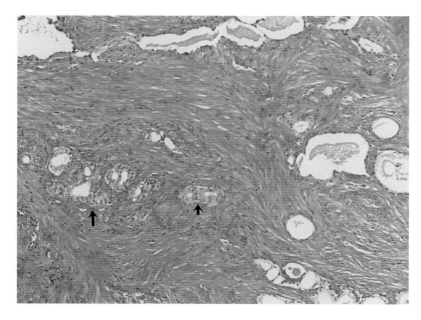

FIGURE 3–81 ▮▮▮ Adenocarcinoma, recurrent after radiation therapy. Infiltrating malignant glands are present *(arrows).* The stroma is fibrotic, and native benign glands show atrophic changes.

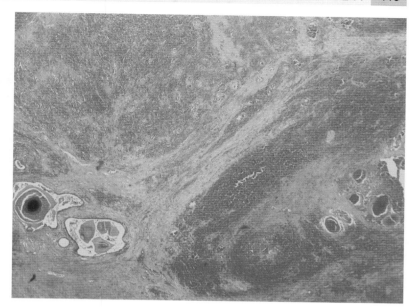

FIGURE 3–82 |█|| Prostate tissue after cryoablation therapy. The ghostly outlines of acinar structures are seen at upper left. Corpora amylacea mark the sites of some ducts. There is extensive stromal hemorrhage and coagulative necrosis.

similar to those after conventional external-beam therapy.

Expression of PSA, PAP, and keratin 34βE12 in the prostatic epithelium is not altered by radiation therapy and is often of value in separating treated adenocarcinoma and its mimics.

Persistent cancer in needle biopsy specimens after radiation therapy has a significant impact on patient management, because positive needle biopsies portend a worse prognosis. Patients with positive biopsies are more likely to have local recurrence, distant metastases, and death from prostate cancer than those with negative biopsies. Cancer grade usually shows little or no evidence of "dedifferentiation" after radiation therapy.

The severity and extent of radiation changes in the prostate may be of prognostic value in patients treated by external-beam therapy and brachytherapy and appear to vary according to radiation dose. No definitive method exists for assessment of tumor viability after irradiation.

Ultrasound Hyperthermia, Microwave Hyperthermia, Laser Therapy, and Hot Water Balloon Thermotherapy

All forms of hyperthermia for nodular hyperplasia result in sharply circumscribed hemorrhagic coagulative necrosis that soon organizes with granulation tissue; the pattern and extent of injury is determined by the method of thermocoagulation employed, the duration of treatment, tissue perfusion factors, and the ratio of epithelium to stroma in the tissue being treated. Confluent coagulation necrosis occurs when multiple laser lesions are created in a single transverse plane.

Cryoablation Therapy (Cryosurgery)

After cryosurgery, the prostate shows typical features of repair, including marked stromal fibrosis and hyalinization, basal cell hyperplasia with ductal and acinar regeneration, squamous metaplasia, urothelial metaplasia, and stromal hemorrhage and hemosiderin deposition. Coagulative necrosis is present between 6 and 30 weeks of therapy, but patchy chronic inflammation is more common. Focal granulomatous inflammation is associated with epithelial disruption due to corpora amylacea. Biopsy after cryosurgery may reveal no evidence of recurrent or residual carcinoma, even in some patients with elevated PSA levels (Fig. 3–82).

PREDICTIVE FACTORS IN PROSTATE CANCER

Multifactorial analysis improves prediction of all outcome variables, including pathologic stage, cancer recurrence, and survival.

Extraprostatic Extension

By international agreement, the term *extraprostatic extension* (EPE) replaces other terms, including capsular invasion, capsular penetration, and capsular perforation. Extension of cancer beyond the edge or capsule of the prostate is diagnostic of EPE. There are three criteria for EPE, depending on the site and composition of the extraprostatic tissue: (1) cancer in adipose tissue, (2) cancer in perineural spaces of the neurovascular bundles, and (3) cancer in anterior muscle (Fig. 3–83). In patients treated by radical prostatectomy for clinically localized cancer, the frequency of EPE (stage pT3 cancer) is 23% to 52%. There is a strong association of tumor volume with EPE and seminal vesicle invasion. Many patients with EPE also have positive surgical margins, and the combination of EPE and positive margins predicts a worse prognosis than EPE alone (Fig. 3–84).

Lymph Nodes

Sampling error by frozen section accounts for a false-negative rate of lymph node metastases of about 2%. There is a low incidence of micrometastatic occult prostatic carcinoma in pelvic lymph nodes that cannot be detected by routine staining.

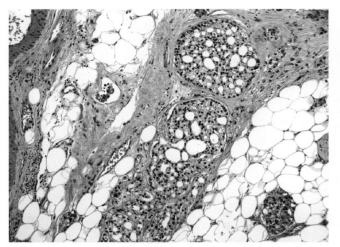

FIGURE 3–83 ▐▌▐▌ Extracapsular extension of adenocarcinoma into soft tissues (fat and fibroconnective tissue) outside the prostate capsule.

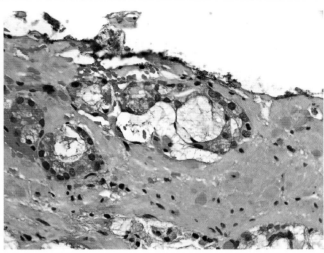

FIGURE 3–84 ▐▌▐▌ Adenocarcinoma present at a yellow-inked resection margin in a radical prostatectomy specimen.

Stage

The TNM system is the international standard for prostatic adenocarcinoma staging (Table 3–1).

PSA-Detected Adenocarcinoma (Clinical Stage T1c)

There is no pathologic stage equivalent for clinical stage T1c, and such tumors are invariably upstaged at surgery, usually to pathologic stage T2 or T3. Clinical stages T1c adenocarcinoma and clinical stage T2a and T2b adenocarcinoma had similar maximum tumor diameters, fre-

quencies of multifocality, tumor grades, DNA content results, pathologic stages, and tumor locations.

Surgical Margins

Positive surgical margins are defined as cancer cells touching the inked surface of the prostate. The frequency of positive surgical margins has steadily declined in the past decade, probably owing to refinements in surgical technique and earlier detection of cancer at smaller volume. Positive margins are located at the apex (48%), rectal and lateral surfaces (24%), bladder neck (16%),

---

TABLE 3–1

TNM PATHOLOGIC STAGING (pT) OF PROSTATIC ADENOCARCINOMA

Primary Tumor (T)

pT2*	Organ confined
pT2a	Unilateral, involving one-half of one lobe or less
pT2b	Unilateral, involving more than one-half of one lobe, but not both lobes
pT2c	Bilateral disease
pT3	Extraprostatic extension
pT3a	Extraprostatic extension**
pT3b	Seminal vesicle invasion
pT4	Invasion of bladder, rectum

Note: There is no pathologic T1 classification.
**Note:* Positive surgical margins should be indicated by an R1 descriptor (residual microscopic disease).

Regional Lymph Nodes (N)

pNX	Regional nodes not sampled
pN0	No positive regional nodes
pN1	Metastases in regional nodes

Used with the permission of the American Joint Committee on Cancer (AJCC), Chicago, Illinois. The original source for this material is the *AJCC Cancer Staging Manual, Sixth Edition* (2002) published by Springer-Verlag New York, www.springer-ny.com.

and superior pedicles (10%). Surgical margin status is an important predictor of patient outcome after radical prostatectomy; it was the only predictor of cancer progression other than Gleason score or DNA ploidy in patients without seminal vesicle invasion or lymph node metastases.

Location of Cancer

The site of origin of cancer appears to be a significant prognostic factor. When cancer arises in the transition zone, it is apparently less aggressive than typical acinar adenocarcinoma arising in the peripheral zone. These adenocarcinomas are better differentiated than those in the peripheral zone, accounting for Gleason primary grade 1 and 2 tumors. The volume of low-grade tumors tends to be smaller than those arising in the peripheral zone, although frequent exceptions are seen. The confinement of transition zone adenocarcinoma to its anatomic site of origin may account in part for the favorable prognosis of clinical stage T1 tumors. The transition zone boundary may act as a relative barrier to tumor extension, because malignant acini appear to frequently fan out along this boundary before invasion into the peripheral and central zones. The World Health Organization recommends that prostate biopsy specimens be submitted separately, that the anatomic site of each prostate biopsy be labeled, and that pathologists report each specimen separately.

Cancer Volume

Biopsy cancer volume depends on multiple factors, including prostate volume, cancer volume, cancer distribution, number of biopsy cores obtained, the cohort of patients being evaluated, and the technical expertise of the investigator. The biopsy extent of tumor provides some predictive value for extent in radical prostatectomy specimens and probably should be reported, although its predictive value for an individual patient is limited. This correlation is greatest for large cancers. High cancer burden on needle biopsy is strongly suggestive of large-volume, high-stage cancer. Unfortunately, low tumor burden on needle biopsy does not necessarily indicate low-volume, low-stage cancer. Cancer volume is a critical element in definitions of clinically significant and insignificant prostate cancer.

Perineural Invasion

Perineural invasion is common in adenocarcinoma, present in up to 38% of biopsy specimens, and may be the only evidence of malignancy in a needle core. Only half of patients with intraprostatic perineural invasion on biopsy have extraprostatic extension. In univariate analysis, perineural invasion was predictive of extraprostatic extension, seminal vesicle invasion, and pathologic stage in patients treated by radical prostatectomy. However, in multivariate analysis, perineural invasion had no predictive value after consideration of Gleason grade, serum PSA, and amount of cancer on biopsy.

Vascular/Lymphatic Invasion

Microvascular invasion is a strong indicator of malignancy, and its presence correlates with histologic grade, tumor progression, and survival.

DNA Ploidy

DNA ploidy analysis of prostate cancer provides important predictive information that supplements histopathologic examination. The 5-year cancer-specific survival is about 95% for diploid tumors, 70% for tetraploid tumors, and 25% for aneuploid tumors.

Genetic Instability in Prostate Cancer

Prostate carcinogenesis apparently involves multiple genetic changes, including loss of specific genomic sequences that may be associated with inactivation of tumor suppressor genes and gain of some specific chromosome regions that may be associated with activation of oncogenes. The most common genetic alterations in PIN and carcinoma are gain of chromosome 7, particularly 7q31; loss of 8p and gain of 8q; and loss of 10q, 16q, and 18q.

VANISHING CANCER PHENOMENON

In some radical prostatectomy specimens, there is minimal or no residual cancer within the specimen. This "vanishing cancer phenomenon" is increasing in incidence as more low-stage cancers are being treated by radical prostatectomy. The inability to identify cancer in a prostate removed for needle biopsy–proven carcinoma does not necessarily indicate technical failure, although it is important to exclude the possibility of improper patient identification. DNA "fingerprinting" has been used as a research tool to compare the formalin-fixed, paraffin-embedded biopsy and prostatectomy tissues.

PROSTATIC SOFT TISSUE TUMORS

BENIGN SOFT TISSUE TUMORS

Leiomyoma and Fibroma

These benign soft tissue tumors are often confused with nodular hyperplasia, and the distinction may be impossible in biopsy or transurethral resection specimens. Leiomyoma is defined as a circumscribed solitary smooth muscle nodule greater than 1 cm in diameter. It is histologically identical to leiomyoma occurring in the uterus and other sites. Fibroma is a similar nodule composed of collagen with few fibroblasts; fibroma may be indistinguishable from a pure stromal nodule of nodular hyperplasia.

Postoperative Spindle Cell Nodule (Postsurgical Inflammatory Myofibroblastic Tumor)

This rare benign reparative process occurs within months of surgery and consists of nodules of spindle cells arranged in fascicles with occasional or numerous mitotic figures (up to 25 mitotic figures/10 high-power fields). The cells have central elongate to ovoid nuclei, small prominent nucleoli, and abundant cytoplasm (see Fig. 2–34).

Inflammatory Myofibroblastic Tumor (Inflammatory Pseudotumor)

This rare benign pathologic entity of unknown etiology occurs in the bladder, prostate, urethra, and other sites without a history of prior surgery. Patients range in age

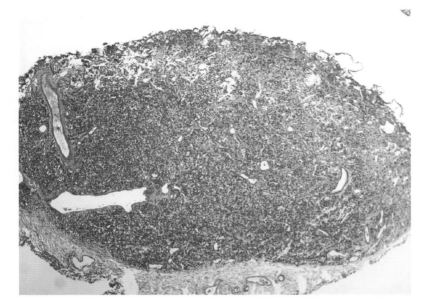

FIGURE 3–85 ▐▐▐▐ Paraganglioma, discovered incidentally in several chips in this specimen obtained by transurethral resection. The tumor eventually metastasized to bone.

from 16 to 73 years (mean, 41 years), with a slight female predilection when it occurs in the bladder. Mean tumor size is 3.6 cm, but it can measure up to 8 cm in diameter. The stroma is loose, edematous, and myxoid, with abundant small slitlike blood vessels resembling granulation tissue. Mitotic figures are infrequent, with fewer than 3 per 10 high-power fields; none is atypical. Ulceration and focal necrosis is present in most cases but is not prominent.

Other Benign Soft Tissue Tumors

Other benign tumors arise in the prostate, including hemangioma, lymphangioma, neurofibroma, neurilemoma, chondroma, hemangiopericytoma, and solitary fibrous tumor. Paraganglioma (pheochromocytoma) rarely arises in the prostate and sometimes metastasizes (Fig. 3–85).

MALIGNANT SOFT TISSUE TUMORS

Sarcoma of the prostate accounts for less than 0.1% of prostatic neoplasms. One third occur in children, and most of these are rhabdomyosarcoma; leiomyosarcoma is most common in adults.

Rhabdomyosarcoma

Rhabdomyosarcoma has a peak incidence between birth and 6 years of age, but sporadic cases have been reported in men as old as 80 years. The prostate, bladder, and vagina account for 21% of cases in children, second only to head and neck origin. Serum PSA and PAP concentration is normal. The tumor is large and bulky, with a mean diameter up to 9 cm. It usually involves the prostate, bladder, and periurethral, perirectal, and perivesicular soft tissues. Urethral involvement may not be apparent cytoscopically. Symptoms include acute or chronic urethral obstruction, bladder displacement, and rectal compression. The prostate may be palpably normal, although large tumors often fill the pelvis and can be palpated suprapubically. Most are embryonal rhabdomyosarcoma, and the remainder are alveolar, botryoid, and spindle cell

subtypes (Fig. 3–86). Tumor cells are arranged in sheets of immature round to spindle cells set in a myxoid stroma. Polypoid tumor fragments ("botryoid pattern") may fill the urethral lumen, covered by intact urothelium with condensed underlying tumor cells creating a distinctive cambium layer. Nuclei are usually pleomorphic and darkly staining. Scattered rhabdomyoblasts may be present, with eosinophilic cytoplasmic processes containing cross striations. Tumor cells display immunoreactivity for myoglobin, desmin, and vimentin but are negative for PSA and PAP. All tumors appear to be aneuploid by flow cytometry.

Leiomyosarcoma

Leiomyosarcoma presents as a large bulky mass that replaces the prostate and periprostatic tissues. It is the most common sarcoma in adults and accounts for 26% of all prostatic sarcomas. Patients range in age from 40 to 71 years (mean, 59 years), with sporadic reports in younger patients. Tumors range in size from 3.3 to 21 cm (mean, 9 cm). The criteria for separating leiomyoma from low-grade leiomyosarcoma have not been precisely defined in the prostate, but they are probably similar to those in other organs, including degree of cellularity, cytologic anaplasia, number of mitotic figures, amount of necrosis, vascular invasion, and size (Fig. 3–87). Tumor cells usually display intense cytoplasmic immunoreactivity for smooth muscle–specific actin and vimentin and weak desmin immunoreactivity. Most are negative for cytokeratin (AE1/AE3) and S-100 protein.

Phyllodes Tumor (Cystosarcoma Phyllodes)

Phyllodes tumor of the prostate is a rare lesion that should be considered a neoplasm rather than atypical hyperplasia owing to the frequent early recurrences, infiltrative growth, and potential for extraprostatic spread in some cases. Dedifferentiation with multiple recurrences in some cases is further evidence of the potentially aggressive nature of this tumor. A benign clinical course has been emphasized in some reports, but the cumulative evi-

Chapter 4

TESTIS

EMBRYOLOGY

Testicular development begins at 4 to 5 weeks of gestation. Genital ridges develop from coelomic epithelium adjacent to the paired mesonephric ducts. Primordial *sex cords* infiltrate the genital ridges. These are cordlike structures derived from the mesonephros; they form seminiferous tubules and the rete testis. They give rise to *Sertoli cells* that populate the seminiferous tubules. A basement membrane separates the seminiferous tubules from the *gonadal stroma*, which gives rise to *Leydig cells*. During the fifth week, seminiferous tubule colonization by *primordial germ cells (gonocytes)* begins. Gonocytes appear in the extraembryonal mesoderm in the posterior wall of the yolk sac in the third week and migrate to the genital ridges. By the end of the eighth week, the testis has assumed an oval shape, is covered by a thin layer of coelomic epithelium, and is composed of gonadal stromal cells and abundant seminiferous tubules populated by germ cells and Sertoli cells. The testis has begun to separate from the mesonephros, which subsequently regresses and is replaced by the metanephros (the definitive kidney). Elements of the mesonephros persist, however, forming the ductuli efferentes, the ductus epididymis, the ductus deferens, the seminal vesicles, and the ejaculatory duct. Germ cell proliferation occurs in the seminiferous tubules in three distinct waves, the last wave beginning between 9 and 12 years of age.

NORMAL ANATOMY AND HISTOLOGY

The testis is suspended in the scrotum by the spermatic cord. It is enclosed within the tunica albuginea, a fibrous capsule partially lined by mesothelium (tunica vaginalis) (Fig. 4–1). Adjacent to the testis is the tunica sac, a cavity lined by mesothelium. Blood vessels, lymphatics, and nerves from the spermatic cord enter the testis posteriorly at the mediastinum testis. Fibrous septa divide the testis into about 250 compartments, each containing one to four seminiferous tubules. Between the compartments lie vascular spaces, nerves, and Leydig cells (Fig. 4–2). Leydig cells are polyhedral and measure about 20 μm in diameter; they have eosinophilic cytoplasm, round uniform nuclei with conspicuous nucleoli, and occasional crystals of Reinke within the cytoplasm.

Seminiferous tubules in the adult testis are surrounded externally by myoid cells and lined internally by multiple layers of germ cells, which are least mature near

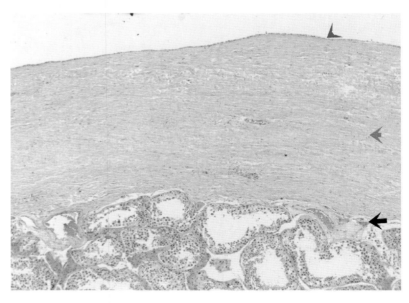

FIGURE 4–1 ▮▮▮ Normal testis. A capsule encloses the testicular parenchyma. It consists of the outer tunica vaginalis (a thin layer of mesothelial cells) *(blue arrow)*, the thick fibrous tunica albuginea *(red arrow)*, and the inner tunica vasculosa, a loose fibroconnective tissue layer containing blood vessels and lymphatics *(black arrow)*. The septa dividing the testis into lobules arise from the tunica vasculosa.

Several images in this chapter are courtesy of Mayo Clinic Foundation, Rochester, MN.

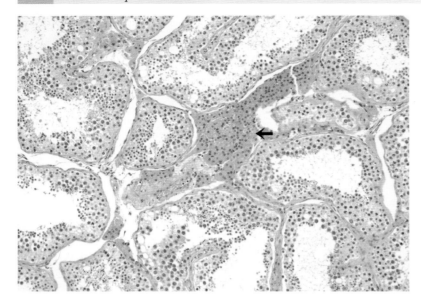

FIGURE 4–2 ▎▎▎▎ Normal testis. Closely packed seminiferous tubules containing Sertoli cells and germ cells. Clusters of pink-staining Leydig cells *(black arrow)* and a small blood vessel lie in the interstitial space between the tubules.

the basement membrane and most mature at the luminal surface. Interspersed between the germ cells are perpendicularly oriented Sertoli cells (Fig. 4–3). Convergence of the seminiferous tubules occurs at the rete testis (Fig. 4–4) (see Chapter 5).

BENIGN TUMORS AND TUMOR-LIKE LESIONS OF THE TESTIS

SPLENOGONADAL FUSION

Splenic and gonadal tissue sometimes fuse during fetal development. As the testis descends, a fibrous cord may maintain a connection between the testis and the normal spleen (continuous splenogonadal fusion). The cord may be composed largely of splenic tissue or may contain small nodules of splenic tissue. In some cases, no connecting cord is present (discontinuous splenogonadal

fusion). The affected testis is undescended in one sixth of cases, and an inguinal hernia is present in one third of cases. Most cases present as palpable inguinal or scrotal masses or are noted incidentally at the time of orchiopexy or hernia repair.

The splenic tissue forms a circumscribed red nodule adjacent to the testis, most often at the upper pole, less often at the lower pole, and, infrequently, within the testis (Fig. 4–5). Nodules are rarely larger than 1.0 cm in diameter. The nodules consist of normal splenic tissue, separated from the normal testicular parenchyma by a fibrous interface (Fig. 4–6).

ADRENOCORTICAL REST

Nodules of ectopic adrenocortical tissue may be found in the spermatic cord or adjacent to the epididymis or rete testis. Some are located between the epididymis and the testis. Most are less than 0.5 cm in diameter and are

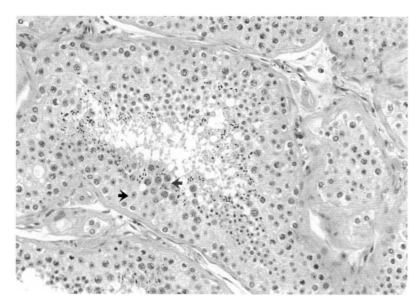

FIGURE 4–3 ▎▎▎▎ Normal testis. A seminiferous tubule containing germ cells in various phases of maturation *(blue arrow)*, interspersed with Sertoli cells *(black arrow)*.

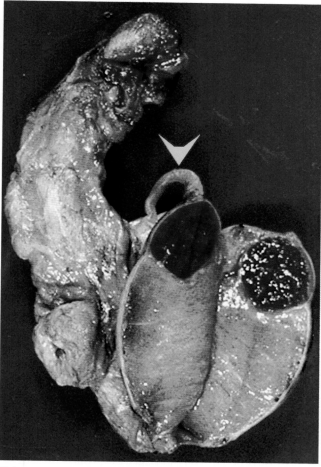

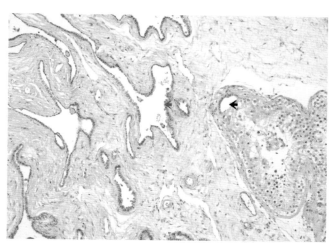

FIGURE 4–4 |▌|| Normal testis. A seminiferous tubule *(black arrow)*, joining the rete testis *(blue arrow)*, a cavernous network of interconnecting channels lined by low columnar epithelium.

FIGURE 4–5 |▌|| Splenogonadal fusion. Ectopic splenic tissue forms a circumscribed red nodule within the testis. *Arrow* indicates a fibrous cord, indicative of the "continuous" type of splenogonadal fusion. (Courtesy of Kavitha Rao, MD, Cleveland, OH.)

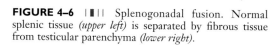

FIGURE 4–6 |▌|| Splenogonadal fusion. Normal splenic tissue *(upper left)* is separated by fibrous tissue from testicular parenchyma *(lower right)*.

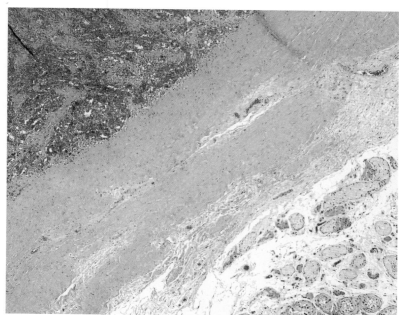

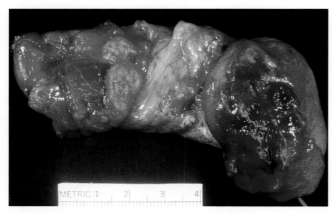

FIGURE 4–7 |▮|| Testicular "tumor" of adrenogenital syndrome. Brown nodules of hyperplastic steroid-type cells distort the surface of the testis *(at right)*.

clinically inapparent. A peritesticular nodule large enough to be detected clinically is usually treated as a testicular neoplasm. Adrenocortical rest is usually yellow-orange and well circumscribed. It consists of normal zonated adrenal cortical tissue confined within a fibrous pseudocapsule.

TESTICULAR "TUMOR" OF THE ADRENOGENITAL SYNDROME

Males with untreated or incompletely treated adrenogenital syndrome, most often the salt-losing variety associated with 21-hydroxylase deficiency, may present in adolescence or young adulthood with bilateral testicular masses composed of hyperplastic steroid-type cells, probably derived from hilar pluripotential cells. The hyperplasia is ACTH-dependent, and tumor size diminishes with ACTH suppression. These tumors can be managed by careful observation.

The nodules may measure up to 10 cm in diameter, may be single or multiple, are bilateral in 83% of cases,

and are various shades of brown, without hemorrhage or necrosis (Fig. 4–7). Microscopically, steroid-type cells form expansile sheets and circumscribed nodules with intersecting fibrous bands (Fig. 4–8). Crystals of Reinke (found in one third of Leydig cell neoplasms) are absent. Abnormal mitotic figures and nuclear atypia are uncommon.

EPIDERMOID CYST

The majority of epidermoid cysts are detected in adolescents and young adults. Their origin has been variously attributed to monodermal development of a teratoma, inclusion of scrotal skin elements, or squamous metaplasia of mesothelial inclusions derived from the tunica vaginalis. Testicular epidermoid cysts are not associated with intratubular germ cell neoplasia and are benign.

Epidermoid cysts are filled with yellow-white amorphous friable debris (Fig. 4–9). Most are 2 to 3 cm in diameter. The microscopic appearance is that of a fibrous-walled cyst lined by keratinizing squamous epithelium (Fig. 4–10). The cyst wall does not contain skin adnexal structures (eccrine glands, hair follicles, sebaceous units).

TESTICULAR INFARCTION AND HEMORRHAGE

Testicular infarction caused by spermatic cord torsion affects the entire testis, which develops red to black discoloration with a hemorrhagic cut surface (Fig. 4–11). Microscopically, the remnants of seminiferous tubules are evident in a background of diffuse interstitial hemorrhage; no viable intratubular cells are evident (Fig. 4–12).

Limited vascular occlusion causes infarction of only part of the testis. Polycythemia, trauma, sickle cell disease, and vasculitis predispose to partial infarction. Limited infarcts may mimic cancer clinically and on gross examination. The cut surface of an infarct may appear hemorrhagic or pale gray-tan. Microscopic findings depend on the age of the infarct. Recent infarcts

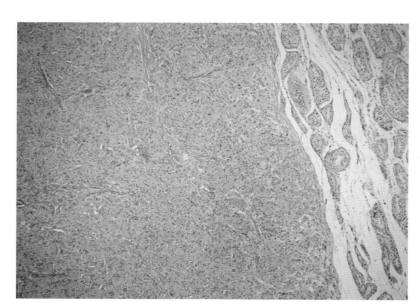

FIGURE 4–8 |▮|| Testicular "tumor" of adrenogenital syndrome. On the left are closely packed hyperplastic steroid-type cells; on the right is normal testicular parenchyma.

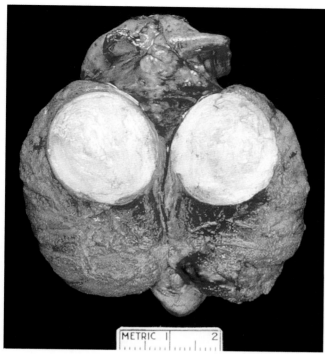

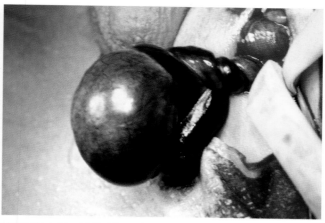

FIGURE 4–11 I∎II Testicular infarction secondary to spermatic cord torsion. (Courtesy of Jack Elder, MD, Cleveland, Ohio.)

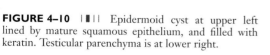

FIGURE 4–9 I∎II Epidermoid cyst. The white material filling the cyst cavity is desquamated keratin.

show the same findings as described for torsion, whereas fibrosis, calcifications, and cholesterol deposits ("clefts") may be the predominant findings in infarcts of longer duration.

Testicular hemorrhage in the absence of trauma is usually caused by a testicular neoplasm or infarct. Rare instances are secondary to vascular disease (arteritis) such as polyarteritis nodosa. Rupture of a large artery produces hematoma in the testis or paratesticular soft

tissues. The gross appearance of hematoma may be similar to that of choriocarcinoma; microscopically, only extravasated blood is found.

ORCHITIS

Orchitis is classified as bacterial orchitis, malakoplakia, viral orchitis, granulomatous orchitis secondary to specific infectious agents, granulomatous orchitis of idiopathic type, and granulomatous orchitis due to sarcoidosis. In some forms of orchitis, epididymitis is a common or constant feature.

Bacterial orchitis is nearly always accompanied by, and preceded by, bacterial epididymitis, most commonly caused by *Escherichia coli*. In the acute phase of infection, edema and abscess formation may be noted grossly (Fig. 4–13); microscopically, neutrophils dominate, filling the interstitium and the seminiferous tubules and

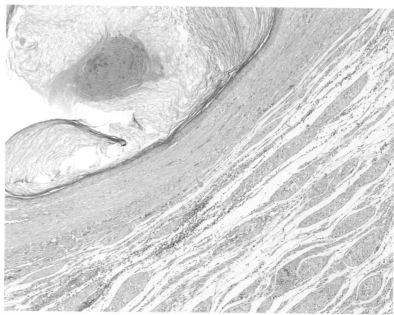

FIGURE 4–10 I∎II Epidermoid cyst at upper left lined by mature squamous epithelium, and filled with keratin. Testicular parenchyma is at lower right.

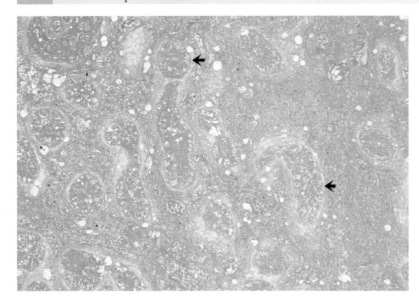

FIGURE 4–12 ▐ ▌▐ ▐ Testicular infarction. The outlines of seminiferous tubules and some of the tubular cells are discernible *(arrows);* no viable tissue is present.

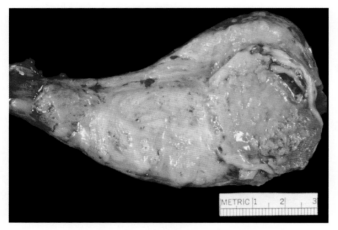

FIGURE 4–13 ▐ ▌▐ ▐ Testicular abscess. The majority of the testicular parenchyma *(at right)* is replaced by purulent exudate.

forming abscesses (Fig. 4–14). In the chronic phase, walled-off abscesses and fibrosis predominate. Lymphocytes, plasma cells, macrophages, and eosinophils are plentiful. Areas of infarction due to small vessel occlusion may be observed.

Malakoplakia is characterized by incomplete processing of the breakdown products of bacteria by macrophages. The testis is affected in 12% of cases of genitourinary malakoplakia. It becomes enlarged, and the parenchyma is yellow-brown and may contain abscesses. The seminiferous tubules and interstitial spaces are infiltrated by macrophages with abundant eosinophilic cytoplasm (Fig. 4–15). Michaelis-Gutmann bodies may be present in some macrophages.

Viral epididymo-orchitis may be caused by numerous viruses. Mumps virus and coxsackievirus B are the most frequent offenders. Mumps orchitis is uncommon in

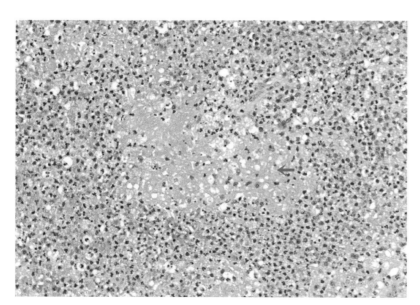

FIGURE 4–14 ▐ ▌▐ ▐ Testicular abscess. Fibrinous exudate forms a central abscess cavity *(arrow),* surrounded by inflammatory cells, predominantly neutrophils and macrophages.

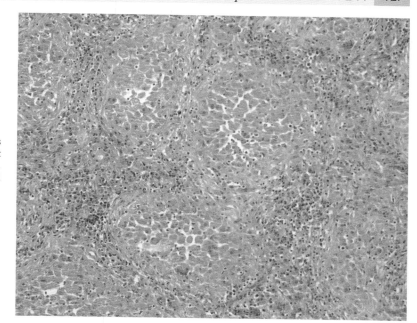

FIGURE 4–15 ❙▌❙❙ Malakoplakia of testis. The cells in the tubules are macrophages with abundant eosinophilic cytoplasm ("von Hansemann histiocytes"). Similar cells, as well as lymphocytes, fill the interstitial spaces.

childhood but develops in up to 35% of adults with mumps, and up to 25% of patients have bilateral involvement. Pathologic changes in the testis include multiple foci of acute inflammation of the seminiferous tubules and interstitial spaces, with loss of tubular cell populations. Resolution of the inflammation leaves a small soft testis with hyalinized, unpopulated tubules and scattered clusters of Leydig cells.

Granulomatous epididymo-orchitis of specific etiology is caused by infection with tuberculosis, syphilis, leprosy, brucellosis, fungal organisms, and parasites. In adults (in whom most cases occur), *tuberculous epididymo-orchitis* usually is associated with tuberculosis elsewhere in the genitourinary tract; in children, the infection arrives via the bloodstream from the lungs. The testis contains caseating and noncaseating granulomas (Fig. 4–16). *Syphilitic orchitis* is characterized by interstitial inflammation with abundant plasma cells and lymphocytes or by

gumma formation (well-delineated areas of necrosis surrounded by chronic inflammatory cells).

In *idiopathic granulomatous orchitis*, the testis becomes enlarged and firm, suggesting cancer. The cut surface appears granular or nodular, with areas of necrosis (Fig. 4–17). Chronic inflammation is concentrated either in the interstitium or within and around tubules (Fig. 4–18). Blood vessels are commonly inflamed and occluded by thrombi. Tubular atrophy and interstitial fibrosis develop. Involvement by *sarcoidosis* is rare and usually is unilateral. The testis is nodular and contains noncaseating granulomas (Fig. 4–19).

INFERTILITY

The evaluation of infertile men is complex, requiring consideration of a wide spectrum of possible etiologic

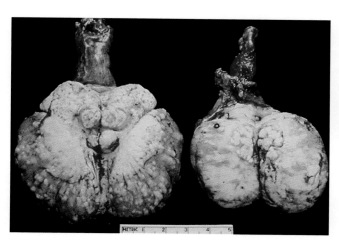

FIGURE 4–16 ❙▌❙❙ Tuberculosis involving both testes. Very little normal parenchyma remains. There is extensive parenchymal fibrosis, and nodules of caseous necrosis are evident. The process involves the epididymis of the testis on the left.

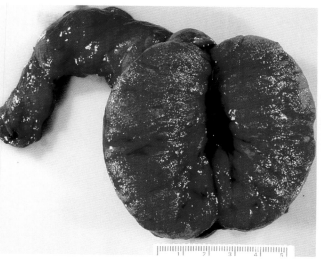

FIGURE 4–17 ❙▌❙❙ Granulomatous orchitis. The testis is edematous and bulging, and widespread areas of pale granularity of the parenchymal surface are evident.

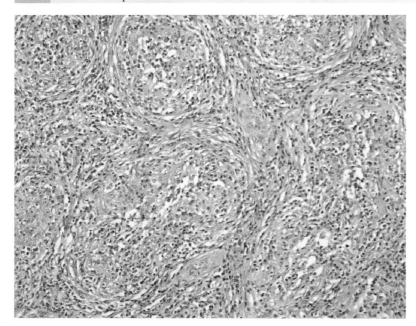

FIGURE 4–18 ▏▐ ▏▏ Nonspecific granulomatous orchitis. The tubular epithelium is replaced by chronic inflammatory cells, which also extensively infiltrate the interstitium.

factors, including congenital anomalies, chromosomal abnormalities, endocrine dysfunction, and iatrogenic injuries. This section is limited to the pathologic findings commonly observed in cases in which testicular biopsy is undertaken to evaluate azoospermia or oligospermia. Because findings differ between the testes in 28% of cases, both testes should be sampled.

HYPOSPERMATOGENESIS

Patients with hypospermatogenesis usually have oligospermia. There are numerous causes for this disorder, including diminished gonadotropin stimulation, dietary deficiencies, injurious agents, and aging. In some patients, no cause is apparent. In this condition, all stages of spermatogenesis are represented in testicular biopsies but there is an overall reduction in spermatogenic activity. Sper-

matogonia, spermatocytes, spermatids, and spermatozoa are present in normal proportions in the seminiferous tubules, but in diminished numbers, resulting in generalized thinning of the germinal cell layer (Fig. 4–20). Spermatozoa are scarce in most tubules and absent in some.

MATURATION ARREST

Patients with this disorder have oligospermia or azoospermia. In most cases, the cause is not identifiable. Testicular biopsy shows interruption of the normal progression of germ cell maturation. The most common finding is spermatogenic arrest at the spermatocyte stage; the tubules contain Sertoli cells, spermatogonia, and variable numbers of primary spermatocytes, but no spermatids or spermatozoa are present. Arrest at earlier or later stages changes the germ cell populations observed,

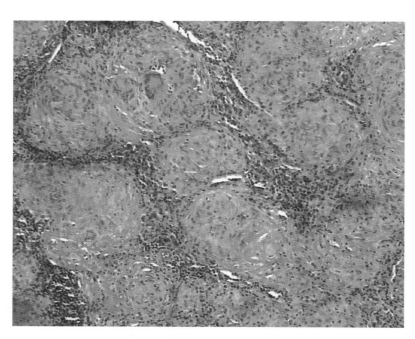

FIGURE 4–19 ▏▐ ▏▏ Sarcoidosis. Numerous noncaseating granulomas composed of aggregates of epithelioid histiocytes and multinucleated giant cells and surrounded by lymphocytes.

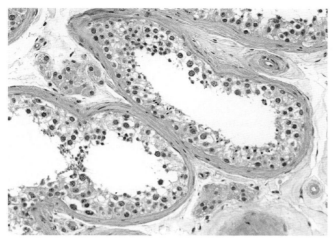

FIGURE 4–20 Hypospermatogenesis. Germ cells proceed through all stages of maturation, forming mature spermatozoa; however, the overall number of germ cells is diminished and the germinal epithelium is thin.

but, regardless of the stage of arrest, mature spermatozoa are sparse or absent (Fig. 4–21).

GERM CELL APLASIA (SERTOLI CELL–ONLY SYNDROME)

Patients with germ cell aplasia are azoospermic. They have slightly small testes and elevated serum follicle-stimulating hormone (FSH) levels but are otherwise normal males. In this pattern of infertility, the seminiferous tubules are populated only by tall columnar Sertoli cells, which contain "windswept" cytoplasmic vacuoles and, sometimes, coarse eosinophilic granules (Fig. 4–22).

KLINEFELTER'S SYNDROME

Men with Klinefelter's syndrome account for up to 10% of patients seen at infertility clinics. They are azoospermic.

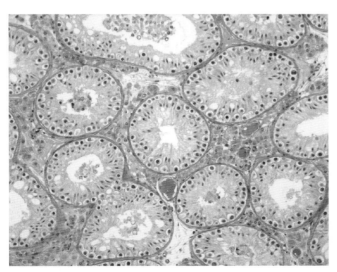

FIGURE 4–21 Maturation arrest. The tubules are populated only by Sertoli cells and immature germ cells, predominantly spermatogonia. No spermatids or spermatozoa are seen.

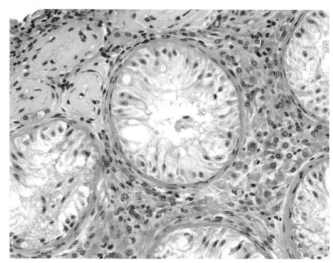

FIGURE 4–22 Germ cell aplasia. The tubules are lined only by Sertoli cells, some of which contain cytoplasmic vacuoles. No germ cell elements are present. Adjacent tubules *(upper left)* are hyalinized.

The seminiferous tubules are small, with thick, hyalinized walls; and most tubules do not contain Sertoli cells, germ cells, or patent lumens (although scattered tubules may contain Sertoli cells and rare spermatogonia) (Fig. 4–23). Similar microscopic findings are seen in *cryptorchid testes* that remain in the abdomen or inguinal canal through puberty (Fig. 4–24). In both conditions, Leydig cells form large interstitial aggregates that suggest hyperplasia, although the absolute number of Leydig cells is diminished (Fig. 4–25).

TESTICULAR NEOPLASMS

Most testicular tumors are derived from germ cells and sex cord/stromal cells. Much less commonly, tumors arise from interstitial mesenchymal cells. Involvement of the testis by extratesticular malignancies accounts for a small percentage of cases. The origin of epidermoid and dermoid cysts of the testis is not clearly understood; they are either derived from germ cells (similar to mature teratoma) or invaginated skin elements. At present, there is lack of uniformity in the classification of testicular tumors. The classification shown in Table 4–1 is based on the World Health Organization (WHO) system.

GERM CELL NEOPLASMS

Incidence

Germ cell neoplasms are the most common malignancy in males between 15 and 44 years old and account for about 1% of male cancers. In prepubertal males, they are not associated with intratubular germ cell neoplasia, are usually of one histologic type, and are biologically less aggressive than those arising after puberty. After puberty, the incidence rises rapidly, peaks between 25 and 35 years, then slowly declines, leveling off by age 60.

Risk Factors

The following factors pose significant risk for the development of germ cell neoplasm: cryptorchidism, previous

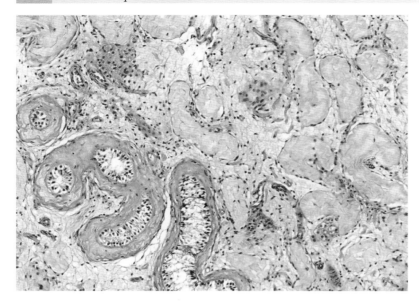

FIGURE 4–23 ▌▌▌▌ Klinefelter's syndrome. Some tubules have patent lumens but show marked hyaline thickening of their basement membranes and absence of germ cell elements; they are lined only by Sertoli cells. Other tubules are completely occluded by hyalinization.

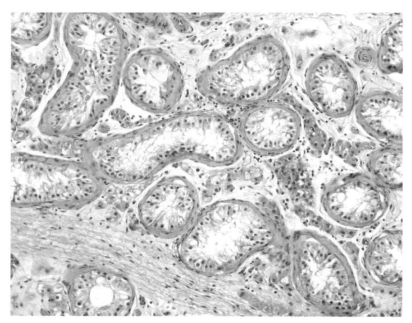

FIGURE 4–24 ▌▌▌▌ Cryptorchid testis. Hyalinized tubules lined almost exclusively by Sertoli cells. Germ cell elements are scant or absent in these tubules.

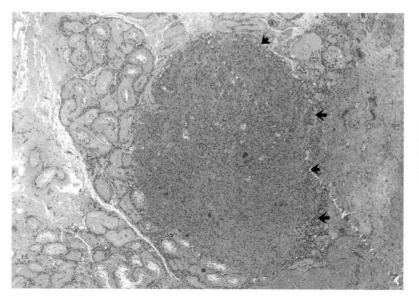

FIGURE 4–25 ▌▌▌▌ Cryptorchid testis excised from a 43-year-old patient. Tubules are extensively hyalinized, and a large aggregate of Leydig cells is present *(outlined by arrows).* Similar findings are common in patients with Klinefelter's syndrome.

TABLE 4–1

CLASSIFICATION OF TESTICULAR NEOPLASMS

Germ Cell Neoplasms
Intratubular germ cell neoplasia (IGCN) and its derivatives
    Seminoma
    Embryonal carcinoma
    Yolk sac tumor
    Teratoma
    Choriocarcinoma
    Mixed germ cell tumor
Germ cell neoplasms not associated with IGCN
    Spermatocytic seminoma
    Pediatric yolk-sac tumor
    Pediatric teratoma

Sex Cord/Stromal Tumors
Leydig cell tumor
Sertoli cell tumor
Granulosa cell tumor, adult and juvenile types
Fibroma thecoma
Mixed and unclassified sex cord/stromal tumor

Mixed Germ Cell and Sex Cord/Stromal Tumors
Gonadoblastoma
Other mixed germ cell and sex cord stromal tumors

Neoplasms of the Rete Testis

Hematopoietic Tumors

Miscellaneous Tumors and Tumor-like Lesions

Adapted from Ulbright TM, Amin MB, Young RH: Atlas of Tumor Pathology, Third Series, Fascicle 25. Tumors of the Testis, Adnexa, Spermatic Cord, and Scrotum. Washington, D.C.: Armed Forces Institute of Pathology, 1999.

---

testicular germ cell neoplasm, family history of testicular germ cell neoplasm, and certain intersex syndromes (gonadal dysgenesis in patients with a Y chromosome, true pseudohermaphrodites, androgen insensitivity syndrome).

Histogenesis

Germ cells transform into seminoma cells, the template for subsequent development of nonseminomatous germ cell tumors. Neoplastic changes in germ cells most often result in the development of intratubular germ cell neoplasia (IGCN). IGCN is commonly found in intact seminiferous tubules at the periphery of postpubertal germ cell tumors and is considered the precursor of these cancers. IGCN, seminoma, and non-seminomatous germ cell tumors share a marker chromosome (isochrome 12p), which results in excess copies of genes derived from the short arm of chromosome 12. Seminoma is the invasive counterpart of IGCN, and additional genetic alterations in seminoma cells result in the development of embryonal carcinoma, teratoma, choriocarcinoma, and/or yolk-sac tumor. Intratubular embryonal carcinoma, choriocarcinoma, and yolk sac tumor are rare.

Pediatric teratoma, pediatric yolk-sac tumor, and spermatocytic seminoma probably result from genetic changes in germ cells different from those of IGCN. These tumors usually are not accompanied by IGCN, do not manifest the isochrome (12p) alteration, and are less aggressive than tumors derived from IGCN.

TABLE 4–2

TNM STAGING OF GERM CELL AND SEX CORD–GONADAL STROMAL TUMORS OF TESTIS

Primary Tumor (T)

pTX	Primary tumor cannot be assessed
pT0	No evidence of primary tumor (e.g., histologic scar in testis)
pTis	Intratubular germ cell neoplasia
pT1	Tumor limited to the testis and epididymis without vascular/lymphatic invasion; tumor may invade into the tunica albuginea but not the tunica vaginalis
pT2	Tumor limited to the testis and epididymis with vascular/lymphatic invasion, or tumor extending through the tunica albuginea with involvement of the tunica vaginalis
pT3	Tumor invades the spermatic cord with or without vascular/lymphatic invasion
pT4	Tumor invades the scrotum with or without vascular/lymphatic invasion

Note: Except for pTis and pT4, extent of primary tumor is classified by radical orchiectomy. TX may be used for other categories in the absence of radical orchiectomy.

Regional Lymph Nodes (N)
Clinical

NX	Regional lymph nodes cannot be assessed
N0	No regional lymph node metastasis
N1	Metastasis with a lymph node mass 2 cm or less in greatest dimension; or multiple lymph nodes, none more than 2 cm in greatest dimension
N2	Metastasis with a lymph node mass more than 2 cm but not more than 5 cm in greatest dimension; or multiple lymph nodes, any one mass greater than 2 cm but not more than 5 cm in greatest dimension
N3	Metastasis with a lymph node mass more than 5 cm in greatest dimension

Pathologic (pN)

pNX	Regional lymph nodes cannot be assessed
pN0	No regional lymph node metastasis
pN1	Metastasis with a lymph node mass 2 cm or less in greatest dimension and less than or equal to 5 nodes positive, none more than 2 cm in greatest dimension
pN2	Metastasis with a lymph node mass more than 2 cm but not more than 5 cm in greatest dimension; or more than 5 nodes positive, none more than 5 cm; or evidence of extranodal extension of tumor
pN3	Metastasis with a lymph node mass more than 5 cm in greatest dimension

Distant Metastasis (M)

MX	Distant metastasis cannot be assessed
M0	No distant metastasis
M1	Distant metastasis
M1a	Non-regional nodal or pulmonary metastasis
M1b	Distant metastasis other than to non-regional lymph nodes and lungs

Note: Additional categories (S0 to S3) are defined by serum levels of lactate dehydrogenase, α-fetoprotein (AFP), and human chorionic gonadotropin (hCG).

Used with the permission of the American Joint Committee on Cancer (AJCC), Chicago, Illinois. The original source for this material is the *AJCC Cancer Staging Manual, Sixth Edition* (2002) published by Springer-Verlag New York, www.springer-ny.com.

INTRATUBULAR GERM CELL NEOPLASIA AND ITS DERIVATIVES

Intratubular Germ Cell Neoplasia

Testes involved by intratubular germ cell neoplasia (IGCN) without an invasive component may appear atrophic, fibrotic, or grossly unremarkable. Microscopically, some seminiferous tubules contain abnormal

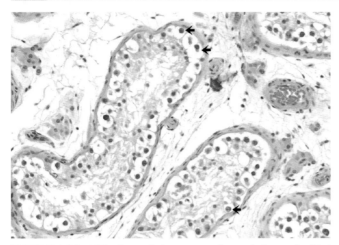

FIGURE 4–26 ▕▐▕▕ Intratubular germ cell neoplasia, unclassified (IGCNU). Neoplastic germ cells *(arrows)* hug the basement membrane, displacing the Sertoli cells.

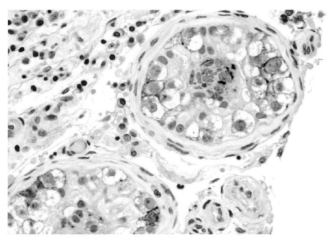

FIGURE 4–27 ▕▐▕▕ IGCNU, immunostained with antibodies against placental-like alkaline phosphatase. The neoplastic cells show brown (positive) immunostaining.

cells adjacent to the basement membrane, replacing or undermining the Sertoli cells. These abnormal cells usually resemble primitive gonocytes: they have large hyperchromatic nuclei, one or two prominent nucleoli, abundant clear cytoplasm, and distinct nuclear and cell membranes (Fig. 4–26). This form of IGCN is designated IGCN, unclassified (IGCNU). The cells of IGCNU almost always demonstrate positive immunostaining for placental-like alkaline phosphatase (PLAP) (Fig. 4–27). Rarely, the intratubular proliferation may be of a specific cell type, such as intratubular embryonal carcinoma (Fig. 4–28).

Seminoma

Approximately half of all germ cell neoplasms are pure seminoma. The average patient age is 40 years; seminoma is uncommon in adolescents and very rare in males younger than 10 years of age. Presenting symptoms include testicular enlargement and/or discomfort, gynecomastia, or symptoms related to metastatic cancer. Serum hCG levels are modestly elevated in up to 25% of patients with pure seminoma, reflecting the fact that 10% to 20% of these tumors have a small component of syncytiotrophoblasts mingling with the seminoma cells. Significant elevation of serum AFP level cannot be attributed to pure seminoma. If a testicular neoplasm consists entirely of seminoma in a patient with elevated serum AFP, one should assume the presence of yolk sac tumor, either undetected in the primary tumor or in distant metastases.

Seminoma averages 5 cm in diameter. It is usually well circumscribed; multinodular and bulging; cream, pink, or tan; with focal hemorrhage (Fig. 4–29). Some show necrosis, fibrous septa, extensive fibrosis, or invasion of adjacent soft tissues.

Microscopically, seminoma usually consists of sheets and nests of cells separated by thin fibrovascular septa but sometimes arrayed in linear cords or ribbons. The fibrovascular septa are typically infiltrated by abundant lymphocytes (Fig. 4–30). Granulomatous inflammation is

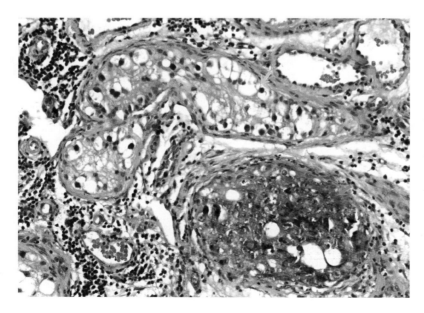

FIGURE 4–28 ▕▐▕▕ IGCNU and intratubular germ cell neoplasia, embryonal type. Tubule at top contains IGCNU *(yellow arrow)*. Tubule at bottom right is filled with cells typically seen in embryonal carcinoma, with necrosis and microcalcifications *(green arrow)*. Invasive embryonal carcinoma formed a clinically evident testicular tumor.

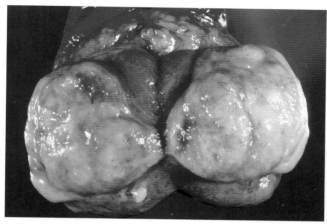

FIGURE 4–29 ❘▌❘❘ Seminoma.

seen in 50% to 60% of seminomas. Necrosis is present in 50% of cases, and vascular invasion is sometimes evident. Tumor cells are round to polygonal, with clear or light pink cytoplasm. The cells have large central nuclei with finely granular chromatin and one or more conspicuous nucleoli. Cell membranes are usually quite distinct (Fig. 4–31). Mitotic figures are readily observed. Syncytiotrophoblasts may be present, singly or in small clusters (Fig. 4–32).

Embryonal Carcinoma

Embryonal carcinoma is a component in 87% of mixed germ cell tumors, so it is present in nearly 40% of all germ cell tumors. In pure form, it accounts for only 2% to 3% of all germ cell tumors. The neoplasm is so named because its cells resemble early embryonic epithelial cells.

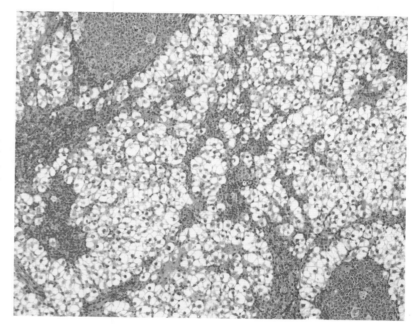

FIGURE 4–30 ❘▌❘❘ Seminoma. Clusters of pale-staining seminoma cells intersected by delicate vascular channels. Numerous lymphocytes are present, with a tendency to congregate along the course of the blood vessels.

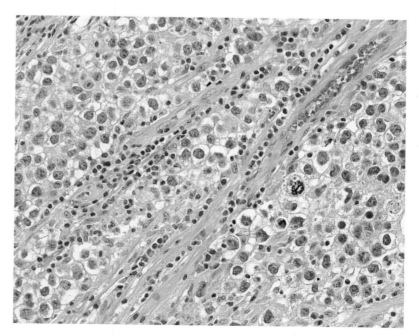

FIGURE 4–31 ❘▌❘❘ Seminoma. The tumor cells in this example have lightly eosinophilic cytoplasm. Cell membranes are distinct, and there is little, if any, cell overlap. Lymphocytes infiltrate the fibrovascular septa.

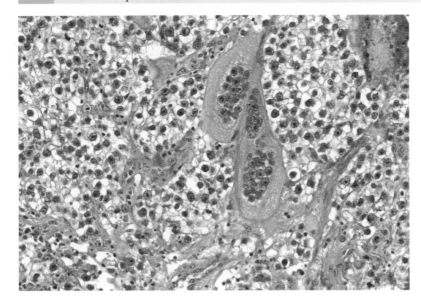

FIGURE 4–32 |▮|| Seminoma. Multinucleated syncytiotrophoblasts *(arrows)* mingling with seminoma cells. No "blood lake" is present, excluding a diagnosis of choriocarcinoma.

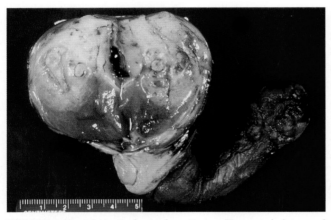

FIGURE 4–33 |▮|| Embryonal carcinoma. Tumor is bulging and poorly circumscribed and has areas of necrosis. This example had no other germ cell elements.

Patients with embryonal carcinoma average 32 years of age. Presenting symptoms include testicular enlargement with or without pain, gynecomastia, or symptoms attributable to metastases. Pure embryonal carcinoma does not cause elevation of serum AFP. Serum hCG level is elevated in 60% of patients with this tumor.

Embryonal carcinoma is typically pink-tan to gray-white, bulging, friable, hemorrhagic, and extensively necrotic (Fig. 4–33). Average tumor size is 2.5 cm. Most are poorly circumscribed, and 25% invade extratesticular soft tissues.

Microscopically, tumor cells are arranged in sheets, tubules, and papillae. In solid areas, the cells are large, round or polygonal, with abundant cytoplasm, which may be clear, pink, or basophilic. Cell nuclei are large and irregular, with coarsely clumped chromatin and one or more prominent nucleoli. Cell membranes tend to

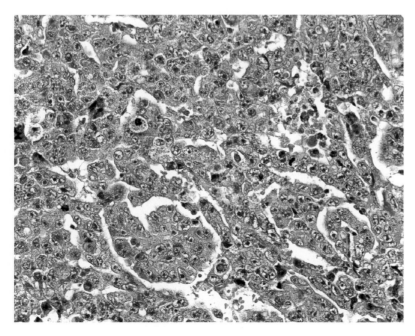

FIGURE 4–34 |▮|| Embryonal carcinoma. Tumor grows in sheets, with poorly formed glandlike spaces. Cytoplasm is basophilic. Single cell apoptosis and focal necrosis are evident. Cells overlap one another, and cell membranes are indistinct. Frequent mitotic figures are present.

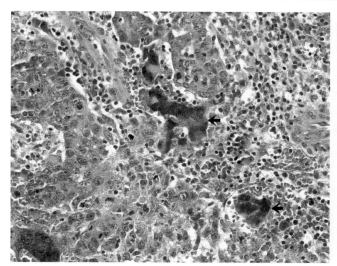

FIGURE 4–35 I ▮ I I Embryonal carcinoma. Dark-staining multinucleated syncytiotrophoblasts are scattered among the embryonal carcinoma cells *(arrows)*. There is considerable background hemorrhage.

be indistinct, and nuclei are crowded and overlapping (Fig. 4–34). In tubules and papillae, tumor cells are cuboidal or columnar. Abundant mitotic figures and areas of necrosis are usually present. Vascular invasion is commonly observed. Syncytiotrophoblasts are often present in embryonal carcinoma, singly or in small clusters, accounting for the high frequency of serum hCG elevation in these patients (60%) (Fig. 4–35).

Yolk Sac Tumor

Also known as *endodermal sinus tumor*, this germ cell neoplasm derives its names from its resemblance to developing extraembryonic mesenchyme in humans; its glomeruloid structures resemble the endodermal sinuses of the rat placenta.

Despite histologic similarities, yolk sac tumors in children differ from the adult counterpart in many respects and are discussed separately. Here the discussion is limited to yolk sac tumor in postpubertal males. In this population, yolk sac tumor is virtually always a component of a mixed germ cell tumor rather than a pure neoplasm.

Most postpubertal males with yolk sac tumor are between 25 and 30 years old; the tumor is rare after age 45. Patients usually note painless testicular enlargement. Serum AFP level is usually elevated.

Because yolk sac tumor in adults is usually a component of a mixed germ cell tumor, the gross findings are quite variable. Most are poorly circumscribed, soft to firm, and gray-white to tan, with considerable necrosis, hemorrhage, and cystic degeneration. Some have a mucoid cut surface (Fig. 4–36).

Yolk sac tumor shows numerous architectural and cytologic patterns microscopically. The *reticular* (microcystic) pattern is most common, consisting of a meshwork network of variably sized empty spaces representing cytoplasmic vacuoles and microcysts (Fig. 4–37). The *endodermal sinus* pattern is distinctive for yolk sac tumor, consisting of papillary fibrovascular structures lined by cuboidal or columnar cells, situated within circumscribed cystic spaces; these structures are called *Schiller-Duval*

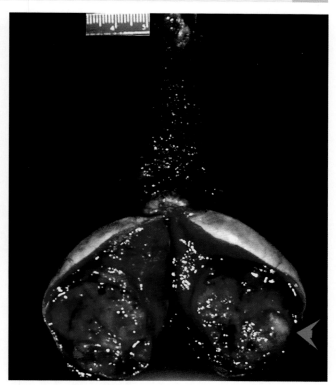

FIGURE 4–36 I ▮ I I Yolk sac tumor. This example is extensively hemorrhagic. Part of the tumor has a glistening, gray, mucoid cut surface *(arrow)*.

bodies (Fig. 4–38). In some tumors, larger "macrocysts" are noted. Tumor cells may be arranged in sheets, acini, or anastomosing villoglandular structures. Some tumors have vesicular spaces with constrictions, resembling the embryonic yolk sac. Cells containing pink hyaline globules of AFP are another distinctive finding in yolk sac tumor; such globules are rarely seen in other germ cell tumors (Fig. 4–39).

Teratoma

Teratoma is a germ cell tumor composed of somatic-type tissues. Although similar histologically, teratoma in children differs from adult teratoma in many respects; childhood teratoma is discussed later. Pure testicular teratoma in postpubertal males is uncommon; teratoma in these patients is usually a component of a mixed germ cell tumor and is present in over half of such tumors. Mature teratoma may not have metastatic potential, but the precursor cells that give rise to teratoma are capable of metastasizing and giving rise to mature teratoma at the metastatic site or, alternatively, giving rise to other types of germ cell tumor. For this reason, a postpubertal male with pure mature teratoma is at risk for metastatic germ cell tumor of any type.

Postpubertal males with teratoma present with testicular enlargement or with symptoms related to metastatic cancer, usually in the second to fourth decade of life. Modest serum AFP elevation may be caused by AFP production by endodermal glandular components in the teratoma; more often, elevations of AFP or hCG result from yolk sac elements or syncytiotrophoblasts in a mixed germ cell tumor.

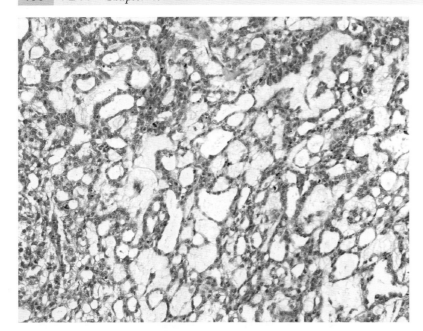

FIGURE 4–37 ▮▮▮ Yolk sac tumor. This is an example of microcystic architecture, one of the most common of the many architectural variations seen in yolk sac tumor.

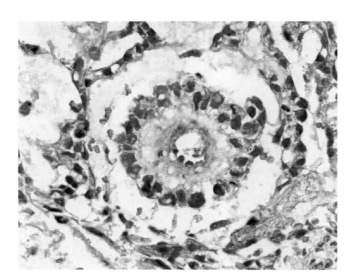

FIGURE 4–38 ▮▮▮ Yolk sac tumor. This is a Schiller-Duval body, one of the architectural variants seen in yolk sac tumor. It consists of a fibrovascular core lined by neoplastic cells that lies within a circumscribed cystic space.

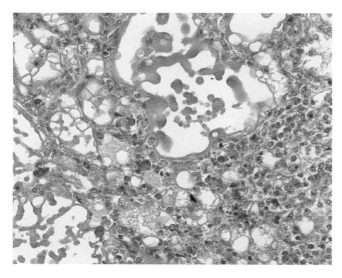

FIGURE 4–39 ▮▮▮ Yolk sac tumor. Hyaline globules of variable size, staining light pink to dark red, are seen in up to 85% of yolk sac tumors. The globules typically contain α-fetoprotein or α_1-antitrypsin. They are rarely seen in other types of germ cell tumor.

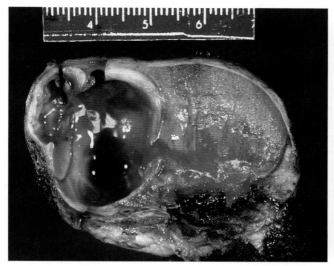

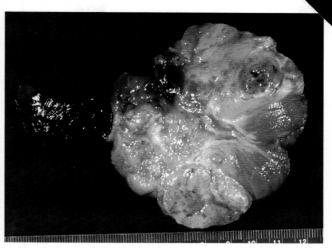

FIGURE 4–40 ▮▮▮▮ Teratoma. Tumor is well circumscribed, solid at the periphery, and centrally cystic. Cyst contents in this example appear mucoid.

FIGURE 4–42 ▮▮▮▮ Immature teratoma. Numerous small cysts are present. (Courtesy of Jie-Gen Jiang, MD, Cleveland, Ohio.)

Pure teratoma varies considerably in size; some of the largest arise in intra-abdominal undescended testes. It is typically solid and cystic, without apparent infiltration of paratesticular structures (Fig. 4–40). Cysts contain mucoid fluid, serous fluid, or keratinous debris. Solid areas may be composed of cartilage or fibrous tissue, sometimes with areas of hemorrhage or necrosis.

Teratoma is composed of somatic-type elements resembling postnatal tissues derived from ectoderm, endoderm, and/or mesoderm, such as cartilage, muscle, neuronal tissue, squamous or urothelial islands, and respiratory or gastrointestinal type glands (Fig. 4–41). Teratoma that contains embryonic tissue such as immature neuroepithelium, embryonic tubules, blastema, or immature soft tissues is designated *immature teratoma* (Figs. 4–42 and 4–43). The significance of the presence

of immature components in a teratoma has not been ascertained. It is also unknown whether grading the degree or the extent of immaturity in a teratoma is of prognostic importance.

Rarely, nongerminal malignancies arise within teratoma in adults. The most common example is rhabdomyosarcoma (Fig. 4–44); others include squamous cell carcinoma, primitive neuroectodermal tumor (PNET), enteric-type adenocarcinoma, and angiosarcoma. Metastases from secondary malignancies tend to be resistant to chemotherapy directed at the primary germ cell neoplasm.

Dermoid cyst is a subset of teratoma. It appears grossly as a unilocular cyst containing milky fluid, keratinous debris, and hair. Nodular projections are often present in the cyst wall. The cyst wall is lined by keratinizing squamous epithelium. Skin appendages (hair

FIGURE 4–41 ▮▮▮▮ Teratoma. Non-neoplastic testis is at right side. The tumor contains an ectodermal element (squamous epithelium shedding keratin debris—*black arrow*), an endodermal element (glandular space at upper left lined by columnar epithelium—*red arrow*), and supporting mesoderm (fibroconnective tissue—*blue arrow*).

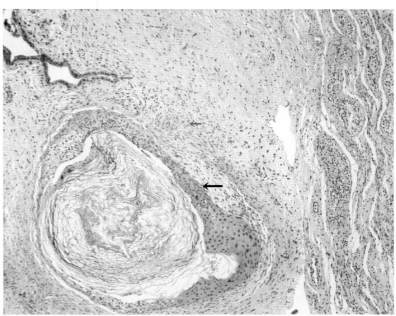

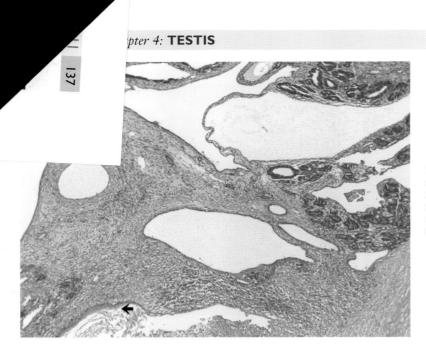

FIGURE 4–43 ▌▐▐▌ Immature teratoma. Although mature squamous epithelium is present *(black arrow)*, the majority of this tumor consisted of immature mesenchymal-type tissue *(yellow arrow)* and a large component of immature neuroepithelium, forming sheets and tubular structures *(red arrows)*.

follicles and sebaceous glands) are present in the dermal layer. Immature elements are, by definition, never present. Dermoid cyst is not associated with IGCN and does not metastasize.

Choriocarcinoma

Choriocarcinoma is composed of an intimate aggregate of cytotrophoblasts and syncytiotrophoblasts. In its pure form, it accounts for 0.3% of testicular neoplasms. It can be identified in approximately 8% of mixed germ cell tumors. Rather than causing symptoms related to testicular enlargement, it tends to metastasize early and widely by hematogenous routes, causing symptoms related to metastatic cancer, such as hemoptysis, gastrointestinal

bleeding, or neurologic symptoms. Most patients are in their second or third decade of life; no prepubertal patients have been reported. About 10% of patients have gynecomastia, a reflection of markedly elevated levels of hCG in most patients.

Testes involved by pure choriocarcinoma may be grossly unremarkable. The tumor creates hemorrhagic necrotic nodules of variable size; they are usually small but sometimes replace much or all of the testis (Fig. 4–45). Occasionally, complete tumor regression leaves only a scar.

Microscopically, choriocarcinoma typically consists of limited foci of viable tumor at the periphery of a pool of blood, fibrin, and necrotic tissue (Fig. 4–46). Viable tumor is composed of variable proportions of multinucleated syncytiotrophoblasts and mononuclear cytotrophoblasts. Syncytiotrophoblasts have dark pink

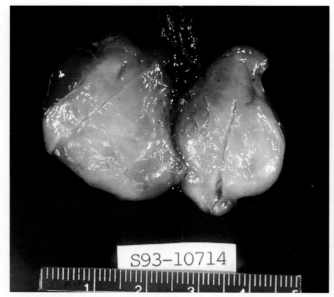

FIGURE 4–44 ▌▐▐▌ Rhabdomyosarcoma. No teratomatous elements were identified; however, rhabdomyosarcoma is one of the most common secondary malignancies arising in teratoma.

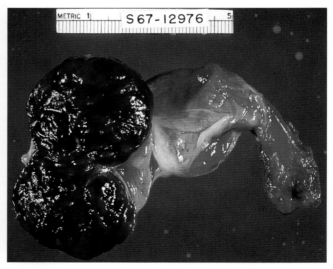

FIGURE 4–45 ▌▐▐▌ Choriocarcinoma. Tumor is diffusely and extensively hemorrhagic.

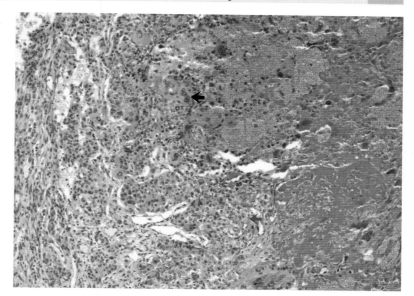

FIGURE 4–46 ▯▮▯▯ Choriocarcinoma. A lake of blood is rimmed by multinucleated syncytiotrophoblasts *(black arrow)* and mononuclear cytotrophoblasts *(blue arrow).*

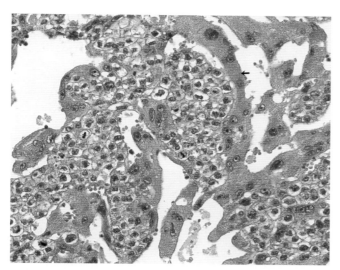

FIGURE 4–47 ▯▮▯▯ Choriocarcinoma. Syncytiotrophoblasts *(black arrow)* forming a mantle over mononuclear cytotrophoblasts *(blue arrow).*

Regressed ("Burnt-Out") Testicular Germ Cell Tumor

Extragonadal germ cell neoplasms are occasionally encountered in patients with clinically normal testes. Isolated germ cell tumors in the pineal region or the mediastinum probably result from aberrant germ cell migration during fetal development. Isolated retroperitoneal germ cell tumor is more likely to represent metastasis from an occult testicular primary tumor that has undergone partial or complete regression. Although any type of germ cell tumor may undergo regression, this behavior is most common in choriocarcinoma.

A testis with a regressed germ cell tumor usually has one or more ill-defined areas of parenchymal scarring, consisting microscopically of dense fibrous tissue, usually with infiltrates of lymphocytes and scattered hemosiderin-laden or lipid-laden macrophages and occasionally with

cytoplasm; their multiple nuclei are hyperchromatic, irregular, often smudged, and devoid of mitotic figures. They form a mantle over clusters of cytotrophoblasts, but more often the two cell types are randomly distributed (Fig. 4–47). Cytotrophoblasts are fairly uniform, with distinct cell membranes, light eosinophilic cytoplasm, and irregular nuclei with frequent mitotic figures. Vascular invasion is usually evident.

Mixed Germ Cell Tumor

This neoplasm contains more than one type of germ cell tumor and is included in the category of nonseminomatous germ cell tumor. Virtually any combination of germ cell tumor may be present. The most common combinations are embryonal carcinoma with teratoma and embryonal carcinoma with seminoma (Figs. 4–48 and 4–49).

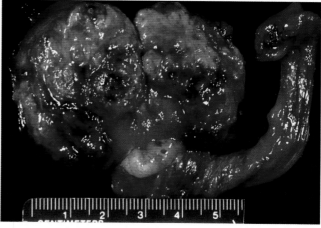

FIGURE 4–48 ▯▮▯▯ Mixed germ cell tumor. The tumor had a mixture of embryonal carcinoma, yolk sac tumor, teratoma, and choriocarcinoma.

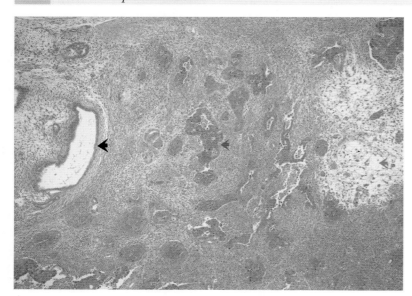

FIGURE 4–49 ▮▮▮ Mixed germ cell tumor. Teratoma with glandular spaces in a mesenchymal background at left *(black arrow);* dark-staining embryonal carcinoma forming sheets and abortive glandular spaces centrally *(blue arrow);* and yolk sac tumor with microcystic architecture at right *(red arrow).*

areas of dystrophic calcification (Figs. 4–50 and 4–51). Residual IGCN or foci of viable germ cell tumor may be present.

GERM CELL NEOPLASMS NOT ASSOCIATED WITH IGCN

Germ cells may undergo cytogenetic changes different from those that result in IGCN. These alternate neoplastic changes result in the development of spermatocytic seminoma and pediatric teratoma and yolk sac tumors, none of which is associated with IGCN.

Spermatocytic Seminoma

This germ cell neoplasm derived its name from the observation that the three cell populations that comprise the tumor resemble the polymorphous cell populations involved in spermatogenesis.

Spermatocytic seminoma differs from classic seminoma in many ways. It does not arise outside the confines of the testis, and it does not have a haploid DNA content. It is not associated with cryptorchidism or with IGCN and does not display the isochrome (12p) cytogenetic abnormality that is common to germ cell tumors. It occurs in men in their mid to late 50s and does not occur in men younger than 30. Patients complain of testicular enlargement, occasionally associated with pain. Serum levels of AFP and hCG are normal. Bilateral asynchronous tumors occur in 9% of patients, a frequency much higher than that observed in patients with classic seminoma.

Spermatocytic seminoma is usually well circumscribed, multinodular, gray to tan, soft, and friable (Fig. 4–52). Cut surfaces may appear mucinous, and cysts are sometimes present. Necrosis and hemorrhage are absent or minimal.

The cells of spermatocytic seminoma form large sheets in an edematous background, intersected by broad fibrous bands. Three cell types (small, medium, and large) are present (Fig. 4–53). The small cells resemble mature lymphocytes. Medium cells, 15 to 20 μm in diameter, are the most numerous cell type. They have pale nuclei and finely granular cytoplasm. The large cells can be up to 100 μm in diameter and sometimes contain multiple nuclei. In some medium and large cells, the

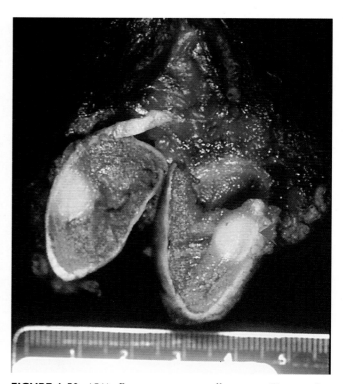

FIGURE 4–50 ▮▮▮ Burnt-out germ cell tumor. Biopsy of a retroperitoneal mass in this 37-year-old man showed seminoma. Clinical examination of testes was inconclusive, but ultrasound disclosed this lesion, prompting orchiectomy. (Courtesy of Rosemary Farag, MD, Cleveland, Ohio.)

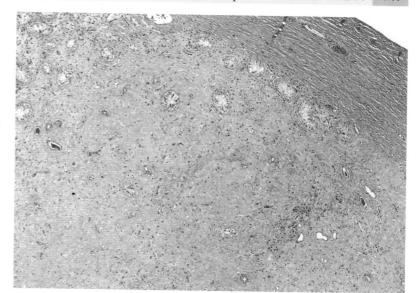

FIGURE 4–51 ❙▊❙❙ Burnt-out germ cell tumor. The nodule shown in Figure 4–50 was submitted entirely for histologic evaluation. The nodule consists of a fibrous scar; no germ cell cancer was identified. A few residual seminiferous tubules are seen at the periphery of the nodule.

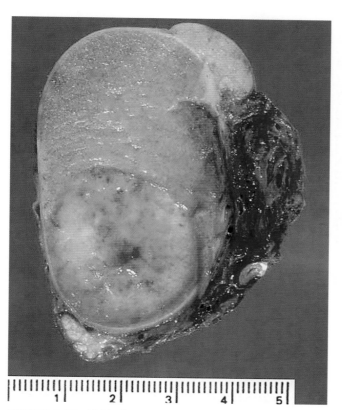

FIGURE 4–52 ❙▊❙❙ Spermatocytic seminoma. Tumor is well circumscribed, with focal hemorrhage and without necrosis.

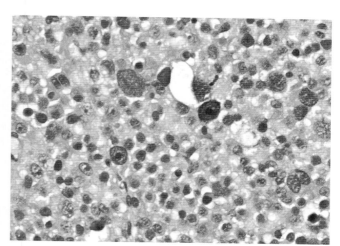

FIGURE 4–53 ❙▊❙❙ Spermatocytic seminoma. Cells with very large nuclei, mingled with cells with small dark nuclei and cells with intermediate-sized nuclei. The largest cell shows filamentous ("spireme") chromatin. Immunostaining was helpful in excluding lymphoma.

nuclear chromatin appears filamentous, similar to that of primary spermatocytes in meiotic prophase. Cell membranes of all cell types are indistinct. Abundant mitotic figures are usually present. Lymphocytic infiltrates and granulomatous reactions are absent. Special stains for glycogen and placental-like alkaline phosphatase (PLAP) are negative (stains are positive in classic seminoma).

Sarcoma develops in 6% of spermatocytic seminomas. Most are undifferentiated, but some show features of rhabdomyosarcoma.

Yolk Sac Tumor in Prepubertal Males

In prepubertal males, yolk sac tumor accounts for 82% of germ cell neoplasms. Patients range in age from newborn to 9 years old, but more than half are younger than 2 years old. In these patients, yolk sac tumor is nearly always pure, is not associated with cryptorchidism or isochrome (12p), and is only rarely associated with IGCN.

Patients have painless testicular enlargement. Serum AFP levels are elevated in only 75% to 80% of patients and are of limited value in children younger than

8 months of age, because serum AFP is physiologically higher in this age group than in older individuals. At the time of diagnosis, 84% to 94% of patients have clinically localized disease.

Pediatric yolk sac tumor is usually circumscribed, homogeneous, and solid tan or gray white, with little or no hemorrhage or necrosis. Cut surfaces may have a mucoid consistency. The microscopic findings are the same as those described in yolk sac tumors arising after puberty.

Yolk sac tumor in prepubertal males behaves much less aggressively than its postpubertal counterparts. However, lymphatic spread to retroperitoneal nodes and hematogenous spread to the lungs occur in up to 14% of patients. Ninety percent of patients survive 5 years.

Teratoma in Prepubertal Males

Teratoma accounts for up to 18% of germ cell neoplasms in prepubertal males. More than half of patients are younger than 24 months old, and nearly all are younger than 5 years old; median patient age is 20 months. Patients often have associated congenital anomalies. Teratomas in these patients are not associated with IGCN or isochrome (12p).

Patients have painless testicular enlargement. Serum AFP and hCG levels are normal. The gross and microscopic pathologic findings are the same as in postpubertal pure teratoma. Most are "completely mature" histologically. Pure testicular mature teratoma in prepubertal males is benign, adequately treated by orchiectomy.

SEX CORD/STROMAL TUMORS

These neoplasms account for 8% of testicular tumors in prepubertal males and 4% of all testicular neoplasms. Their names are derived from the resemblance of the component cells to cells native to the testis (Sertoli cells, Leydig cells, and supporting stromal cells).

Leydig Cell Tumor

Leydig cell tumor accounts for 2% to 3% of all testicular neoplasms. It occurs in patients of any age older than 2 years, but the average age at onset is 40 years old. This tumor is capable of secreting sex hormones. Virilization is noted in virtually all children with Leydig cell tumor, and gynecomastia occurs in about 10%. Adults report testicular enlargement, gynecomastia (30%), and, sometimes, diminished libido or impotence.

Most Leydig cell tumors are between 2 and 5 cm in diameter. They are usually solid, yellow or brown, and sharply circumscribed (Fig. 4–54). Hemorrhage and necrosis are minimal or absent. About 10% are locally invasive.

Microscopically, the tumor cells form sheets with a myxoid or edematous background and intersecting fibrous septa (Fig. 4–55). Tumor cells are large and polygonal, with abundant eosinophilic finely granular cytoplasm and small round uniform nuclei, most of which have conspicuous nucleoli (Fig. 4–56). In one third of cases, rod-shaped intracytoplasmic crystals of Reinke may be observed (Fig. 4–57).

Approximately 10% of Leydig cell tumors are malig-

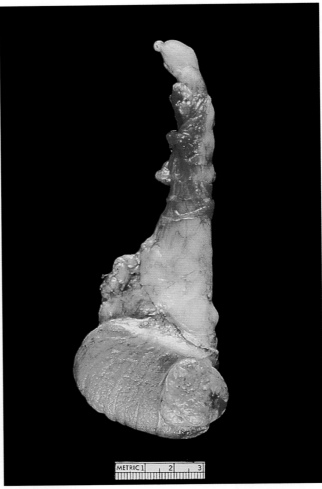

FIGURE 4–54 ▐▌▐▐ Leydig cell tumor. It is sharply circumscribed and yellow, with focal hemorrhage.

nant. Patients with malignant Leydig cell tumor average 63 years of age. Pathologic findings that correlate with malignancy include large size (malignant tumors average 6.9 cm in diameter), infiltrative tumor borders, angiolymphatic invasion, necrosis, pronounced nuclear atypia, and increased mitotic activity (Figs. 4–58 and 4–59).

Sertoli Cell Tumor

Fewer than 1% of testicular neoplasms are Sertoli cell tumor. It develops in patients of any age but occurs predominantly in middle-aged men. Most arise sporadically, but Sertoli cell tumor may be associated with androgen insensitivity syndrome, Peutz-Jeghers syndrome, and Carney's syndrome. Sertoli cell tumor occurring in patients with Peutz-Jeghers syndrome is benign. Patients usually present with testicular enlargement, but some complain of gynecomastia or impotence related to estrogen production by the tumor.

Sertoli cell tumor is usually solid, gray-white or yellow-tan, and well circumscribed (Fig. 4–60). Mean tumor diameter is 3.0 cm. Cyst formation or hemorrhage is noted in some, but necrosis is unusual.

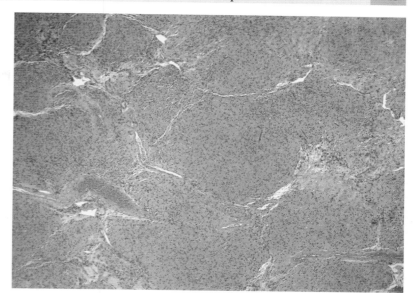

FIGURE 4–55 |▌|| Leydig cell tumor. Sheets and nodules of darkly eosinophilic tumor cells separated by broad fibrovascular bands.

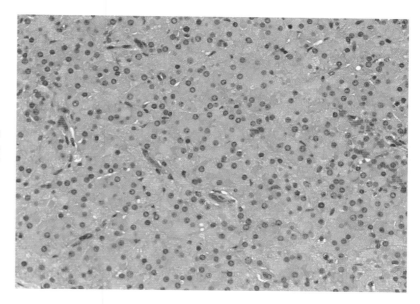

FIGURE 4–56 |▌|| Leydig cell tumor. Tumor cells have abundant darkly eosinophilic cytoplasm and round, uniform nuclei with small nucleoli. Mitotic figures and necrosis are absent.

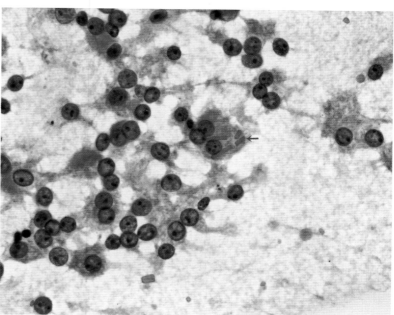

FIGURE 4–57 |▌|| Leydig cell tumor. About one third have Reinke's crystals in the cytoplasm of some cells, as demonstrated by the *blue arrow.*

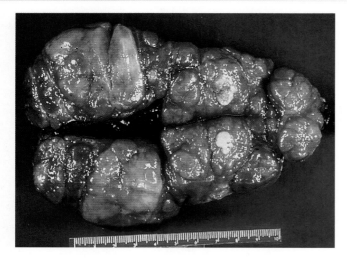

FIGURE 4–58 ▐▐▌▐ Leydig cell tumor. Features correlating with malignant potential (large size and areas of necrosis) are evident.

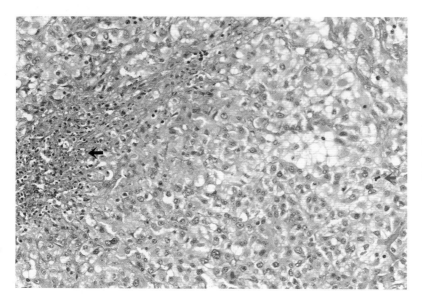

FIGURE 4–59 ▐▐▌▐ Leydig cell tumor. A section from the tumor illustrated in Figure 4–58. Cell nuclei vary considerably in shape and size; necrosis is present *(black arrow)*; a mitotic figure is also seen *(blue arrow)*; all these features suggest malignancy.

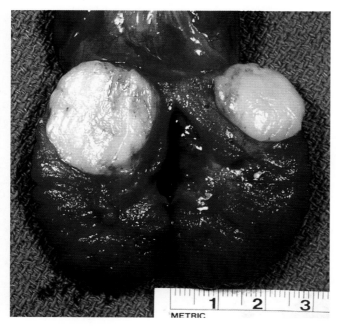

FIGURE 4–60 ▐▐▌▐ Sertoli cell tumor. Lesion is solid and sharply circumscribed, without necrosis.

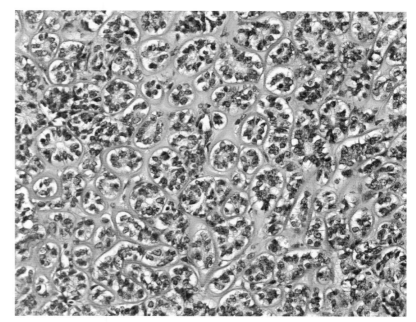

FIGURE 4–61 ▮▮▮▮ Sertoli cell tumor. Round or elongate tubules, lined by uniform cells, in a sclerotic background.

Microscopically, several architectural patterns are seen. Most commonly, round or elongate tubules are present, sometimes in a collagenous background (Fig. 4–61). Cell nuclei are small and uniform, without nucleolar prominence or significant mitotic activity. Some cells have minimal cytoplasm, and others have abundant pale cytoplasm due to the presence of lipid.

Sclerosing Sertoli cell tumor occurs only in adults and is not associated with hormonal symptoms or malignant behavior. It is microscopically distinctive because the background stroma is densely collagenized.

Large cell calcifying Sertoli cell tumor occurs sporadically and in Carney's syndrome. Most patients are in late adolescence or early adulthood. Some have hormonal symptoms. The tumor is usually white or yellow-tan and well circumscribed, with a gritty consistency. It consists of large cells with abundant pink finely granular cytoplasm, arranged in small nests, cords, sheets, ribbons, or solid tubules. Cell nuclei are small and round, with conspicuous nucleoli. Widespread calcific deposits are present in the stroma (Fig. 4–62). About 17% are malignant.

Mixed and Unclassified Sex Cord/ Stromal Tumors

These tumors occur in adults and children, and some cause gynecomastia. They are well circumscribed, gray, yellow, or tan. Microscopically, the tumor cells show both stromal and sex cord differentiation. A tumor composed of adult granulosa cell tumor mixed with tubules containing

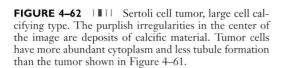

FIGURE 4–62 ▮▮▮▮ Sertoli cell tumor, large cell calcifying type. The purplish irregularities in the center of the image are deposits of calcific material. Tumor cells have more abundant cytoplasm and less tubule formation than the tumor shown in Figure 4–61.

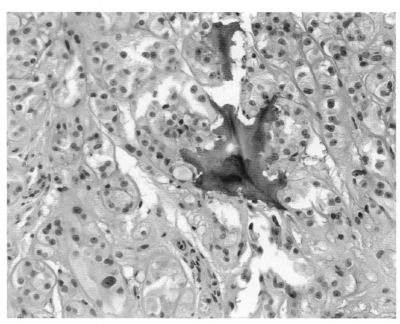

Sertoli cells is an example of a mixed sex cord/stromal tumor. Unclassified tumors are those in which the Sertoli cell and stromal components do not form readily recognizable patterns. Tumors of this type are usually benign in children; in adults, 25% are malignant.

MIXED GERM CELL/SEX CORD/ STROMAL TUMORS

Tumors composed of neoplastic germ cell elements mixed with neoplastic sex cord/stromal elements are usually either gonadoblastoma or "unclassified" germ cell/sex cord/stromal tumor.

Gonadoblastoma

Most gonadoblastomas arise in dysgenetic gonads in patients with intersex syndromes associated with the presence of a Y chromosome. The great majority are phenotypic females, and a minority are phenotypic males with cryptorchidism, hypospadias, and gynecomastia; some have ambiguous genitalia. One or both gonads are "streak gonads" or "streak testes" (Fig. 4–63). Phenotypic males with dysgenetic gonads often have müllerian duct remnants (uterus and fallopian tubes). Gonadoblastoma is bilateral in at least one third of cases. A fourth of gonadoblastomas are found only by microscopic examination. Larger tumors are solid, gritty, yellow, tan, or gray and measure up to 8 cm in diameter.

Gonadoblastoma is composed of seminoma-like germ cells and immature Sertoli cells admixed in round nests. Sex cord cells surround single germ cells or small clusters of germ cells, and they also encircle round deposits of pink basement membrane material. Calcification is present in 80% of tumors and may be extensive.

In about 50% of cases, seminoma is also present and a small number have nonseminomatous germ cell cancer. Bilateral gonadectomy is warranted in patients diagnosed with gonadoblastoma and in patients at high risk for developing it.

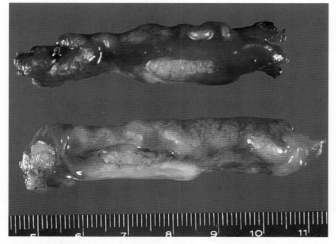

FIGURE 4–63 ▐ ▌▐ ▐ Streak gonads. The patient had gonadal dysgenesis. The gonads consist mainly of adnexal structures, with small nodules of gonadal tissue. A gonadoblastoma was found in one of the gonadal nodules. (Courtesy of Beverly Dahms, MD, Cleveland, OH.)

Other Mixed Germ Cell/Sex Cord/ Stromal Tumors

These are rare, hormonally inactive, benign tumors composed of both neoplastic germ cells and sex cord cells but microscopically unlike gonadoblastoma. They occur in adults sporadically, rather than in a setting of gonadal dysgenesis or intersex syndrome.

CARCINOMA OF THE RETE TESTIS

This is a rare malignancy limited to white men older than 30 years old who present with scrotal swelling and discomfort; it is often of long duration. Hydrocele formation accompanies about half of the tumors, and scrotal skin metastases are sometimes present. This tumor is aggressive and is lethal in approximately two thirds of cases.

Tumors are white, solid, and firm, sometimes with cystic degeneration, and measure up to 10 cm in diameter. If small, they are near the rete testis. Nodules of metastatic cancer may be present on the tunica surface, and spermatic cord invasion is evident in one third.

Microscopically, tumor cells form solid nodules and nests, papillae, and elongate slitlike tubules lined by malignant cells, in a fibrous stroma (Fig. 4–64). Tumor cells are cuboidal and small, with scant cytoplasm and dark nuclei. Frequent mitotic figures, areas of necrosis, and tumor invasion into cord structures, the tubules or stroma of the rete testis, or the parenchyma of the testis are commonly present.

HEMATOPOIETIC TUMORS OF THE TESTIS

Lymphoma

Lymphoma accounts for approximately 5% of all testicular neoplasms, and its frequency increases with patient age. In men older than 60 years old, at least half of testicular neoplasms are lymphomas. The incidence of bilateral involvement (usually metachronous) ranges up to 38%. Most testicular lymphomas reflect systemic cancer. Patients present with testicular enlargement accompanied by fever, night sweats, or weight loss. Five-year disease-free survival in patients with testicular lymphoma is approximately 35%.

Testes involved by lymphoma average 6 cm in diameter and show partial or complete effacement of normal architecture by a diffuse, firm, homogeneous pink-tan, yellow, or cream-colored infiltrate (Fig. 4–65). The border between the infiltrate and normal parenchyma is indistinct. Focal necrosis is sometimes present.

Lymphoma appears microscopically as a diffuse cellular infiltrate in the interstitium, surrounding and sparing seminiferous tubules (Fig. 4–66). Tumor cell infiltration of the epididymis, spermatic cord structures, and vascular channels is common. Approximately 80% of testicular lymphomas are of diffuse large cell type, and nearly all are of B-cell phenotype. The cellular findings are typical of lymphoma encountered at other sites.

Plasmacytoma and Multiple Myeloma

Testicular infiltration by malignant plasma cells occurs in approximately 2% of patients with multiple myeloma,

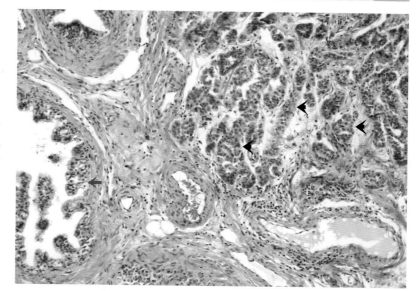

FIGURE 4–64 | ▌ | | Rete testis adenocarcinoma. Normal rete structures are at lower left *(blue arrow)*. Tumor *(upper right)* forms tubules and small nests *(black arrows)*. Tumor cells have scant cytoplasm, and hyperchromatic nuclei with prominent nucleoli.

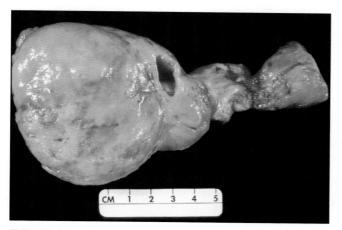

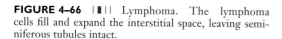

FIGURE 4–65 | ▌ | | Lymphoma. Testicular parenchyma is diffusely effaced by the malignant cellular infiltrate.

but most of these infiltrates are not clinically evident. At least half of patients diagnosed with plasma cell tumors of the testis have a known history of multiple myeloma. Plasma cell malignancy confined to the testis (plasmacytoma) is rare (Figs. 4–67 and 4–68).

Leukemia

Approximately two thirds of patients with acute leukemia have testicular infiltrates of leukemic cells, and a fourth of patients with chronic leukemia are similarly affected. Fewer than 10% of these infiltrates are clinically apparent. Testicular enlargement caused by leukemic infiltration is rarely the presenting symptom in such cases. In testes involved by leukemia, the malignant lymphoid or myeloid cells show patterns of infiltration similar to those observed in lymphoma and plasmacytoma.

FIGURE 4–66 | ▌ | | Lymphoma. The lymphoma cells fill and expand the interstitial space, leaving seminiferous tubules intact.

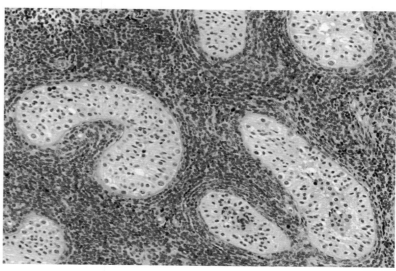

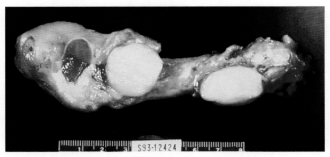

FIGURE 4–67 ▮▮▮ Plasmacytoma. Residual normal testis is seen on the left. These firm white nodular tumors were composed entirely of malignant plasma cells. Patient was not known to have systemic plasma cell malignancy.

MISCELLANEOUS NEOPLASMS

Soft Tissue Neoplasms

A small number of testicular neoplasms are derived from interstitial mesenchymal cells, endothelial cells, and peritubular myoid cells. These tumors are morphologically and biologically similar to their counterparts in other body sites (Fig. 4–69).

Metastases to the Testis

Nonhematopoietic metastases involve the testis in as many as 3.6% of men dying of cancer. Testicular enlargement is the first symptom of cancer in 6% of cases of testicular metastasis diagnosed during life. The majority of

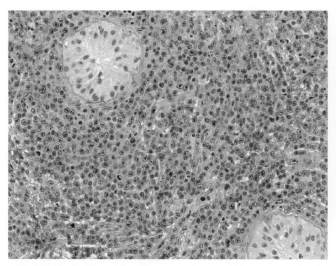

FIGURE 4–68 ▮▮▮ Plasmacytoma. Intact tubules surrounded by malignant plasma cells. The tumor cells are poorly differentiated, requiring ancillary studies to confirm the diagnosis.

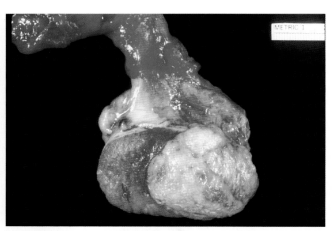

FIGURE 4–70 ▮▮▮ Metastatic prostate cancer, forming a large circumscribed nodule.

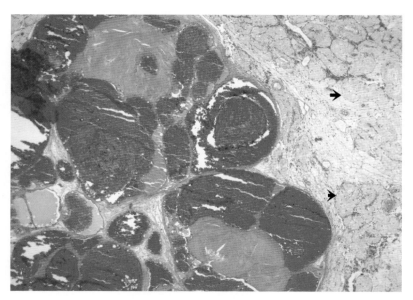

FIGURE 4–69 ▮▮▮ Hemangioma. This small benign soft tissue tumor was found incidentally in a testis excised therapeutically for treatment of prostate cancer. Lakes of blood are separated by fibrovascular septa. The adjacent testicular parenchyma *(arrows)* shows marked atrophic changes.

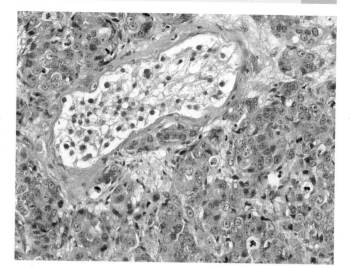

FIGURE 4–71 | ▌ | | Metastatic prostate cancer. The tumor is poorly differentiated; no well-formed acinar structures are seen (compare with Figure 4–68). Immunostain for prostate-specific antigen assisted in confirming the diagnosis.

patients are older than 50 years old, but patients younger than 40 years old account for one third of the total. Common primary sites are prostate (33% of cases) and lung (20% of cases). Malignant melanoma, renal carcinoma, and gastrointestinal carcinoma are other common primary sites.

Testes involved by metastatic cancer often show one or more nodules of tumor (Fig. 4–70). In testes excised for treatment of prostate cancer, the metastases may only be microscopic. Metastases can mimic a variety of primary testicular neoplasms, including embryonal carcinoma, carcinoid, and Leydig cell tumor (Fig. 4–71).

Chapter 5

SPERMATIC CORD AND TESTICULAR ADNEXAE

The paratesticular region includes the testicular tunics, efferent ductules, epididymis, spermatic cord, and vas deferens. Numerous rare and interesting lesions arise in this region, including cysts, "celes," inflammatory diseases, embryonic remnants, neoplasms, and neoplasm-like proliferations. In children, one of the common neoplasms is paratesticular rhabdomyosarcoma. In adults, the most common pathologic conditions in order of frequency are epididymitis, lipoma of the spermatic cord, adenomatoid tumor of the epididymis, and sarcoma of the spermatic cord.

EMBRYOLOGY AND NORMAL ANATOMY

The paratesticular region contains numerous anatomically complex epithelial and mesenchymal structures, often within embryonic remnants (Fig. 5–1). The rete testis of the mediastinum of the testis, the first element of the wolffian collecting system, connects the seminiferous tubules and efferent ductules.

The most common abnormalities of the paratesticular region are benign, including hydrocele, lipoma, and inflammatory conditions such as epididymitis, but a variety of cystic and proliferative lesions also occur and are diagnostically challenging.

EMBRYOLOGY

The embryology of the testis is described in Chapter 4; a brief summary of significant events in development of paratesticular tissues is provided here. The testis and head of the epididymis arise from the genital ridge. The wolffian ducts, the male genital ducts, are paired tubes that are associated with the developing gonads and degenerating mesonephric tubules. The body and tail of the epididymis, the vas deferens, and the ejaculatory duct arise from the mesonephric tubules; other degenerating tubules often persist as embryonic remnants, including the appendix epididymis, paradidymis, and cranial and caudal aberrant ductules (see Fig. 5–1). The paired vasa deferentia connect to the ejaculatory ducts within the prostate, which, in turn, have their outlets in the prostatic urethra adjacent to the müllerian tubercle. Blind diverticula of the distal vas deferens form the seminal vesicles. The müllerian duct, or paramesonephros, regresses in men but may persist as embryonic remnants, such as the appendix testis and prostatic utricle.

ANATOMY

Scrotum and Testicular Tunics

The scrotum is divided by a partial median septum into two compartments, each of which contains a testis and epididymis and the lower portion of the spermatic cord. The scrotal wall consists of six layers, from the inside outward: the tunica vaginalis, the internal spermatic fascia, the cremasteric muscle, the external spermatic fascia, the dartos muscle, and the skin. The tunica vaginalis is a thin mesothelium-covered layer of the parietal peritoneum that also covers the white fibrous tunica

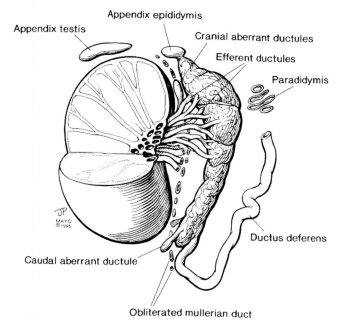

FIGURE 5–1 ▌▌▌ Anatomy of the testis and paratesticular adnexae, including embryonic remnants. (From Bostwick DG: Spermatic cord and testicular adnexae. In Bostwick DG, Eble JN [eds]: Urologic Surgical Pathology. St. Louis, Mosby, 1997, p. 648.)

albuginea of the testis and epididymis; it is initially in contact with the peritoneal cavity from which it arises, but it becomes isolated with regression of the processus vaginalis. The internal spermatic fascia is a continuation of the transversalis fascia, and the external fascia is a continuation of the external oblique aponeurosis. The cremasteric muscle consists of incomplete slips of muscle, usually in the upper part of the scrotal wall. The dartos muscle consists of smooth muscle embedded in loose areolar tissue. The scrotum is supplied by the external and internal pudendal, cremasteric, and testicular arteries. Lymphatic drainage is to the superficial inguinal lymph nodes.

Rete Testis

The rete testis is formed by the convergence of the seminiferous tubules. The tubules follow a cranial and dorsal course through the fibrous connective tissue of the mediastinum testis, eventually merging into 12 to 20 ducts (the efferent ductules, or ductuli efferentes [Fig. 5–2]), which perforate the tunica vaginalis and form the head of the epididymis at the upper pole of the testis. After

puberty, elastic fibers are present in the muscular coat of the ductules, epididymis, and vas deferens.

Epididymis

The epididymis is a highly convoluted tubule that is attached to the dorsomedial portion of the testis, connecting the efferent ductules of the rete testis with the vas deferens. It is about 6 meters long. The head consists of a series of conical masses, the lobules, each of which contains a single duct measuring 15 to 20 cm long; it is lined by tall columnar epithelium and invested with a thick layer of smooth muscle. The body of the epididymis is a single highly convoluted tube that increases in diameter distally to form the tail. The tail distally merges with the vas deferens.

Vas Deferens (Ductus Deferens) and Spermatic Cord

The vas deferens is about 46 cm long, traversing the spermatic cord and inguinal canal to connect the tail of the epididymis with the ejaculatory ducts. In the spermatic cord it is invested with a thick muscular coat that

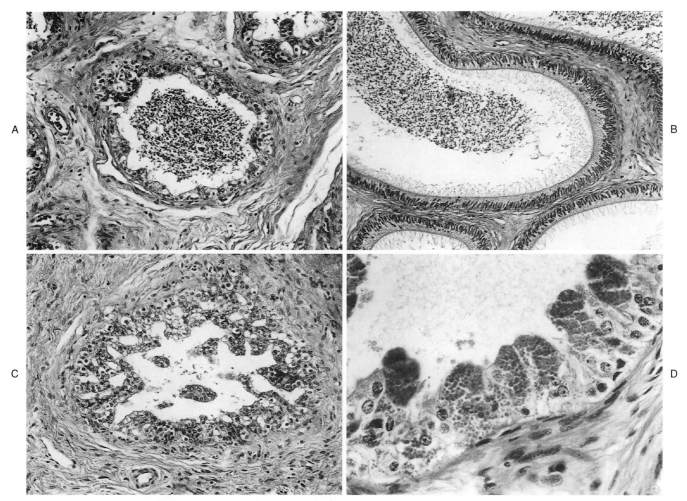

FIGURE 5–2 ▮▮▮ *A,* Normal efferent ductules with luminal sperm. *B,* Normal epididymis with luminal sperm. *C,* Cribriform hyperplasia of the efferent ductules. *D,* Coarse granular cytoplasmic change of the vas deferens (From Schned AR, Memoli VA: Coarse granular cytoplasmic change of the epididymis: An immunohistochemical and ultrastructural study. J Urol Pathol 2:213–222, 1994.)

includes the internal spermatic, cremasteric, and external spermatic fasciae; other structures of the spermatic cord include the pampiniform plexus, the testicular artery, lymphatics, and nerves. On exiting the spermatic cord, the vas deferens passes extraperitoneally, upward, and laterally in the pelvis it passes medial to the distal ureter and the posterior wall of the bladder, terminating at an acute angle in a dilated ampulla that, with the duct of the seminal vesicle, forms the ejaculatory duct. The vas deferens is supplied by its own artery, the artery of the vas deferens, which is usually a branch of the internal iliac or umbilical artery.

The vas deferens is lined by columnar epithelium in low folds. The wall of the vas deferens consists of three layers of smooth muscle: the inner longitudinal, middle circular, and outer longitudinal layers. Elastic fibers appear in the muscular wall after puberty.

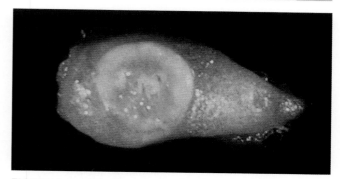

FIGURE 5–3 ¦▌¦¦ Heterotopic adrenal cortical tissue in the left spermatic cord forming a discrete yellow-orange nodule. (From Bostwick DG: Spermatic cord and testicular adnexae. In Bostwick DG, Eble JN [eds]: Urologic Surgical Pathology. St. Louis, Mosby, 1997, p. 650.)

CONGENITAL ANOMALIES

Abnormal development of the paratesticular region may result in a variety of anomalies, including embryonic remnants, agenesis, atresia, ectopia, and cysts. There is an increased frequency of anomalies in boys with cryptorchidism and congenital rubella. Bilateral anomalies result in sterility.

Agenesis and atresia of the testis, epididymis, and vas deferens result from failure of development of the genital ridge, often with anomalies of other wolffian derivatives and renal ectopia, agenesis, or dysplasia. Congenital absence of the vas deferens may be autosomal recessive and is often associated with cystic fibrosis (see later). Duplications may involve any structure of the adnexae but are rare. Ectopic insertion of the ureteric bud in the epididymis, vas deferens, or seminal vesicles also may occur. Congenital or developmental cysts of the epididymis are extremely rare and may be associated with intrauterine exposure to diethylstilbestrol. The cysts are usually solitary but may be multiple and bilateral.

Ectopic epididymis may be found anterior to the testis, in the retroperitoneum, and within the kidney.

SPLENOGONADAL FUSION

Splenogonadal fusion is a rare congenital anomaly in which there is fusion of the splenic and gonadal anlage. This condition is discussed and illustrated in Chapter 4.

ADRENAL HETEROTOPIA AND RENAL ECTOPIA

Adrenal cortical tissue may be present anywhere along the route of descent of the testis from the abdomen to the scrotum. It is usually an incidental finding at inguinal herniorrhaphy or epididymo-orchiectomy, present in up to 1% of children undergoing such operations. Adrenal cortical tissue has been identified in inguinal hernia sac, spermatic cord (see Fig. 5–3), epididymis, and the rete testis. It may present as a small palpable tumor and appears as small yellow-orange nodules, usually near the

inguinal ring. The lesions almost always consist of adrenal cortical tissue resembling zona glomerulosa and fasciculata. Rarely, they may contain medullary tissue. Involution during childhood is the rule, but exceptional cases persist and become functional, rarely harboring neoplasms.

Ectopic renal tissue has rarely been observed in the scrotum, consisting of tubules and immature glomeruli.

WOLFFIAN AND MÜLLERIAN REMNANTS

Numerous embryonic remnants are found in the paratesticular area, including the appendix testis (hydatid of Morgagni), appendix epididymis, paradidymis, and vasa aberrantia.

Appendix Testis (Hydatid of Morgagni)

The appendix testis is present on more than 90% of testes at autopsy. This structure is located at the superior pole of the testis adjacent to the epididymis. Grossly, it varies from 2 to 4 mm, appearing as a polypoid or sessile nodular excrescence. Microscopically, it contains a fibrovascular core of loose connective tissue covered by simple cuboidal or low columnar müllerian-type epithelium that is in continuity with the tunica vaginalis at the base. The fibrovascular core may contain tubular inclusions lined by similar cuboidal epithelium. Torsion of the appendix testis may be painful and may mimic testicular torsion.

Appendix Epididymis (Vestigial Caudal Mesonephric Collecting Tubule)

The appendix epididymis is present on about 35% of testicles examined at autopsy. Grossly, it is a pedunculated spherical cystic or elongate structure arising from the anterosuperior pole of the head of the epididymis. Microscopically, it is lined by cuboidal to low columnar epithelium, which may be ciliated and show secretory activity. The wall consists of loose connective tissue and is covered on its outer surface by flattened mesothelial cells that are continuous with the visceral tunica vaginalis. The appendix epididymis may become dilated by serous fluid and, when enlarged, may mimic a tumor. Torsion may occur, sometimes in cryptorchidism.

Paradidymis (Organ of Giraldés)

This wolffian duct embryonic remnant consists of clusters of tubules lined by cuboidal to low columnar epithelium within the connective tissue of the spermatic cord, superior to the head of the epididymis.

Vasa Aberrantia (Organ of Haller)

These wolffian duct remnants appear as clusters of tubules that are histologically similar to the paradidymis. They arise within the groove between the testis and epididymis. Torsion of the vas aberrans is rare.

Other Lesions Associated with the Epididymis

Other rare epididymal lesions have been described, including epididymal cyst (Fig. 5–4), duplication, and ectopic epididymal tissue associated with inguinal hernia. Cyst and duplication may arise from the caudal vasa aberrantia.

Walthard Rest

This remnant, probably of müllerian origin, consists of solid and cystic nests of uniform epithelial cells with ovoid nuclei and characteristic longitudinal grooves.

CYSTIC FIBROSIS

Cystic fibrosis is a genetic abnormality that often affects the testicular adnexae, resulting in infertility owing to agenesis or atresia of mesonephric structures or anomalies of the testes. Patients with congenital bilateral absence of vas deferens often have cystic fibrosis, although this finding may occur in patients without cystic fibrosis.

NON-NEOPLASTIC DISEASES OF THE SPERMATIC CORD AND TESTICULAR ADNEXAE

"CELES" AND CYSTS

Hydrocele

This mesothelial-lined cyst results from accumulation of serous fluid between the parietal and visceral tunica vaginalis of the testis (Fig. 5–5A). Congenital hydrocele occurs when a patent processus vaginalis allows communication between the tunica sac and the peritoneal cavity. The prevalence of congenital hydrocele is about 6% at birth and 1% in adulthood. Most cases of hydrocele are of uncertain etiology, but some are associated with inguinal hernia, scrotal trauma, epididymo-orchitis, or tumors of the testis or paratesticular region. Possible causes of idiopathic hydrocele include excessive secretion within the testicular tunics by parietal mesothelial cells, decreased reabsorption, and congenital absence of efferent lymphatics.

Hydrocele is lined by a single layer of cuboidal or flattened mesothelial cells, with underlying connective tissue stroma. The luminal fluid is usually clear and

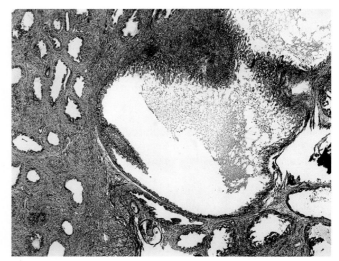

FIGURE 5–4 ▮▮▮ Small epididymal cyst that formed a palpable paratesticular mass. (From Bostwick DG: Spermatic Cord and testicular adnexae. In Bostwick DG, Eble JN [eds]: Urologic Surgical Pathology. St. Louis, Mosby, 1997, p. 651.)

serous unless complicated by infection or hemorrhage. The surface is often covered by fibrinous adhesions and inflammation, and subepithelial chronic inflammation and fibrosis may be present. In some cases, progressive fibrosis narrows or obliterates the cyst lumen, creating adhesions and multiple cysts. Spermatocele may rupture into the hydrocele sac.

Hematocele (Hematoma)

Hematocele refers to the accumulation of blood in the space between the parietal and visceral tunica vaginalis, often in association with hydrocele (see Fig. 5–5B). Longstanding hematocele becomes calcified and fibrotic, with numerous hemosiderin-laden macrophages. The causes of hematocele are similar to those for hydrocele.

Idiopathic hematoma may arise in the spermatic cord or epididymis.

Varicocele

Varicocele is a mass of dilated tortuous veins of the pampiniform venous plexus of the spermatic cord that occurs posterior and superior to the testis, sometimes extending into the inguinal ring (see Fig. 5–5C). The venous plexus normally empties into the internal spermatic vein near the internal inguinal ring; poor drainage and progressive dilatation and elongation result from incompetent valves of the left internal spermatic vein that empties into the renal vein. The right internal spermatic vein is less likely to be involved with varicocele because it drains directly into the inferior vena cava and is less likely to have incompetent valves.

Varicocele results from a number of conditions, but most cases are idiopathic. Unilateral varicocele in older men may indicate the presence of a renal tumor that has invaded the renal vein and occluded the spermatic vein drainage. Varicocele has been reported in association with maternal exposure to diethylstilbestrol. Patients with varicocele sometimes present with testicular pain associated with sexual activity.

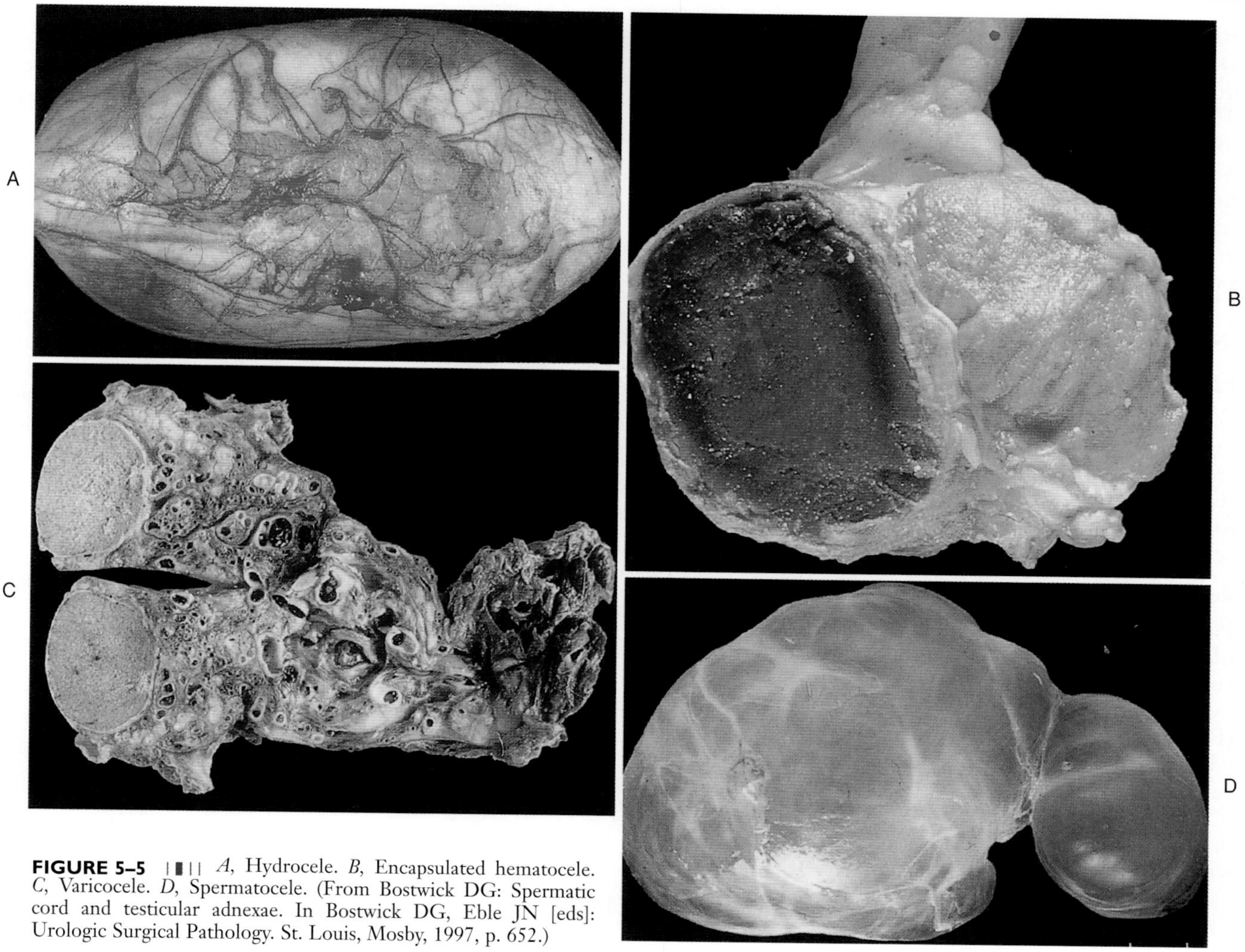

FIGURE 5–5 ▮▮▮ *A,* Hydrocele. *B,* Encapsulated hematocele. *C,* Varicocele. *D,* Spermatocele. (From Bostwick DG: Spermatic cord and testicular adnexae. In Bostwick DG, Eble JN [eds]: Urologic Surgical Pathology. St. Louis, Mosby, 1997, p. 652.)

Long-standing varicocele causes testicular atrophy and infertility in the affected testis. Treatment consists of ligation of the internal spermatic vein at the level of the internal inguinal ring.

Spermatocele (Acquired Epididymal Cyst)

Spermatocele is a dilatation of an efferent ductule in the region of the rete testis or caput epididymis. The inner lining consists of a single layer of cuboidal to flattened epithelial cells, which are often ciliated. The wall is composed of fibromuscular soft tissue, often with chronic inflammation. The cyst may be unilocular or multilocular and usually contains spermatozoa (see Fig. 5–5D). Torsion is a rare complication of spermatocele.

Mesothelial Cyst

Mesothelial cyst is a rare lesion that may involve the tunica sac, the epididymis, or the spermatic cord.

Mesothelial cyst of the tunica sac most often occurs in men older than 40 years of age, but all ages are affected. It is usually unilateral and situated on the anterolateral surface of the testis and may measure up to 4.0 cm in greatest dimension. The cyst is filled with clear or blood-tinged serous fluid, and the lining consists of typical mesothelial cells with a wall composed of hyalinized fibrous tissue. Rarely, the lining epithelium shows focal squamous metaplasia.

Unilocular and multilocular mesothelial cyst of the spermatic cord is rare and probably arises from embryonic mesothelial remnants of the processus vaginalis.

Epidermoid Cyst (Epidermal Cyst)

Epidermoid cyst is common in the testis, comprising about 1% of testicular tumors, but it may also rarely arise in the paratesticular area and epididymis. Epidermoid cyst consists of a lining of benign keratinizing squamous epithelium and a wall composed of fibrous connective tissue, often with inflammation. The cyst cavity contains desquamated keratin. Cutaneous adnexal structures, such as eccrine or apocrine glands and hair follicles, are absent, as are teratomatous elements. Paratesticular epidermoid cyst may arise from squamous metaplasia of wolffian duct structures, displacement of squamous epithelium from the scrotal skin to paratesticular structures during embryogenesis, or squamous metaplasia of mesothelial cyst. Epidermoid cyst in the paratesticular area does not recur after surgical excision.

Dermoid Cyst (Mature Teratoma)

Dermoid cyst most often involves the testis and paratesticular structures, but it may occur in the spermatic cord. This cyst measures up to 4 cm in diameter and contains soft cheesy yellow-white amorphous material with or without hair and calcifications. The cyst is lined by keratinized squamous epithelium, and the wall contains typical dermal adnexal structures such as pilosebaceous units. Dermoid cyst does not recur or metastasize after excision.

INFLAMMATORY AND REACTIVE DISEASES

Epididymitis

Epididymitis may be acute or chronic, depending on the inciting agent and the duration of infection. Most cases result from retrograde spread by vesicoepididymal urine reflux, but hematogenous and lymphatic spread account for some cases. Congenital anomalies such as ureteral ectopia may cause epididymitis in infants.

Acute Epididymitis

Patients with acute epididymitis usually present with unilateral painful enlargement of the epididymis, more commonly on the right side, often involving the testis (50% of cases have epididymo-orchitis) and vas deferens (Fig. 5–6). The epididymis is thickened, congested, and edematous, with white fibrinopurulent exudate in the tubules and stroma. Microabscesses and fistulas may occur, but rupture is uncommon. The tubules may be damaged or destroyed by the inflammation, sometimes with squamous metaplasia and regenerative changes.

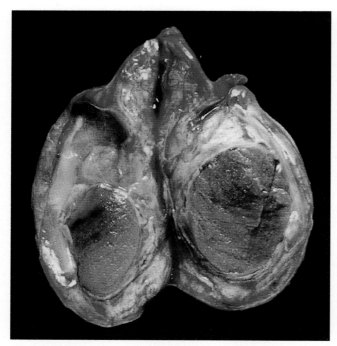

FIGURE 5–6 ▮▮▮ Acute epididymitis with associated testicular infarction. (From Bostwick DG: Spermatic cord and testicular adnexae. In Bostwick DG, Eble JN [eds]: Urologic Surgical Pathology. St. Louis, Mosby, 1997, p. 654.)

Acute epididymitis is commonly caused by bacteria. Coliforms account for most cases in children, whereas *Neisseria gonorrhoeae* and *Chlamydia trachomatis* are most frequent in young men and *Escherichia coli* and *Pseudomonas* predominate in older men. Other bacteria that may cause acute epididymitis include *Klebsiella*, *Staphylococcus*, *Streptococcus pneumoniae*, *Neisseria meningitidis*, *Aerobacter aerogenes*, and *Haemophilus influenzae*. The epididymis is a reservoir for *Neisseria gonorrhoeae*, and although infection may be asymptomatic, microabscesses and edema are common, usually without extensive necrosis.

Clinical and histopathologic findings allow separation of some cases of chlamydial and bacterial epididymitis. *Chlamydia trachomatis*–positive cases are clinically indolent, with minimally destructive periductal and intraepithelial inflammation with epithelial regeneration. Lymphoepithelial complexes and squamous metaplasia are sometimes present. *Escherichia coli*–positive cases are characterized by scrotal pain, pyuria, leukocytosis, and highly destructive epididymitis with abscesses and xanthogranulomas.

Viral causes of acute epididymitis include mumps and cytomegalovirus, similar to those causing orchitis. Mumps epididymitis, present in 85% of cases of mumps orchitis, occurs before testicular involvement, usually appearing as unilateral scrotal swelling after parotitis. The epididymis shows vascular congestion, edema, and interstitial lymphocytic inflammation; neutrophils are usually not a prominent feature. Cytomegaloviral epididymitis may occur in patients with the acquired immunodeficiency syndrome (AIDS).

Traumatic acute epididymitis is characterized by vascular congestion, petechial hemorrhages, and hematocele. Drugs such as amiodarone may also cause epididymitis.

Chronic Epididymitis

Although many cases of acute epididymitis resolve, some become chronic. The epididymis in chronic epididymitis is indurated and scarred, with cystically dilated tubules, marked fibrosis, chronic inflammation, and sperm granulomas (see later). The epithelium shows reactive or metaplastic changes, often with cytoplasmic vacuolization and luminal hyaline aggregates. Epididymitis nodosa, a proliferative lesion of the epididymis, may result from chronic inflammation or trauma, reminiscent of vasitis nodosa. Calcification is common in chronic epididymitis, and there may be a foreign body giant cell reaction. Xanthogranulomatous epididymitis may also occur. Special stains for bacteria and fungi may be of value.

Causes of chronic epididymitis include infectious agents, sarcoidosis, and sperm granuloma. The epididymis is the reservoir for tuberculous involvement in the male genital tract, with secondary testicular involvement and other local sites of involvement in about 80% of cases; for example, 40% of cases of renal tuberculosis are accompanied by epididymal infection. Patients usually present with painless scrotal swelling, but other signs and symptoms include unilateral or bilateral mass, infertility, and scrotal fistula. Caseating granulomatous inflammation is prominent, with fibrous thickening and enlarge-

TABLE 5–1

COMPARISON OF BACTERIAL AND CHLAMYDIAL EPIDIDYMITIS*

	Bacterial Epididymitis[†]	Chlamydial Epididymitis
Clinical Features		
Patient age (yr)	59.8 (39–79)	42.8 (22–74)
Pain	Yes	Infrequent
Laboratory Features		
Pyuria	Frequent	Infrequent
Elevated erythrocyte sedimentation rate	Yes	No
Elevated C-reactive protein	Yes	No
Pathologic Features		
Tissue destruction	Yes	Minimal
Xanthogranulomas	Yes	Minimal
Abscesses and necrosis	Yes	Minimal
Cytoplasmic location of antigens	Histiocytes	Epithelial cells

From Bostwick DG: Spermatic cord and testicular adnexae. In Bostwick DG, Eble JN (eds): Urologic Surgical Pathology. St. Louis, Mosby, 1997.
*For details see Hori S, Tsutsumi Y: Histologic differentiation and bacterial epididymitis: Nondestructive and proliferative versus destructive and abscess forming—immunohistochemical and clinicopathologic finding. Hum Pathol 26:402–407, 1995.
[†]Usually *Escherichia coli.*

ment of the epididymis and adjacent structures (Fig. 5–7). Rarely, miliary tuberculosis causes small punctate white lesions. Epididymitis may also result from other fungi (*Histoplasma capsulatum, Coccidioides immitis, Blastomyces dermatitidis*), parasites (*Schistosoma hematobium, Treponema pallidum, Wuchereria bancrofti*), leprosy, and viruses.

Malakoplakia of the epididymis is uncommon, usually occurring with testicular involvement. Patients are asymptomatic or present with painful scrotal swelling or hydrocele. The histologic findings are similar to those of malakoplakia at other sites.

Sarcoidosis involves the genital tract in about 5% of cases at autopsy but is rarely symptomatic. The epididymis is the most common site of genital involvement. Patients present with painful or painless scrotal swelling, which is bilateral in about 33% of cases. Non-necrotizing granulomatous inflammation is typical, similar to involvement at other sites.

Sperm Granuloma

Sperm granuloma is an exuberant foreign body giant cell reaction to extravasated sperm. Experimental injection of ceroid pigment produces granulomatous inflammation, suggesting that destruction of sperm initiates the process. An autoimmune reaction has been proposed but is not favored. In more than 40% of cases, there is a history of vasectomy. Patients may have no symptoms but often present with pain and swelling of the upper pole of the epididymis, spermatic cord, and, rarely, testis. Others have a history of trauma, epididymitis, or orchitis.

Sperm granuloma appears as a solitary yellow nodule or multiple small indurated nodules measuring up to 4 cm in diameter. Foreign body-type granulomas are present, with necrosis in the early stages and progressive fibrosis in late stages (Fig. 5–8). Extravasated sperm are often present in large numbers but are engulfed by macrophages (referred to as spermiophages) and eventually disappear. Yellow-brown ceroid pigment, a lipid degradation product of sperm, may persist. Vasitis nodosa (see next) occurs in about one third of cases of sperm granuloma.

Vasitis and Vasitis Nodosa

Inflammation of the vas deferens (vasitis or deferentitis) usually occurs in association with epididymitis or posterior urethritis. Vasitis nodosa is a benign ductular proliferation that produces nodular and fusiform enlargement of the vas deferens, often after vasectomy.

In vasitis nodosa, the vas deferens may be more than 1 cm in diameter, with diffuse enlargement or rounded indurated masses punctuated by small lumens. The ductular proliferation is prominent and may be mistaken histologically for metastatic prostatic adenocarcinoma (Fig. 5–9). Chronic inflammation and fibrosis are always observed, although in variable amounts, and are sometimes accompanied by muscular hyperplasia of the wall. The ductules vary from discrete round acinar structures to plexiform masses of irregular

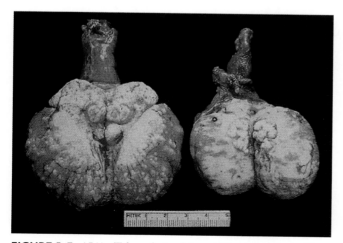

FIGURE 5–7 | ▌| | Tuberculosis of the epididymis and testis. (From Bostwick DG: Spermatic cord and testicular adnexae. In Bostwick DG, Eble JN [eds]: Urologic Surgical Pathology. St. Louis, Mosby, 1997, p. 654.)

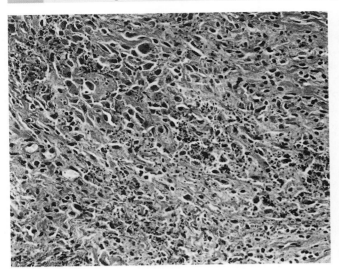

FIGURE 5–8 | ▮ | | Sperm granuloma. (From Bostwick DG: Spermatic cord and testicular adnexae. In Bostwick DG, Eble JN [eds]: Urologic Surgical Pathology. St. Louis, Mosby, 1997, p. 655.)

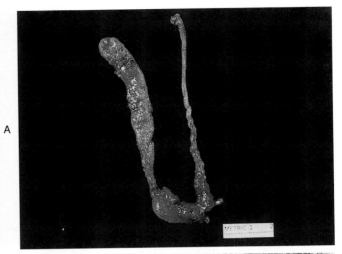

A

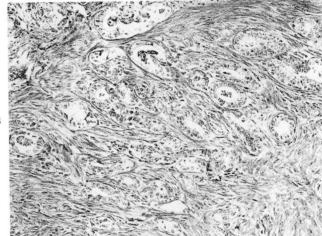

B

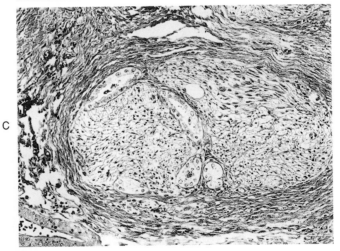

C

FIGURE 5–9 | ▮ | | Vasitis nodosa. *A,* Grossly apparent nodularity in the midportion *(bottom)* of the vas deferens. *B,* Proliferation of small tubules mimicking prostatic adenocarcinoma. *C,* Perineural invasion by vasitis nodosa. (From Bostwick DG: Spermatic cord and testicular adnexae. In Bostwick DG, Eble JN [eds]: Urologic Surgical Pathology. St. Louis, Mosby, 1997, p. 656.)

acini. The cells are cuboidal or low columnar, with a moderate amount of pale granular cytoplasm, central large nuclei with uniform chromatin, and single enlarged nucleoli. Cilia may be present. Perineural invasion is common and often extensive and may be mistaken for malignancy; benign vascular invasion may also occur. Sperm granulomas are present in about 50% of cases, and sperm are often present in the acinar lumens of vasitis nodosa. A histologically similar process may occur in the epididymis (epididymitis nodosa).

Vasitis nodosa is a benign reactive process. Trauma or surgery results in epithelial rupture with release of sperm into the soft tissues of the vas deferens, invoking a prominent fibroinflammatory response. However, some cases have no history of trauma and are idiopathic.

Funiculitis (Inflammation of the Spermatic Cord)

Inflammation of the spermatic cord, or funiculitis, often accompanies vasitis, usually as the result of direct extension from the vas deferens, but isolated involvement may occur by hematogenous spread from other sites of inflammation. Funiculitis appears as enlargement of the spermatic cord. Tuberculous funiculitis is rare, presenting as multiple large discrete masses or diffuse thickening with typical necrotizing granulomatous inflammation. Perforation of an incarcerated hernia may cause extravasation of fecal contents and vegetable fibers, resulting in an exuberant foreign-body giant cell reaction in the cord. Sclerosing endophlebitis and thrombosis of the pampiniform plexus may accompany funiculitis, resulting in necrosis and gangrene.

Meconium-Induced Inflammation

Prenatal or antenatal perforation of the colon may cause meconium leakage through the patent processus vaginalis into the scrotum, resulting in foreign body giant cell reaction, chronic inflammation, and scarring; this is referred to as meconium periorchitis, meconium granuloma, or meconium vaginalisitis. Fewer than 30 cases are reported, rarely in association with cystic fibrosis. Grossly, the tunica vaginalis contains a single mass or is studded with numerous orange or green nodules composed of chronically inflamed myxoid stroma, sometimes containing bile, cholesterol, or lanugo hairs within histiocytes. Hydrocele is often present.

OTHER NON-NEOPLASTIC DISEASES

Torsion of the Spermatic Cord and Embryonic Remnants

Torsion of the spermatic cord results in hemorrhagic infarction of the testis, described in Chapter 4. The following describes torsion of embryonic remnants, which may clinically mimic torsion of the cord.

Torsion is a common abnormality of the appendix testis. Patients complain of acute scrotal pain, often following vigorous exercise. About 90% of patients are boys between 10 and 12 years of age, but males of all ages are affected. Typical histologic features of torsion are present, including severe congestion, edema, and hemorrhagic infarction.

Torsion of the appendix epididymis is much less common than torsion of the appendix testis, and the histologic findings are similar. Torsion of the vasa aberrantia is extremely rare, with fewer than 10 reported cases.

Calculi and Calcification

Acute and chronic epididymitis and vasitis predispose to calculus formation, usually in the epididymis, vas deferens, and scrotum (Fig. 5–10). The calculi are composed of phosphates and carbonates and are brown stones up to 1 cm in diameter.

Idiopathic mural calcification of the vas deferens occurs in up to 15% of diabetics. These deposits in the smooth muscle are focal and variable in appearance, rarely with osseous metaplasia. Inflammation-induced calcifications are scattered throughout the smooth muscle, usually associated with chronic inflammation and fibrosis.

NEOPLASMS

BENIGN NEOPLASMS AND PSEUDOTUMORS

A variety of unusual tumors and tumor-like proliferations arise in the paratesticular region, often of uncertain histogenesis. Because of the rarity of many of these benign tumors, they may be erroneously considered malignant.

Lipoma

Lipoma is the most common paratesticular tumor, accounting for up to 90% of spermatic cord tumors (Fig. 5–11). Lipoma usually occurs in adults, but it may be seen at all ages. Grossly, it is a circumscribed unencapsulated mass of lobulated yellow adipose tissue up to 30 cm in diameter and weighing as much as 3.2 kg. The microscopic appearance is similar to that of lipoma at other sites, consisting of mature adipose tissue.

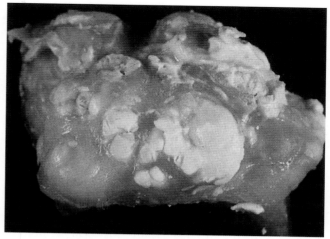

FIGURE 5–10 |▮|| Idiopathic scrotal and epididymal calcinosis in an otherwise healthy 37-year-old-man forming a multinodular mass measuring 3 cm in greatest dimension. (From Bostwick DG: Spermatic cord and testicular adnexae. In Bostwick DG, Eble JN [eds]: Urologic Surgical Pathology. St. Louis, Mosby, 1997, p. 657.)

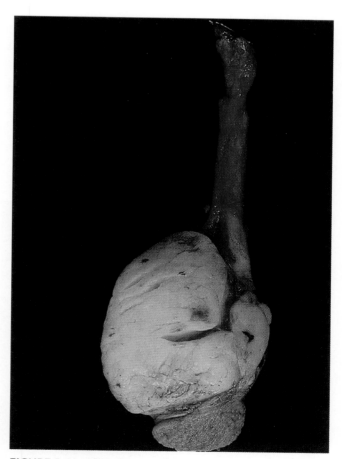

FIGURE 5–11 |▮|| Lipoma of the cord dwarfing the testis. (From Bostwick DG: Spermatic cord and testicular adnexae. In Bostwick DG, Eble JN [eds]: Urologic Surgical Pathology. St. Louis, Mosby, 1997, p. 658.)

Adenomatoid Tumor

Adenomatoid tumor is the most common tumor of the epididymis and cord and second in frequency only to lipoma in the paratesticular area; it accounts for about one third of paratesticular tumors. It also arises in the tunica sac distant from the epididymis and may be present in association with hydrocele. It is a benign neoplasm of mesothelial origin.

Adenomatoid tumor is usually seen in men between 20 and 50 years of age, but it has been reported in men as old as age 79 years. Most are painless and are discovered during routine physical examinations, but some lesions are found incidentally at epididymo-orchiectomy or autopsy. Adenomatoid tumor consists of a firm circumscribed solid mass, up to 5 cm in greatest dimension, but usually less than 2 cm. It is usually located in the head of the epididymis but rarely arises in the lower pole of the epididymis, testicular tunics, or spermatic cord. The cut surface is homogeneous and white-gray (Fig. 5–12*A*). The characteristic microscopic finding is irregular tubules, cell nests, and solid trabeculae of cuboidal to flattened epithelioid or endothelioid cells (see Fig. 5–12*B*). The tumor cells are eosinophilic, with variably sized cytoplasmic vacuoles. Nuclei are small and vesicular with inconspicuous nucleoli. The stroma contains fibroblasts, blood vessels, and smooth muscle. Focal stromal hyalinization may be present, and the tumor may infiltrate the testis.

Although it is rarely locally invasive, adenomatoid tumor does not metastasize. This tumor may recur if incompletely excised, but it does not recur after complete excision.

Well-Differentiated Papillary Mesothelioma

This tumor of the tunica vaginalis is found rarely in young men with hydroceles. Grossly, it consists of a hydrocele sac with papillary excrescences and cystic or

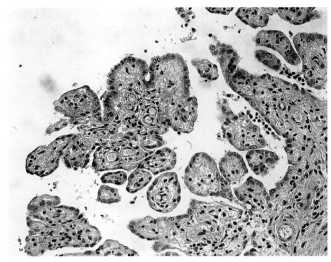

FIGURE 5–13　▌▌▌▌　Benign papillary mesothelioma of the tunica vaginalis. (From Bostwick DG: Spermatic cord and testicular adnexae. In Bostwick DG, Eble JN [eds]: Urologic Surgical Pathology. St. Louis, Mosby, 1997, p. 660.)

solid areas. Microscopically, there are complex papillae covered by cuboidal, columnar, or flattened mesothelial cells with large vesicular nuclei and glassy eosinophilic cytoplasm (Fig. 5–13). There is no significant nuclear atypia. Psammoma bodies are often present.

Well-differentiated papillary mesothelioma is considered a benign neoplasm best treated by complete excision. No recurrences have been reported.

Papillary Cystadenoma of the Epididymis

Papillary cystadenoma of the epididymis is a benign tumor that accounts for about one third of all primary epididymal tumors. It occurs in men between 16 and

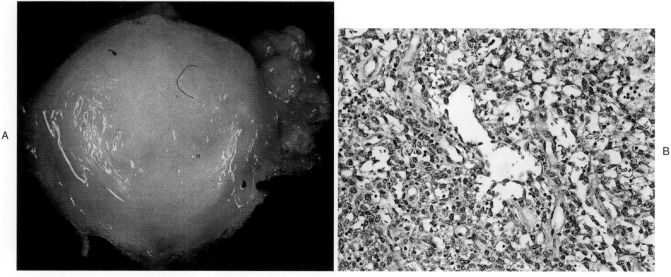

FIGURE 5–12　▌▌▌▌　Adenomatoid tumor of the epididymis. *A,* Grossly, the tumor was a firm white-gray mass. *B,* Anastomosing tubules lined by cells with small nuclei and punctuated by thin-walled vessels. (From Bostwick DG: Spermatic cord and testicular adnexae. In Bostwick DG, Eble JN [eds]: Urologic Surgical Pathology. St. Louis, Mosby, 1997, p. 659.)

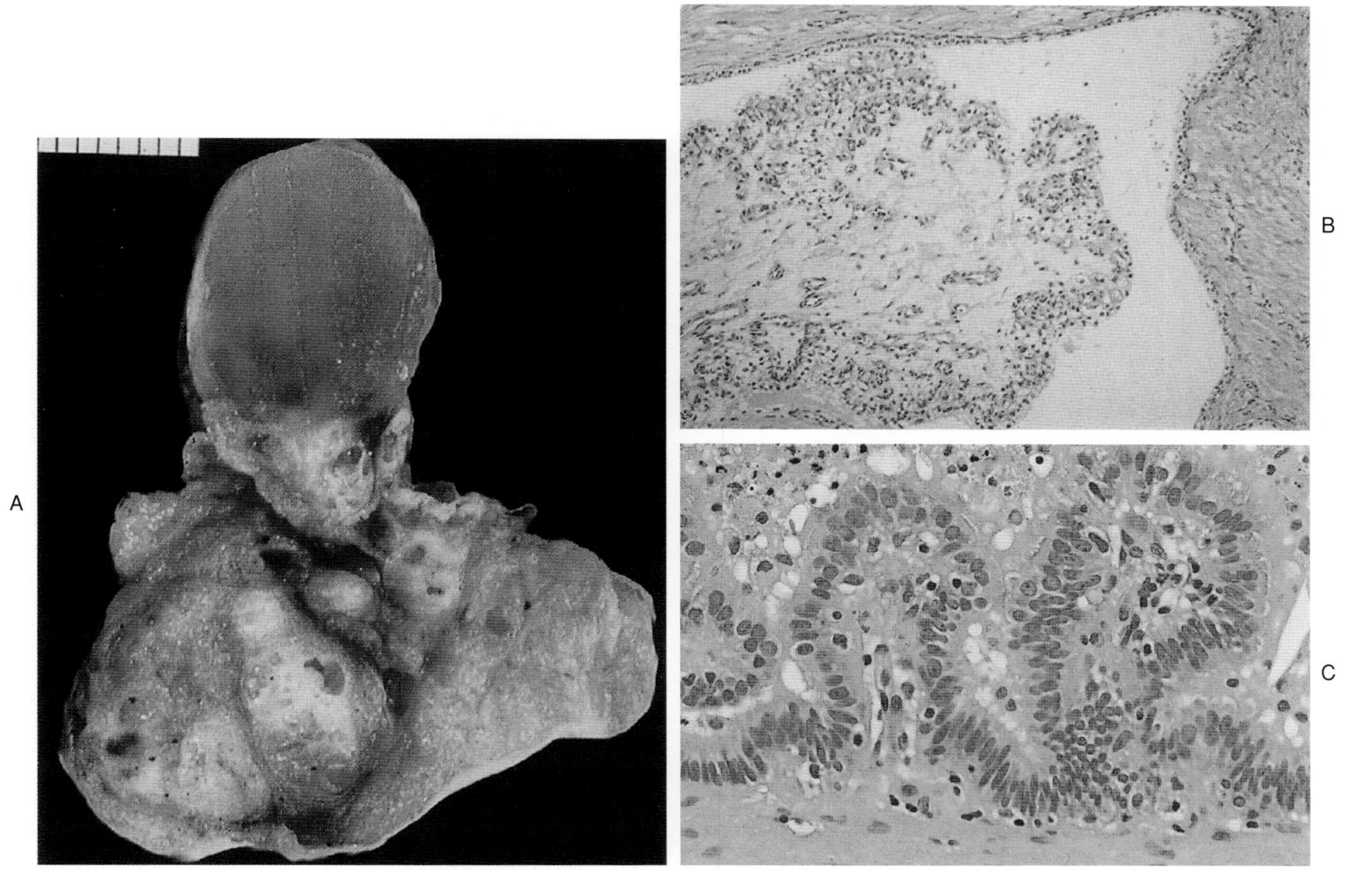

FIGURE 5–14 I▌II Papillary cystadenoma of the epididymis. *A*, Grossly, the tumor consisted of a papillary mass. *B*, Cystic space containing well-formed papillae. This 35-year-old man had a history of von Hippel–Lindau syndrome, including bilateral renal cell carcinoma and cerebellar and retinal hemangioblastomas. *C*, Another case of papillary cystadenoma from a patient without a history of von Hippel–Lindau syndrome. (Cases in *A* and *B* courtesy of Dr. Bernd Scheithauer, Rochester, MN; from Bostwick DG: Spermatic cord and testicular adnexae. In Bostwick DG, Eble JN [eds]: Urologic Surgical Pathology. St. Louis, Mosby, 1997, p. 660.)

81 years of age, with a mean of 36 years. More than 50 cases have been reported. About 40% of cases of papillary cystadenoma of the epididymis are bilateral, and these appear as cystic masses in the head of the epididymis that measure up to 6 cm in diameter. The cut surface is gray-brown with yellow foci and often contains cyst fluid that varies from clear and colorless to yellow, green, or blood-tinged (Fig. 5–14*A*). Microscopically, papillary cystadenoma consists of dilated ducts lined by papillae with a single or double layer of cuboidal to low columnar epithelium (see Fig. 5–14*B*). The cells have characteristic clear glycogen-filled cytoplasm with secretory droplets and cilia at the surface. The papillary cores and cyst walls consist of fibrous connective tissue that may be hyalinized or inflamed. About two thirds of cases of papillary cystadenoma of the epididymis occur in patients with von Hippel-Lindau syndrome (see Fig. 5–14*C*) and are more frequently bilateral in this syndrome.

Inflammatory Pseudotumor and Fibrous Pseudotumor

These terms encompass a wide variety of non-neoplastic fibroinflammatory lesions of the testicular tunics, epididymis, and spermatic cord, lesions variously designated

chronic periorchitis, fibrous proliferation of the tunics, fibroma, nonspecific paratesticular fibrosis, nodular fibrous periorchitis, nodular fibropseudotumor, reactive periorchitis, and pseudofibromatous periorchitis. It is probable that all such lesions are part of a spectrum of inflammation and repair, and the findings in an individual case represent the stage of evolution of the inflammatory, vascular, myofibroblastic, and fibroblastic reparative responses to injury. Lesions diagnosed as fibrous pseudotumor are second only to adenomatoid tumor as causes of testicular adnexal masses.

These lesions clinically mimic testicular and paratesticular neoplasms. Patients are usually in the third decade of life, but age ranges from 7 to 95 years. Most lesions involve the tunics and may be associated with hydrocele, hematocele, or both. Less commonly, the epididymis or spermatic cord is involved. A history of infection, surgery, trauma, or inflamed hydrocele is often elicited, but in many cases no such history is forthcoming.

Tumors may be single, multiple, or plaquelike and may be up to 8 cm in greatest dimension (Fig. 5–15). They are usually white, gray, or yellow and sometimes are focally calcified. Consistency ranges from gelatinous to stony hard.

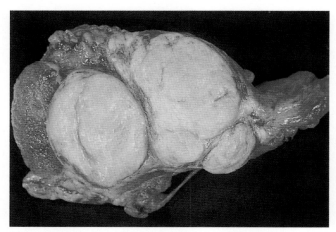

FIGURE 5–15 ▌▐ ▏▏ Fibrous pseudotumor of the testicular tunics. (From Bostwick DG: Spermatic cord and testicular adnexae. In Bostwick DG, Eble JN [eds]: Urologic Surgical Pathology. St. Louis, Mosby, 1997, p. 661.)

Histologic findings are diverse. Inflammatory pseudotumor consists of a cellular irregular proliferation of spindle, stellate, and oval cells in a loose collagenous and often focally myxoid background, usually with prominent vascularity. Fibrous pseudotumor consists of paucicellular hyalinized fibrous connective tissue with varying degrees of chronic inflammation, and rarely calcification and ossification. In all such lesions, features of malignancy, such as brisk mitotic activity, necrosis, and high-grade cytologic atypia, are absent.

Leiomyoma

Men with genital leiomyoma range in age from 25 to 81 years, with a mean of 48 years. Hydrocele or hernia sac is identified in up to 21% of cases, and up to 39% are bilateral. Leiomyoma appears as a round, firm, gray-white mass measuring up to 8 cm in diameter; the cut surface is homogeneous and whorled and bulges from the adjacent soft tissues (Fig. 5–16). It has typical micro-

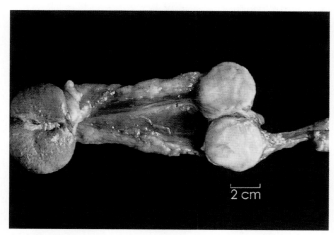

2 cm

FIGURE 5–16 ▌▐ ▏▏ Leiomyoma of the vas deferens. (From Bostwick DG: Spermatic cord and testicular adnexae. In Bostwick DG, Eble JN [eds]: Urologic Surgical Pathology. St. Louis, Mosby, 1997, p. 662.)

scopic features of leiomyoma, including interlacing fascicles of spindled smooth muscle cells with few or no mitotic figures. Surgical excision of epididymal leiomyoma is curative. Leiomyoma is less common in the spermatic cord than the epididymis, with fewer than 20 reported cases.

Gonadal Stromal Tumor

Gonadal stromal tumor accounts for up to 3% of testicular tumors, and rare extratesticular examples have been reported. Embryogenesis of the testis can account for extratesticular nests of germ cells and stromal cells. Microscopic foci of gonadal interstitial cells are occasionally observed in extratesticular sites such as the spermatic cord and epididymis in orchiectomy specimens removed for other reasons, and these may account for gonadal stromal tumor at such sites.

Other Benign Paratesticular Soft Tissue Neoplasms

Other rare benign paratesticular tumors include mucinous adenoid tumor, schwannoma, neurofibroma, and hemangioma of the testicular tunics. Lymphangiectasia, lymphangioma, hemangioma, and neurofibroma may arise in the spermatic cord or epididymis. There have been rare case reports of aggressive angiomyxoma, angiomyofibroblastoma, granular cell tumor, cutaneous myxoma, carcinoid, paraganglioma, solitary fibrous tumor, and rhabdomyoma of the spermatic cord.

MALIGNANT NEOPLASMS

Liposarcoma

The most common sarcoma of the paratesticular region in adults is spermatic cord liposarcoma. The mean patient age is 56 years, with a range from 16 to 90 years. Grossly, liposarcoma is a lobulated mass of yellow tissue that often resembles lipoma (Fig. 5–17A). Microscopically, the most common pattern is well-differentiated liposarcoma (lipoma-like liposarcoma), often with prominent sclerosis. Myxoid liposarcoma and pleomorphic liposarcoma have also been described at this site.

Rhabdomyosarcoma

Paratesticular rhabdomyosarcoma may arise in the testicular tunics, epididymis, or spermatic cord; the paratesticular region is the single most common site of occurrence of this cancer. When the tumor is large or locally invasive, the exact site of origin cannot be determined. Rhabdomyosarcoma is the most common sarcoma of the paratesticular area in children, with a peak incidence at about 9 years, although it occurs at any age.

Grossly, rhabdomyosarcoma is an encapsulated white-gray mass with focal hemorrhage and cystic degeneration that measures up to 20 cm in diameter. Most are embryonal rhabdomyosarcoma, consisting of small round cells with dark nuclei, scant cytoplasm, and variable numbers of cells showing myoblastic differentiation—short spindled cells and large malignant rhabdomyoblasts with copious eosinophilic cytoplasm. The connective tissue stroma may be myxoid. The spindle cell variant of embryonal rhabdomyosarcoma is commonly found in this

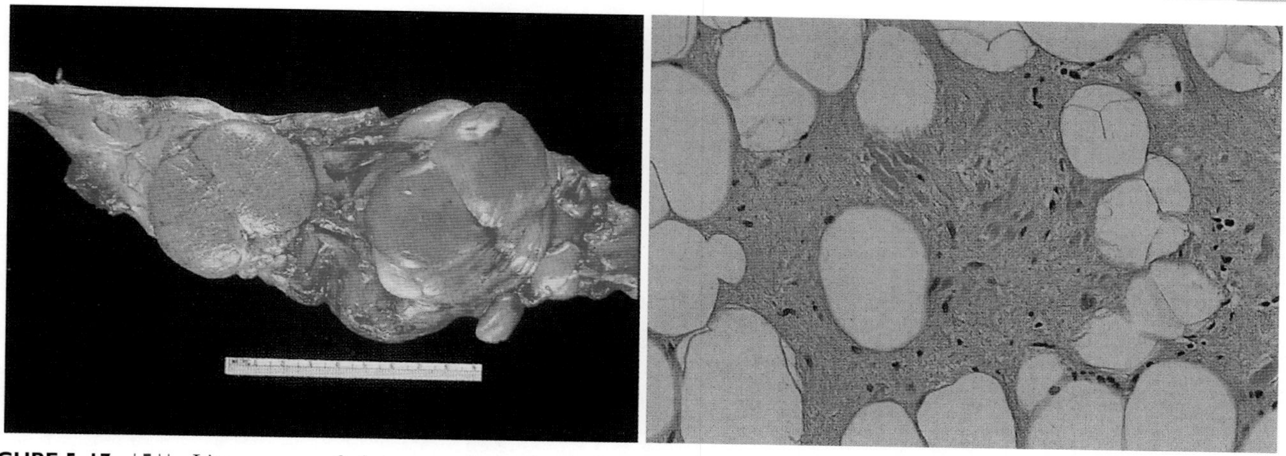

FIGURE 5–17 |▮|| Liposarcoma of the spermatic cord. *A*, Grossly, the tumor consisted of a multinodular mass of firm tan tissue. *B*, Delicate fibrosis and increased cellularity were observed within adipose tissue. (From Bostwick DG: Spermatic cord and testicular adnexae. In Bostwick DG, Eble JN [eds]: Urologic Surgical Pathology. St. Louis, Mosby, 1997, p. 662.)

region. It is composed of intersecting fascicles of spindle cells, some of which show cross striations; it may resemble leiomyosarcoma or fibrosarcoma. It is significant in that it has a much better prognosis than other forms of embryonal rhabdomyosarcoma. Rhabdomyosarcomas of the alveolar and pleomorphic types are highly aggressive tumors; fortunately, they are rare in this site.

Leiomyosarcoma

Leiomyosarcoma is more common in the spermatic cord than in the epididymis, with more than 100 reported cases. It arises in patients of all ages, with a peak in the sixth and seventh decades; more than 80% of patients are older than 40 years of age.

Grossly, leiomyosarcoma is a solid gray-tan mass involving the intrascrotal portion of the spermatic cord or epididymis. Typical cases consist of spindle cell proliferations with features of leiomyosarcoma found at other sites. Some cases show bizarre morphologic features and are diagnosed as leiomyosarcoma chiefly on the basis of immunohistochemical evidence of smooth muscle differentiation. Distinction of a very well-differentiated leiomyosarcoma from leiomyoma may be difficult. However, any level of mitotic activity in a smooth muscle tumor in this area, particularly when nuclear atypia is present, should be considered indicative of malignancy.

Malignant Fibrous Histiocytoma

Fewer than 20 reported cases of malignant fibrous histiocytoma (MFH) involving the spermatic cord and paratesticular area have been reported. Mean patient age is 64 years. Grossly, the tumor is solid gray or yellow-white, has a whorled cut surface, and measures up to 10 cm in diameter. Histologic patterns include myxoid, inflammatory, and pleomorphic MFH. About one third of patients with MFH develop local recurrence or distant metastases.

Other Sarcomas

More than 60 cases of spermatic cord and epididymal fibrosarcoma have been described, but some of these probably represent other forms of sarcoma. Most occur in adults, but all ages may be affected.

The gross and microscopic appearance of fibrosarcoma of the paratesticular area are similar to that at other sites. More than half of patients die of locally recurrent or metastatic tumor.

Most types of sarcoma have been described in the paratesticular area, including neurofibrosarcoma, angiosarcoma, chondrosarcoma, and undifferentiated sarcoma. Primitive neuroectodermal tumor (extraskeletal Ewing's sarcoma) has also been reported.

Malignant Mesothelioma

Paratesticular malignant mesothelioma is rare, with fewer than 70 reported cases. Most occur in the tunica vaginalis, with very few in the spermatic cord and epididymis. Mean patient age is about 55 years and ranges from 12 to 84 years. Primary peritoneal malignant mesothelioma may present as a mass in an inguinal hernia. Malignant mesothelioma of the tunica vaginalis may appear in pipe fitters with asbestos exposure, raising the possibility of asbestos as a contributory factor, similar to pleural and peritoneal mesothelioma. Bilateral mesothelioma of the tunica vaginalis mesothelioma of the tunica vaginalis occurs rarely.

Grossly, malignant mesothelioma appears as multiple friable cystic and solid masses and small nodules studding the lining of a hydrocele, hernia sac, or the peritoneum (Fig. 5–18). Continuity between the tumor and adjacent mesothelium of the tunica vaginalis may be apparent, and there may be invasion of adjacent structures.

Histologically, paratesticular malignant mesothelioma is similar to mesothelioma at other sites and may be epithelial, spindle cell, or biphasic, with a wide morphologic spectrum (see Fig. 5–18). The epithelial pattern is most common, accounting for about 75% of cases, and may be mixed with papillary, tubular, and solid areas. Spindle cells predominate in the sarcomatous pattern and may merge perceptively with solid epithelioid nests. Tumor cells are

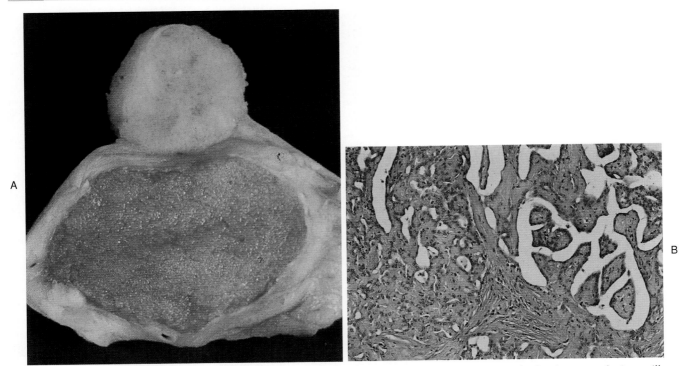

FIGURE 5–18 ❙▮❙❙ Malignant mesothelioma of the tunica vaginalis. *A*, Grossly, the tumor consisted of a large exophytic papillary mass. *B*, Micropapillations are lined by cells flattened to cuboidal tumor cells. (Case courtesy of Dr. Jan Kennedy, Atlanta, GA; from Bostwick DG: Spermatic cord and testicular adnexae. In Bostwick DG, Eble JN [eds]: Urologic Surgical Pathology. St. Louis, Mosby, 1997, p. 664.)

cuboidal or flattened, with variable amounts of eosinophilic cytoplasm and atypical vesicular nuclei, often with prominent nucleoli. Mitotic figures are usually present.

Malignant mesothelioma is aggressive, with a potential for late recurrence or metastasis. It recurs locally along the vas deferens or in the pelvis and usually spreads by lymphatic routes to pelvic, retroperitoneal, or distant lymph nodes. About half of patients remain free of tumor up to 18 years after treatment.

Adenocarcinoma of the Epididymis

Fewer than 30 reported cases of epididymal adenocarcinoma have been reported. The mean patient age is 44 years, with a range from 5 to 78 years. The tumors measure up to 9 cm in diameter and may be multicystic or solid. About half are associated with hydrocele.

Microscopically, there are typical features of adenocarcinoma, including papillary, glandular, mucinous, and solid undifferentiated patterns. Squamous cell carcinoma may also be admixed. Nearly half of reported patients develop metastases.

Germ Cell Tumor

A variety of germ cell tumors have been described in the paratesticular area, including seminoma, embryonal carcinoma, and teratoma. The epididymis is more commonly involved than the spermatic cord, but germ cell tumor at either site is rare. The demographic and pathologic features of paratesticular germ cell tumor are similar to those of the testis. These tumors probably arise from misplaced germinal elements.

Malignant Lymphoma and Hematopoietic Neoplasms

Malignant lymphoma is the most common tumor of the testis in men older than 50 years of age; yet paratesticular

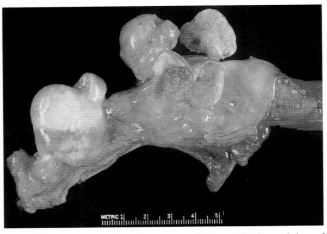

FIGURE 5–19 ❙▮❙❙ Hernia sac containing multiple nodules of metastatic colonic adenocarcinoma. (From Bostwick DG: Spermatic cord and testicular adnexae. In Bostwick DG, Eble JN [eds]: Urologic Surgical Pathology. St. Louis, Mosby, 1997, p. 666.)

lymphoma is uncommon. Rare cases of primary epididymal or spermatic cord lymphoma have appeared. Secondary lymphoma has been described in all sites of the paratesticular area, invariably in association with testicular involvement. Plasmacytoma of the spermatic cord has also been reported.

Metastases

Metastases to the paratesticular area are rare and usually arise from the prostate, kidney, and stomach. Rare cases have originated from colonic adenocarcinoma (Fig. 5–19), pancreatic adenocarcinoma, urothelial carcinoma, ileal carcinoid, and malignant melanoma. Patients with paratesticular metastases usually have a poor outcome.

PENIS AND SCROTUM

with Roy King, MD

Lesions discussed in this chapter are those that are often sampled or excised for diagnostic or therapeutic reasons. Many are lesions that are clinically suggestive of neoplasia. Lesions that are exceptionally rare and that are appropriately diagnosed without requiring histopathologic evaluation are not discussed here.

PENIS

HISTOLOGY

The glans penis consists of squamous epithelium overlying lamina propria and corpus spongiosum (Fig. 6–1). Lamina propria consists of loose fibroconnective tissue 1 to 3 mm thick, lacking skin adnexal structures. The corpora cavernosa terminate in or near the glans. The erectile tissues of the corpus spongiosum and the corpora cavernosa are separated by tunica albuginea, 1 to 2 mm thick.

The foreskin consists of an outer layer of squamous epithelium overlying dermis (containing cutaneous adnexal structures); beneath these layers are dartos muscle, a layer of lamina propria, and, innermost,

mucosal epithelium, which lacks adnexal structures. Mucosal epithelium and underlying lamina propria and dartos muscle line the coronal sulcus, the junction between glans and foreskin.

The body (shaft) of the penis is covered by skin, closely apposed to underlying dartos muscle. Beneath dartos muscle is a thin layer of fibroadipose tissue overlying Buck's fascia, a fibroelastic membrane containing abundant nerves and blood vessels (Fig. 6–2). In cross section, Buck's fascia encircles the corpora cavernosa, the corpus spongiosum, and the urethra. Buck's fascia terminates at the coronal sulcus. The corporal structures are enclosed by tunica albuginea (Fig. 6–3).

Penile melanosis is characterized by macular hyperpigmentation of the penile shaft and/or glans. Lesions may be up to 2 cm in diameter. The main differential diagnosis is with malignant melanoma. A biopsy of the affected site demonstrates hyperpigmentation of the basal layer that is accentuated at the tips of the rete ridges. There is mild acanthosis; however, melanocytes are normal in number. Melanophages may be present in the papillary dermis (Fig. 6–4). There appears to be no relation to mucocutaneous melanoma.

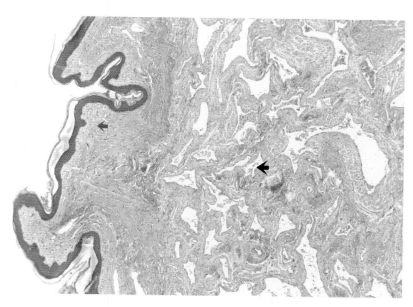

FIGURE 6–1 ▮▮▯▯ Glans penis, normal histology. Squamous epithelium overlying lamina propria *(blue and yellow arrows)* and corpus spongiosum *(black arrow)*.

Several images in this chapter are courtesy of Mayo Clinic Foundation, Rochester, MN.

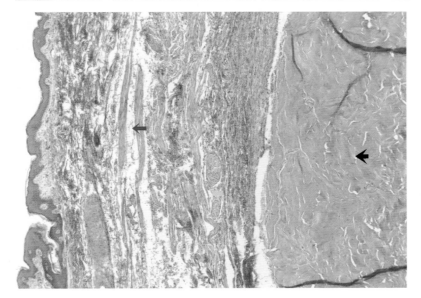

FIGURE 6–2 ▮▮▮ Penis, body, normal histology. Dartos muscle *(blue arrow)*, Buck's fascia *(yellow arrow)*, and tunica albuginea *(black arrow)*.

INFLAMMATORY PENILE DISORDERS

Zoon's Balanitis (Plasma Cell Balanitis)

This lesion is most commonly observed in elderly un-circumcised men. Its etiology is unknown. It appears as a bright red patch on the glans or inner foreskin, clinically mimicking squamous cell carcinoma in situ and prompting biopsy. Microscopically, the upper dermis is infiltrated by a variable number of plasma cells, often arranged in a band. Numerous dilated capillaries are evident in the dermis, and the overlying squamous epithelium is usually thin and sometimes absent (Fig. 6–5).

Balanitis Xerotica Obliterans

Men and women sometimes develop an atrophic disorder of the genital or perianal skin known as lichen sclerosus et atrophicus. This lesion, when it involves the glans

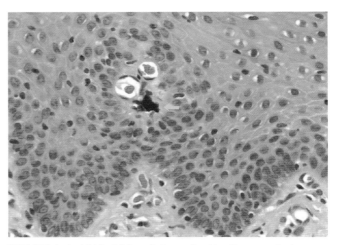

FIGURE 6–4 ▮▮▮ Melanosis in penile skin. Brown melanin granules are present in the basal layer of cells, and a large aggregate of melanin granules is seen in a melanophage *(arrow)*.

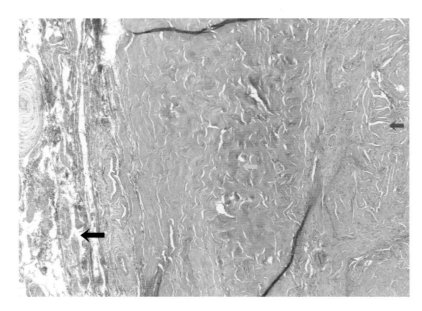

FIGURE 6–3 ▮▮▮ Penis, body, normal histology. Buck's fascia *(black arrow)*, tunica albuginea *(yellow arrow)*, and corpus cavernosum *(blue arrow)*.

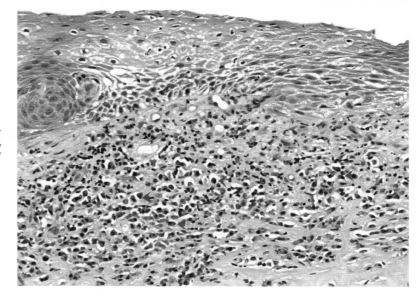

FIGURE 6–5 | ▮ | | Zoon's balanitis. There is a band-like infiltrate of chronic inflammatory cells in the dermis, predominantly plasma cells *(blue arrows)*, with a few lymphocytes.

penis or foreskin, is called balanitis xerotica obliterans (BXO). Its cause is unknown. Occasional cases are associated with squamous cell carcinoma.

BXO results in a circumscribed firm gray-white patch on the foreskin or glans, commonly abutting or even surrounding the urethral meatus. Depending on its location and extent, it can produce symptoms related to phimosis or urethral meatal stenosis.

Microscopically, the epidermis is thin, with overlying hyperkeratosis. The rete pegs become progressively shortened, and the basal layer of the epidermis becomes inconspicuous. The upper dermis is at first edematous, with a prominent bandlike lymphocytic infiltrate. Over time, the dermal edema changes to dermal collagenization and the extent of lymphocytic infiltration diminishes (Fig. 6–6).

Peyronie's Disease

This condition affects men with an average age of 53 years and is uncommon in men younger than 40. When erect, the penis is bent or constricted, and the majority of patients note pain with erection. Plaques are commonly palpable on the dorsum of the penis, sometimes causing concern for malignancy. Although there are numerous theories to explain its occurrence, the cause of Peyronie's disease remains unknown.

The plaques are composed of fibrous tissue localized in the tunica albuginea, sometimes with associated calcification or bone formation (Fig. 6–7). Plaque formation probably begins with fibrin deposition in small blood vessels of the tunica albuginea, followed by

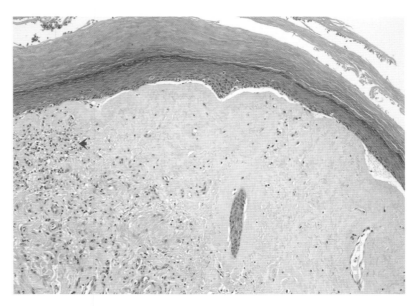

FIGURE 6–6 | ▮ | | Balanitis xerotica obliterans. Epidermis is thin, and rete pegs are short or absent. Hyperkeratosis is evident. At left, there is a scant residual lymphocytic infiltrate *(arrow);* at right, the dermis has become collagenized.

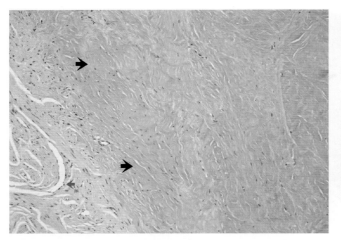

FIGURE 6–7 ▏▌▏▏ Peyronie's disease. Normal corpus cavernosal tissue is at lower left *(blue arrow)*. The plaque *(black arrows)* consists of densely collagenized fibrous tissue, with scattered spindly fibroblasts.

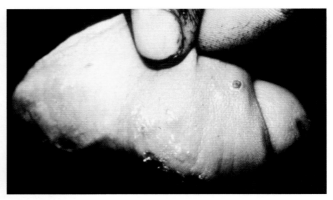

FIGURE 6–9 ▏▌▏▏ Herpes simplex. Vesicles and ulcers in varying phases of healing. (Courtesy of Hernan Valdez, MD, Cleveland, OH.)

perivascular inflammation, fibroblast proliferation, and deposition of collagen. The microscopic findings in mature plaques resemble fibromatosis in other sites, such as Dupuytren's contracture.

Lipogranuloma

This condition results from injection of foreign materials (wax, silicone, or paraffin) into the penis. In some cases, the scrotum is also an injection site. Nodules develop where the foreign material is situated, sometimes causing penile deformity. In the absence of a helpful history, malignancy may be suspected.

Microscopically, excised tissue consists of fibrotic stroma with areas of marked sclerosis, infiltrated by chronic inflammatory cells and foreign body giant cells. Numerous cystic spaces of variable size are present, unlined by epithelial cells or endothelial cells (Fig. 6–8).

INFECTION-RELATED PENILE ULCERATION

The differential diagnosis of infection-related non-neoplastic penile ulceration includes herpes simplex, syphilis, granuloma inguinale, lymphogranuloma venereum, and chancroid.

Herpes Infection

Genital herpes is a sexually transmitted viral infection caused by herpes simplex virus (HSV). HSV type 2 is the major etiologic agent. However, in the United States, 30% of new cases of genital herpes are caused by HSV type 1. In most cases of genital herpes, transmission occurs during times of asymptomatic HSV shedding. Primary genital herpes may occur on the glans, prepuce, shaft, sulcus, and scrotum. The classic presentation is grouped vesicles that evolve to pustules and subsequently become ulcerated (Fig. 6–9). These small ulcerations heal in 2 to 4 weeks. Tender inguinal lymphadenopathy

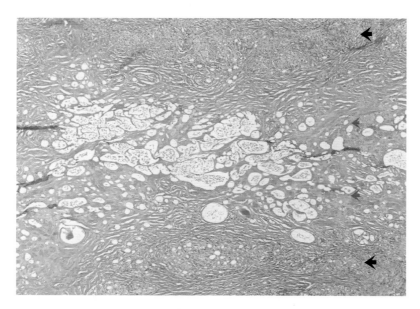

FIGURE 6–8 ▏▌▏▏ Sclerosing lipogranuloma. The central part of the image is sclerotic fibroconnective tissue with numerous unlined cystic spaces of variable size *(blue arrows)*. At top and bottom are aggregates of chronic inflammatory cells, mainly macrophages and multinucleated giant cells *(black arrows)*.

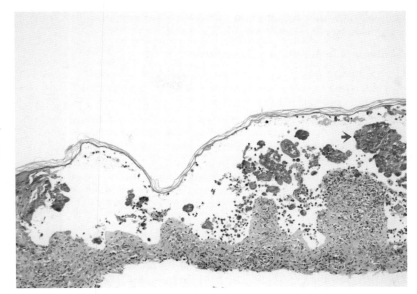

FIGURE 6–10 |▮|| Herpes simplex. A remnant of intact squamous epithelium is seen at far left. A cystic bleb has formed, populated by infected multinucleated squamous cells with viral nuclear inclusions *(arrow)*.

occurs during the second and third weeks of the primary infection. Recurrent genital herpes usually occurs on the penile shaft and glans, and the lesions are similar to those seen in the primary infection, however possibly on a reduced scale.

Diagnosis may be made with a Tzanck smear. Fluid from an intact vesicle is smeared on a slide, dried, and stained with Wright's or Giemsa's stain. Giant keratinocytes and multinucleated giant keratinocytes may be seen. Fluid for direct fluorescent antibody testing will also identify HSV type 1 and HSV type 2. A biopsy will demonstrate ballooning and reticular epidermal degeneration with multinucleated giant keratinocytes with intranuclear inclusions (Fig. 6–10).

Syphilis

Syphilis is a sexually transmitted infection caused by the spirochete *Treponema pallidum* and is characterized by a painless ulcer or chancre at the site of inoculation. The chancre may range from a few millimeters to 2 cm in diameter, with raised borders and a red, meaty color (Fig. 6–11). The chancre is commonly firm with indurated borders and is painless. The chancre is usually located in the prepuce, in the coronal sulcus of the glans, or on the shaft. Regional lymphadenopathy appears within 1 week.

A biopsy of the ulcer will demonstrate a dense plasma cell–rich inflammatory infiltrate and a proliferation of small blood vessels with prominent endothelial cell nuclei (Fig. 6–12). A Warthin-Starry stain may

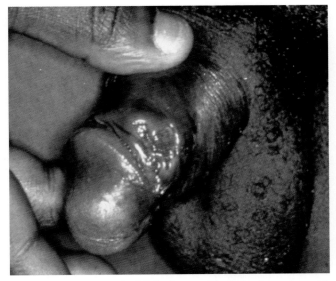

FIGURE 6–11 |▮|| Syphilitic chancre. The lesion is an ulcer with raised, rolled edges. (Courtesy of Hernan Valdez, MD, Cleveland, OH.)

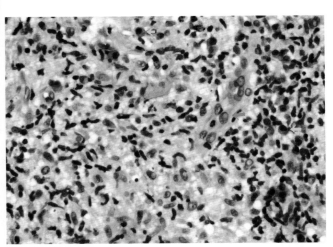

FIGURE 6–12 |▮|| Syphilitic chancre. There is a dense infiltrate of inflammatory cells, including plasma cells *(yellow arrows)*. A capillary with marked endothelial hyperplasia is present *(green arrow)*.

demonstrate the treponemes. Dark-field examination and serology confirm these findings.

Granuloma Inguinale (Donovanosis)

Granuloma inguinale is a destructive bacterial infection characterized by ulceration and caused by *Calymmato-bacterium granulomatis*, an encapsulated gram-negative rod. The disease is rare in the United States. There is usually a history of sexual exposure in endemic areas of tropical countries. The lesions are distributed mainly on the prepuce or glans and the penile shaft. The primary ulcer is characterized by a painless, broad, superficial ulcer with a beefy-red texture and sharply defined edges. There is usually no accompanying inguinal lymphadenopathy.

The diagnosis may be obtained by a crush preparation of a punch biopsy stained with Wright's or Giemsa's stain. Alternatively, histologic examination of a biopsy will demonstrate a dense dermal infiltrate of plasma cells and histiocytes. Identification of large mononuclear cells containing cytoplasmic inclusions (Donovan bodies) is pathognomonic.

Lymphogranuloma Venereum

Lymphogranuloma venereum (LGV) is a sexually transmitted disease caused by *Chlamydia trachomatis*. LGV occurs sporadically in North America and is endemic in certain parts of Africa and Southeast Asia and South America. In the United States, most cases occur in patients who have traveled to endemic areas. The primary lesion presents as a small papule or vesicle that evolves rapidly to painless erosion that heals without scarring. The primary lesion is innocuous, and many patients do not have recollection of the primary lesion. Striking lymphadenopathy, usually unilateral, appears 1 to 4 weeks after the primary lesion heals. The lymph nodes become tender and fluctuant (buboes) and ulcerate, releasing purulent material. In about 20% of patients, there is enlargement of lymph nodes above and below Poupart's ligament, creating the so-called groove sign and considered pathognomonic for LGV.

The most accurate diagnostic serologic assay is the microimmunofluorescent technique. This is highly sensitive and specific for determining individual serotypes of *C. trachomatis*. The complement fixation test is also useful but is not as specific. Culture of *C. trachomatis* is available but is positive only in a third of cases.

Chancroid

Chancroid is a sexually transmitted disease caused by the gram-negative bacillus *Haemophilus ducreyi*. Chancroid occurs sporadically in the United States and is endemic in tropical and subtropical Third World countries. The primary lesion is characterized by a very painful ulcer with sharp, undermined borders; it is not indurated. The lesions can occur on the prepuce, frenulum, coronal sulcus, glans, and shaft. Painful inguinal lymphadenopathy occurs in about half of patients 1 to 2 weeks after the primary ulcer. The ulcers are highly infectious. The lymphadenopathy often results in breakdown with suppuration.

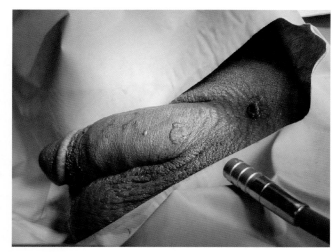

FIGURE 6–13 ▎▎▏▏ Flat condyloma acuminatum in an adult. (Courtesy of Allan Seftel, MD, Cleveland, OH.)

Accurate diagnosis of chancroid is dependent on culture of *H. ducreyi*. The bacteria require specialized growth media, and sensitivity is only 80% using this media. The most reliable results are obtained by inoculation of the exudate directly onto the culture plate.

INFECTION-RELATED PENILE NODULES AND WARTY LESIONS

Condyloma Acuminatum

Condyloma acuminatum is most common in young sexually active males. It may involve any part of the penis but most often appears on the glans and foreskin. It may also appear on the skin of the scrotum or perineum. Some condylomas are flat and inconspicuous, but most have a papillary or cauliflower-like appearance (Figs. 6–13 and 6–14). Most are caused by infection of squamous

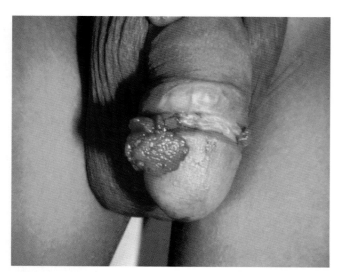

FIGURE 6–14 ▎▎▏▏ Condyloma acuminatum in a 7-year-old boy. There was clinical suspicion of child abuse. (Courtesy of Allan Decter, MD, Winnipeg, Manitoba.)

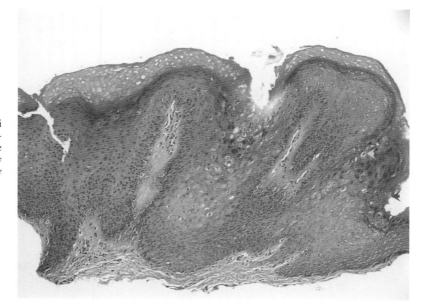

FIGURE 6–15 ▎█▎▎ Condyloma acuminatum. Nuclei remain large in cells near the surface. Nuclei have irregular contours, and cytoplasmic retraction away from the nuclei creates a halo effect—"koilocytic change" *(yellow arrow)*. Parakeratosis and hyperkeratosis are present *(blue arrow)*.

cells by human papillomavirus types 6 and 11; dysplastic lesions are caused by types 16, 18, 31, 33, and 35.

Microscopically, it is a proliferative papillomatous squamous lesion. The squamous epithelium is thickened but shows orderly maturation. Hyperkeratosis and parakeratosis are common. Many of the squamous cells show features collectively known as "koilocytosis": wrinkled, pleomorphic and hyperchromatic nuclei, cytoplasmic retraction away from the nucleus, and frequent binucleation (Fig. 6–15). Mitotic figures are confined to the basal layer. Moderate to severe dysplasia may occur rarely and is characterized by progressive loss of normal maturation toward the surface and by the presence of mitotic figures in the upper levels of the dysplastic epithelium.

Molluscum Contagiosum

Molluscum contagiosum is characterized by the presence of numerous dome-shaped papules, 3 to 6 mm in diameter, on the skin of the penile shaft (Fig. 6–16). The papules often have a central dimple. Lesions are caused by infection of squamous cells by a DNA poxvirus. Most patients are youthful or immunocompromised. Left untreated (except in immunocompromised patients), most lesions disappear spontaneously within 6 to 12 months.

Microscopically, the papule appears as a cup-shaped squamous proliferation that bulges downward into the dermis (Fig. 6–17). The basal cell layer is unremarkable. The cells of the stratum malpighii have cytoplasmic viral inclusions that become larger and change color from eosinophilic to basophilic as they reach the surface. The surface of the papule, where the contents are extruded, resembles a crater. The underlying dermis is unremarkable, unless the contents of the epidermal papule rupture into it.

PENILE CYSTS

Epidermoid Cyst

Epidermoid cyst begins as an epidermal inclusion. It commonly occurs in the skin of the penis and scrotum. It is lined by keratinizing squamous epithelium. The cyst enlarges as desquamated keratin accumulates within the cyst cavity. It rarely exceeds 1.0 cm in diameter. Some become infected or cause a local inflammatory reaction to extravasation of cyst contents into the surrounding soft tissues. Microscopically, the cyst wall (if identifiable) is lined by keratinizing squamous epithelium. Keratin debris is usually present (Fig. 6–18). In some cases, only a residual foreign-body giant cell reaction with evidence of acute and chronic inflammation is evident.

Mucous Cyst

Mucous cyst is seen most often in the glans or the foreskin. It is unilocular, is lined by stratified columnar epithelium with mucus cells, and contains mucinous material.

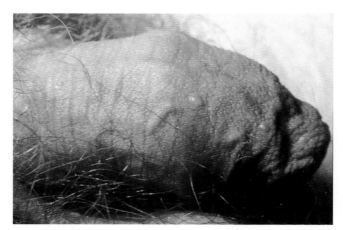

FIGURE 6–16 ▎█▎▎ Molluscum contagiosum. In some papules, a small central dimple may be evident. (Courtesy of Hernan Valdez, MD, Cleveland, OH.)

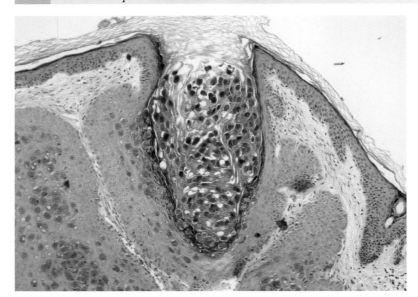

FIGURE 6–17 ▮▮▮▮ Molluscum contagiosum. Basal cells are normal. Malpighian cells acquire eosinophilic cytoplasmic inclusions; the inclusions become basophilic in the upper layers and in the cells extruded into the cup-shaped crater.

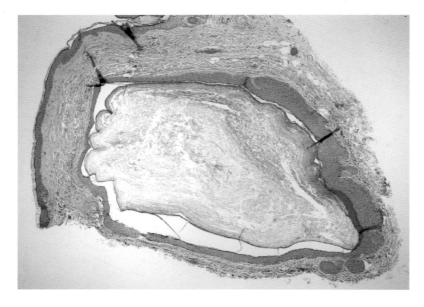

FIGURE 6–18 ▮▮▮▮ Epidermoid cyst. The cyst is lined by squamous epithelium and contains keratin debris.

Median Raphe Cyst

This cyst may be unilocular or multilocular. It is lined by pseudostratified columnar epithelium and contains mucinous material (Figs. 6–19 and 6–20).

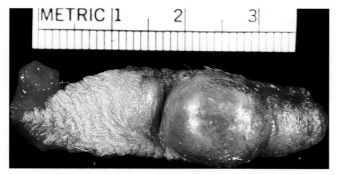

FIGURE 6–19 ▮▮▮▮ Median raphe cyst.

PENILE SQUAMOUS CELL CARCINOMA IN SITU

Squamous cell carcinoma in situ (CIS) involving the glans and foreskin traditionally was called *erythroplasia of Queyrat*, and the traditional name of squamous cell CIS involving the shaft of the penis was *Bowen's disease.* Other synonyms for this condition include *severe dysplasia* and *high-grade squamous intraepithelial lesion.*

Most men with penile CIS are between 40 and 60 years old. Lesions involving the glans or foreskin are usually erythematous, shiny, velvety, and slightly raised. Lesion size in the glans and foreskin varies; some are small and circumscribed, and others are extensive and poorly delineated. Lesions involving the shaft are usually circumscribed, scaly, and gray-white, but they may appear ulcerated (Fig. 6–21). Lesions such as Zoon's balanitis, drug eruption, lichen planus, and psoriasis may clinically mimic CIS. The frequency of progression to invasive squamous cell carcinoma is similar (5% to 10%)

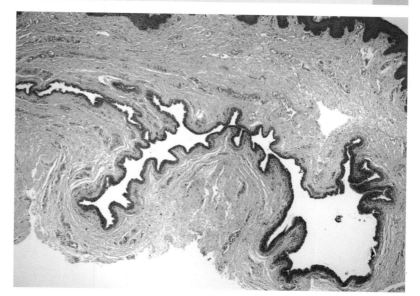

FIGURE 6–20 |▮|| Median raphe cyst, lined by pseudostratified columnar epithelium.

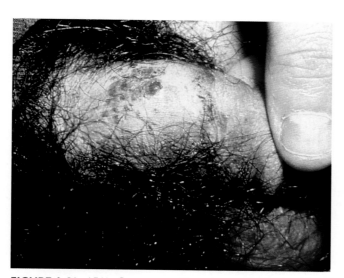

FIGURE 6–21 |▮|| Squamous cell carcinoma in situ in skin of penile shaft (Bowen's disease).

for CIS involving either the penile shaft or the glans and foreskin.

Microscopically, at least two thirds or more of the thickness of the squamous epithelium is cytologically atypical. Cell nuclei are enlarged, hyperchromatic, and pleomorphic. Cells are dyskeratotic and lack polarity (Fig. 6–22). Multinucleation is common, and abundant mitotic figures are usually present, some of which are atypical.

Bowenoid Papulosis

This is a proliferative squamous lesion, probably caused by human papillomavirus infection (types 16 and 18), that is indistinguishable from CIS histologically but differs from CIS clinically and biologically. It occurs in men between 20 and 40 years old and presents as numerous papules, usually on the penile shaft and rarely on the glans, foreskin, or perineum. It is biologically indolent, responding to conservative local therapy or regressing spontaneously if untreated.

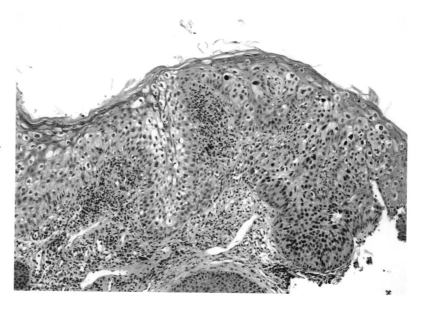

FIGURE 6–22 |▮|| Squamous cell carcinoma in situ, penile shaft. Abnormal squamous cells with marked nuclear pleomorphism and hyperchromasia, and loss of polarity, occupy much of the thickness of the epithelial layer.

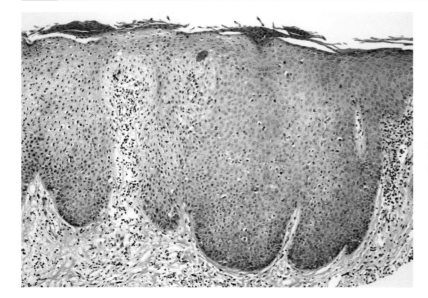

FIGURE 6–23 ▐ ▌ ▌ ▌ Bowenoid papulosis. There is full-thickness abnormality of the squamous epithelium, with delayed maturation, nuclear irregularity, and mitotic activity in the upper cell layers.

Individual papules may measure up to 10 mm; coalesced lesions may be larger. The histologic findings are virtually indistinguishable from those of CIS (Fig. 6–23). The correct diagnosis requires clinical correlation.

PENILE SQUAMOUS CELL CARCINOMA

Etiology

Squamous cell carcinoma accounts for more than 95% of penile cancer; most of the rest are sarcomas. The occurrence of penile squamous cell carcinoma is linked epidemiologically to lack of circumcision, phimosis, poor hygiene, viruses, and tobacco smoking. Epithelial irritation by smegma and epithelial infection by human papillomaviruses 16 and 18 are frequently cited etiologic factors. These factors are enhanced in uncircumcised men, in men with phimosis, and in men without the means or the will to practice good penile hygiene.

Clinical Features

The age range of patients with squamous cell carcinoma is from 20 to 90 years; average age is about 60 years. Patients are commonly concerned by the presence of an exophytic mass, an ulcer, or an area of mucosal erythema (Figs. 6–24 through 6–26). Less common presenting complaints include penile pain, bleeding or discharge, or voiding difficulty. Almost all penile squamous cell carcinomas originate in the mucosal epithelium of the glans (most common), coronal sulcus, or foreskin. Primary carcinoma of the skin covering the shaft and foreskin is rare.

Differentiation and Grading

Microscopically, squamous cell carcinoma consists of malignant squamous cells forming fungating exophytic masses or ulcerative lesions infiltrating underlying structures (Fig. 6–27). Tumor grade is assigned according to the degree of cytologic atypia, the relative abundance of mitotic figures, and the presence or absence of visible intercellular bridges, keratin pearls (aggregates of anucleate keratin), and necrosis.

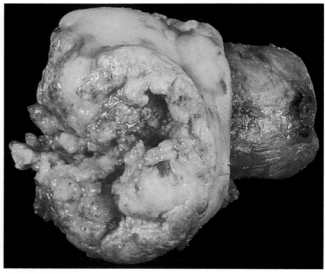

FIGURE 6–24 ▐ ▌ ▌ ▌ Squamous cell carcinoma of the penis, predominantly exophytic.

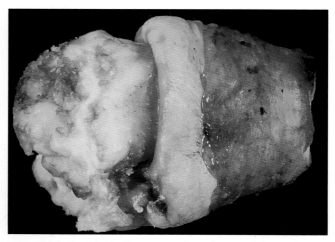

FIGURE 6–25 ▐ ▌ ▌ ▌ Squamous cell carcinoma of the penis, predominantly ulcerative.

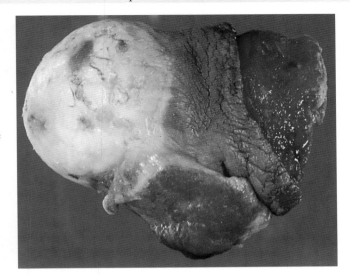

FIGURE 6–26 | ▮ | | Squamous cell carcinoma of the penis, erythematous and superficially ulcerative.

Well-differentiated squamous cell carcinoma (grade 1) has minimal cytologic atypia, rare mitotic figures, abundant keratin pearls, and readily visible intercellular bridges. Tumor cells often have abundant dark pink cytoplasm that sometimes appears glassy. It tends to form papillomatous exophytic structures and infiltrates underlying tissues as delicate finger-like projections. Poorly differentiated carcinoma (grade 3) is characterized by abundant mitotic figures, absence of recognizable intercellular bridges, absence of keratin pearls, and pronounced nuclear atypia. Necrosis may be present. The features of moderately differentiated carcinoma (grade 2) lie between these extremes; intercellular bridges and keratin pearls are present but infrequent, and mitotic activity and nuclear atypia are greater than in well-differentiated tumors but less than in poorly differentiated tumors.

The probability of lymph node metastases increases as the degree of differentiation diminishes. Overall, about 25% of patients with well-differentiated cancer develop lymph node metastases, nearly half with moderately differentiated carcinoma have lymph node metastases, and over 80% with poorly differentiated carcinoma have lymph node metastases.

Growth Patterns

Growth pattern of penile squamous cell carcinoma is variable and prognostically significant because of its influence on tumor stage. *Vertical growth carcinoma* is often high grade and deeply invasive. *Superficial spreading carcinoma* is usually well or moderately differentiated, grows horizontally, and invades minimally. *Verruciform carcinoma* has several well or moderately differentiated subtypes; invasion tends to be limited or sometimes

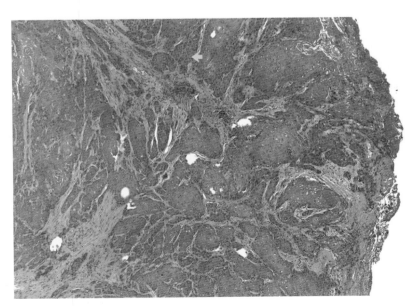

FIGURE 6–27 | ▮ | | Squamous cell carcinoma of the penis, invading in nests and cords, with a desmoplastic stromal reaction. Well-differentiated areas show abundant keratin production *(green arrow)*, which is less apparent in moderately differentiated areas *(yellow arrow)*.

absent in these tumors. Over 80% of vertical growth carcinomas are associated with inguinal lymph node metastases, whereas node metastases in the other growth patterns occur in fewer than half the cases. Prognosis is best for patients with verruciform cancers and worst for those with vertical growth tumors. Prognosis for superficial spreading tumors is intermediate between these extremes.

Staging

The TNM staging system of the American Joint Committee on Cancer and the International Union Against Cancer is given in Table 6–1.

Subtypes of Squamous Cell Carcinoma

Squamous cell carcinoma of the usual type has little or no papillary component. It is typically well or moderately differentiated, composed of irregular fingers and nests of malignant squamous cells that infiltrate underlying tissues. Stromal desmoplasia and infiltrates of chronic inflammatory cells are commonly present. Poorly differentiated carcinoma is rare and more likely to be located on the penile shaft than on the glans or prepuce.

Basaloid carcinoma is an aggressive tumor that accounts for about 10% of penile cancer. It consists of closely packed solid sheets or nests of small cells with minimal cytoplasm and abundant mitotic figures; necrosis is commonly present. It is typically deeply infiltrative, and more than half of patients have inguinal lymph node metastases when first diagnosed.

Warty (condylomatous) carcinoma is a low-grade squamous cell carcinoma, accounting for 6% of penile cancers and for about one third of verruciform carcinomas. It is typically large (up to 7 cm). Microscopically, it

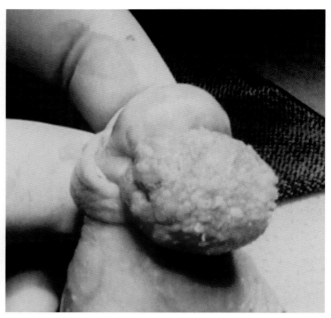

FIGURE 6–28 ▮▮▮ Verrucous carcinoma of penis. (Courtesy of Michael Oefelein, MD, Cleveland, OH.)

consists of a papillary exophytic component and an infiltrative basal component. The papillae are long, undulating, and complex. They are lined by squamous cells with koilocytic changes. The base of the tumor is raggedly infiltrative, commonly into the corpus spongiosum, but rarely involving corpus spongiosum. Lymph node metastasis is uncommon.

Verrucous carcinoma is rare, slow growing, exophytic, and often large when diagnosed (Fig. 6–28). It is composed of straight papillary structures with inconspicuous fibrovascular cores, thickly lined by squamous epithelium with little or no cytologic atypia and no koilocytic features. There is a sharp discrete interface between the base of the tumor and the underlying lamina propria (Fig. 6–29). This lesion does not metastasize, but about one third recur locally.

Papillary carcinoma, not otherwise specified (NOS) is squamous cell carcinoma with both exophytic and endophytic growth. The exophytic component consists of papillary structures with fibrovascular cores of variable length lined by thickened atypical squamous epithelium. Abundant keratin may fill the spaces between the papillae. The tumor cells are usually well or moderately differentiated. Koilocytic changes are absent. The tumor infiltrates structures at its base and is often surrounded by stromal desmoplasia and chronic inflammation. Metastases occur in some cases; the 5-year survival is about 90%.

Sarcomatoid carcinoma is rare (about 1% of penile carcinomas) and biologically aggressive. It is usually large, fungating, and deeply invasive. Satellite tumor nodules may be seen in the corpus cavernosum or in penile skin. Microscopically, it consists of malignant spindle cells, often admixed with bizarre cells or tumor giant cells. Components of recognizable sarcoma (e.g., chondrosarcoma, osteosarcoma) are sometimes present. An in situ or invasive squamous component may be

TABLE 6–1

TNM STAGING OF CARCINOMA OF THE PENIS

Primary Tumor (T)

TX	Primary tumor cannot be assessed
T0	No evidence of primary tumor
Tis	Carcinoma in situ
Ta	Noninvasive verrucous carcinoma
T1	Tumor invades subepithelial connective tissue
T2	Tumor invades corpus spongiosum or cavernosum
T3	Tumor invades the urethra or prostate
T4	Tumor invades other adjacent structures

Regional Lymph Nodes (N)

NX	Regional lymph nodes cannot be assessed
N0	No regional lymph node metastasis
N1	Metastasis in a single superficial inguinal lymph node
N2	Metastasis in multiple or bilateral superficial inguinal lymph nodes
N3	Metastasis in deep inguinal or pelvic lymph nodes(s), unilateral or bilateral

Distant Metastasis (M)

MX	Distant metastasis cannot be assessed
M0	No distant metastasis
M1	Distant metastasis

Used with the permission of the American Joint Committee on Cancer (AJCC), Chicago, Illinois. The original source for this material is the *AJCC Cancer Staging Manual, Sixth Edition* (2002) published by Springer-Verlag New York, www.springer-ny.com.

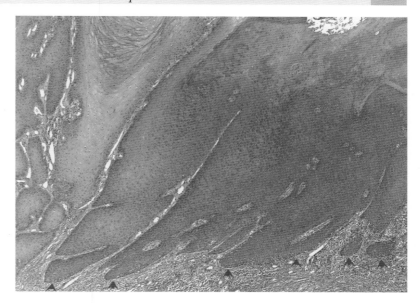

FIGURE 6–29 | ▌| | Verrucous carcinoma of penis. The tumor forms long thick pegs, which form a smooth regular interface with underlying lamina propria *(blue arrows).*

present. Positive immunostaining of tumor cells for keratin is diagnostically useful.

For patients with the various subtypes of penile squamous cell carcinoma, prognosis is best for those with verrucous carcinoma, slightly worse for those with warty carcinoma and papillary squamous cell carcinoma, NOS, more guarded for patients with nonpapillary squamous cell carcinoma of usual type, and worst for patients with basaloid or sarcomatoid carcinoma.

RARE PENILE NEOPLASMS

Basal Cell Carcinoma

Basal cell carcinoma occasionally involves the skin of the penile shaft and, less commonly, the glans or foreskin, usually in older white patients, forming a small nonhealing ulcer. It is an indolent lesion, usually cured by complete excision. Microscopically, it consists of infiltrating nests of uniform small dark epithelial cells, which tend to "palisade" at the periphery of the nest (Fig. 6–30). Intercellular bridges are not apparent, nor is there obvious keratin formation. The stroma around the tumor nests may be desmoplastic or may appear mucinous. Cleftlike spaces are often noted between tumor nests and the surrounding stroma (a tissue-processing artifact).

Melanoma

This lesion occurs mostly in white patients older than 50 years of age. It is most common on the glans, but it also occurs on any other penile location. It forms a dark nodule or ulcer with irregular borders. Its histologic features, and the prognostic implications of the histologic findings, are the same as those for melanoma in other body sites (Fig. 6–31). The prognosis for patients with

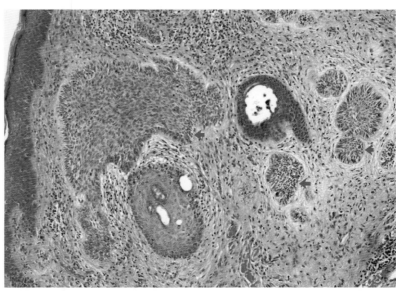

FIGURE 6–30 | ▌| | Basal cell carcinoma, forming nests of tumor cells in the dermis *(blue arrows).* Note the "palisade" arrangement of tumor cells at the periphery of the nests and the paucity of keratin formation.

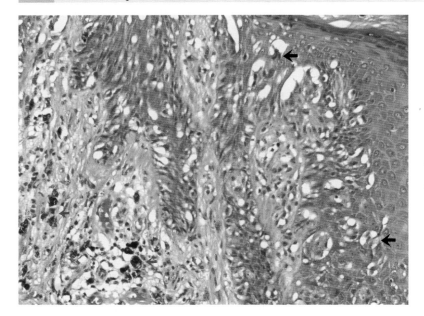

FIGURE 6–31   ▌▌▏▏   Melanoma. Malignant melanocytes form clusters at the base of the epidermis *(red arrow)* and infiltrate the upper levels of the epidermis *(black arrows)*, as well as the underlying dermis *(blue arrows)*.

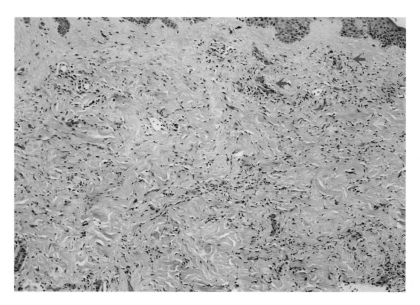

FIGURE 6–32   ▌▌▏▏   Kaposi's sarcoma, AIDS-related. In this "early" lesion, the tiny dark slitlike structures are miniature blood vessels proliferating around larger blood vessels *(blue arrows)* and dissecting bundles of dermal collagen *(yellow arrows)*. The findings are obviously quite subtle and challenging.

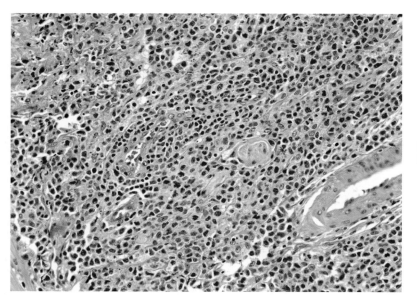

FIGURE 6–33   ▌▌▏▏   Lymphoma. Malignant cells infiltrating soft tissues of penis.

penile melanoma is much worse than for those with squamous cell carcinoma: lymph node metastasis has already occurred in most patients by the time the diagnosis is made.

Sarcoma

The most common sarcomas involving the penis are those of vascular type: angiosarcoma, Kaposi's sarcoma, and epithelioid hemangioendothelioma (Fig. 6–32). Virtually any other type of sarcoma may arise in the penis; most involve the corpora cavernosa. Penile sarcoma is sometimes difficult to distinguish histologically from malignant melanoma and sarcomatoid carcinoma.

Hematopoietic Neoplasms

Lymphoma may involve the penis in rare instances, forming either a mass lesion in the body of the penis or an ulcerating skin lesion. Most cases are of diffuse large cell type (Figs. 6–33 and 6–34).

Leukemia may present with similar penile manifestations.

Cancer Metastatic to the Penis

Penile metastasis from a distant neoplasm is rare and usually occurs late in the course of the primary disease. Prostatic adenocarcinoma and urothelial carcinoma of the bladder account for about 70% of cases; colonic adenocarcinoma and renal cell carcinoma are also common primary sites. Priapism develops in nearly half of cases, owing to malignant infiltration of the corpora cavernosa; other symptoms may include urethral bleeding or voiding difficulty. In the great majority of cases, metastasis from a known primary is suspected, but occasionally the penile metastasis is the initial manifestation of cancer. Survival following diagnosis is usually brief.

Metastases usually develop initially in the corpus cavernosum, forming painless palpable mass lesions (Figs. 6–35 and 6–36). Subsequent involvement of the overlying skin results in ulceration.

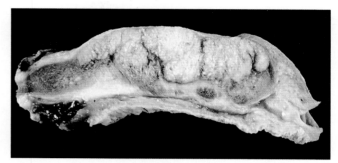

FIGURE 6–35 ▮ Metastatic urothelial carcinoma forming nodules in the corpora cavernosa of the penis.

SCROTUM

NON-NEOPLASTIC CONDITIONS

Hidradenitis Suppurativa

This condition results from obstruction of the drainage systems of apocrine and eccrine glands by follicular hyperkeratosis, for reasons that are not fully understood. It involves skin in the axilla, groin, perineum, areola, and umbilicus. Pilosebaceous units become distended, and infection with a variety of bacteria supervenes. The pilosebaceous units rupture, releasing their contents into the surrounding dermis. This results in necrotizing and granulomatous inflammation with abscess formation. The process spreads to involve deeper subcutaneous tissue, and sinus tracts form to allow drainage to the skin surface (Fig. 6–37).

The inflammation begins with tender red papules, followed by fluctuant small abscesses that drain to the skin through sinuses. The process becomes diffuse as lesions coalesce to form plaques.

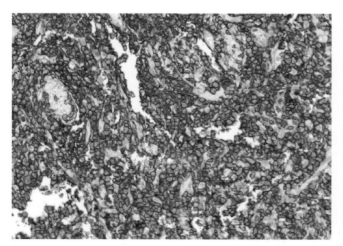

FIGURE 6–34 ▮ Lymphoma. Tumor cells of the lesion illustrated in Figure 6–33 show strong immunoreactivity to antibodies against leukocyte common antigen.

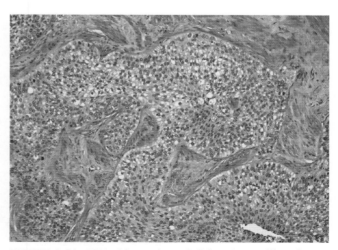

FIGURE 6–36 ▮ Metastatic urothelial carcinoma filling the vascular spaces of the corpus cavernosum.

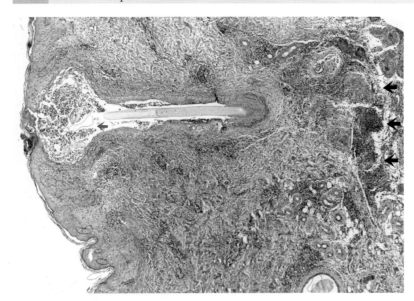

FIGURE 6–37 ||■|| Hidradenitis suppurativa. Acute inflammatory exudate is present in the lumen of the hair shaft *(blue arrow)*. Around the eccrine units at the base of the hair follicle there are chronic inflammatory cell infiltrates *(black arrows)*.

Idiopathic Scrotal Calcinosis

Epidermoid and pilar cysts of the scrotum sometimes become calcified. Calcification of dermal connective tissue of the scrotum without evidence of a preexisting cyst is termed *idiopathic scrotal calcinosis*. Many authorities believe the condition develops within eccrine units, with progressive loss of lining epithelial cells as the calcific deposits slowly accumulate. Most patients are adolescents or young men who note one or more nodules in the scrotal skin measuring up to 3 cm in diameter. The skin overlying the nodules is usually unremarkable but sometimes ulcerates.

Microscopically, rounded aggregates of granular calcific debris are present in the dermis. A foreign-body giant cell reaction may be apparent in surrounding tissues, and, in some instances, the remnants of a cyst wall lining may be present (Fig. 6–38).

Fat Necrosis

Rarely, children or young adolescents may develop fat necrosis in the scrotum. The etiology is unknown; some cases are attributed to exposure to prolonged and intense cold. Fat necrosis presents as a scrotal nodule, sometimes involving both sides of the scrotum. Microscopic findings in excised lesions are those of fat necrosis, often with associated inflammatory infiltrates.

SCROTAL NEOPLASMS

Squamous Cell Carcinoma

Squamous cell carcinoma is the most common scrotal cancer. It has long been linked to exposure to work-related carcinogens, many of them of hydrocarbon type. It is much less common than squamous cell carcinoma of the penis. Most patients are middle-aged or older.

It typically begins as a slow-growing papule, nodule, or wart on the scrotal surface. With enlargement, it develops central ulceration and raised, rolled margins (Fig. 6–39).

Microscopically, it is usually well or moderately differentiated (Fig. 6–40). Squamous cell carcinoma in situ is commonly evident adjacent to the invasive lesion, and koilocytic changes suggestive of human papillomavirus infection may be apparent in some cases.

About 25% of patients have inguinal lymph node metastases at the time of diagnosis. Patients whose cancer is localized to the scrotum, or invasive into local structures, have a survival rate of 70%. Patients with metastatic cancer limited to inguinal nodes have a survival rate of 44%. Metastases to pelvic nodes, or distant organs, are generally incompatible with long-term survival.

Basal Cell Carcinoma

Scrotal basal cell carcinoma is rare. It occurs in middle-aged or older men (average age 65 years), presenting as

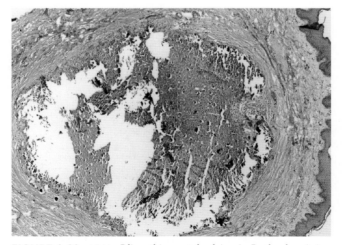

FIGURE 6–38 ||■|| Idiopathic scrotal calcinosis. In the dermis is a cystic space filled with granular calcific debris.

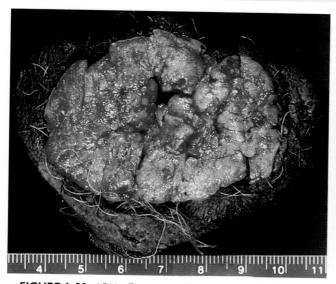

FIGURE 6–39 I ▌I I Squamous cell carcinoma of the scrotum.

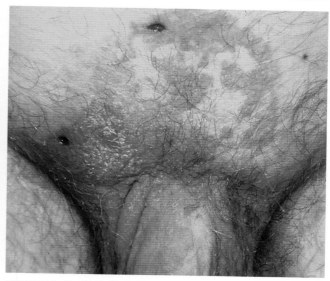

FIGURE 6–41 I ▌I I Extramammary Paget's disease, affecting skin of mons pubis, scrotum, and penis. The small round ulcers are punch biopsy sites.

painless plaque or nodule with ulceration. It has no association with industrial carcinogen exposure or human papillomavirus infection.

Basal cell carcinoma of the scrotum metastasizes to regional lymph nodes or distant organs more commonly than its counterparts in other body sites.

Paget's Disease

Extramammary Paget's disease arises in skin with apocrine glands, including penis and scrotum. Most cases of scrotal Paget's disease are associated with synchronous or metachronous carcinoma of the prostate, urethra, or urinary bladder. It is believed to arise by malignant transformation of epidermal cells programmed for apocrine differentiation. It presents as a scaly eczematous

skin lesion that is often erythematous and sometimes exudative (Fig. 6–41).

Microscopically, the squamous epithelium is infiltrated by large cells with light pink or nearly clear cytoplasm and large vesicular nuclei, situated singly or in small nests along the basal aspect of the epithelium and also congregating at the tips of the rete pegs (Fig. 6–42). Some of these atypical cells are located higher in the epidermis. Rarely, microinvasion into the dermis may be observed. Paget's cells contain intracytoplasmic mucin, a feature demonstrable with mucin stains; this finding distinguishes Paget's cells from squamous cell carcinoma in situ and melanoma (Fig. 6–43). Immunostains are also helpful in this distinction.

FIGURE 6–40 I ▌I I Squamous cell carcinoma, infiltrating soft tissues of scrotum.

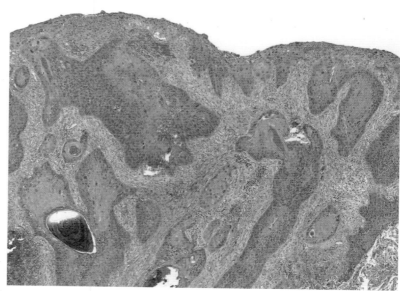

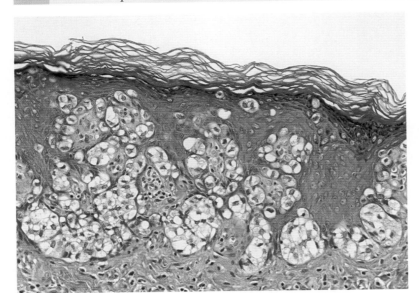

FIGURE 6–42 ▐ ▌▐| | Extramammary Paget's disease. The epidermis is infiltrated by clusters of large cells with abundant clear or lightly eosinophilic cytoplasm and large vesicular nuclei.

Benign Soft Tissue Tumors

A wide assortment of benign soft tissue tumors occur in the scrotum, including tumors of vascular, fibrous, smooth muscle, and neural origin (Fig. 6–44).

Sarcoma

Most cases of primary scrotal sarcoma are leiomyosarcoma, occurring in men older than age 35 years, with an average age near 60 years. Tumor size ranges up to 60 cm. The microscopic findings are the same as those of leiomyosarcoma arising in other sites. Prognosis is guarded, because local recurrence or metastases may appear after long periods of surveillance. Liposarcoma and malignant fibrous histiocytoma also occur rarely in the scrotum.

Metastases to the Scrotum

Most cutaneous scrotal metastases originate from primary carcinoma in the prostate, colon, stomach, or kidney. The tumor histology, correlated with clinical findings, generally allows for accurate diagnosis.

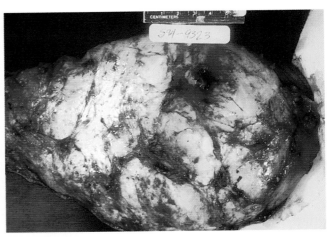

FIGURE 6–44 ▐ ▌▐| | Large scrotal hemangioma.

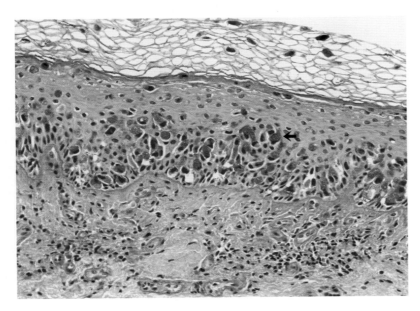

FIGURE 6–43 ▐ ▌▐| | Extramammary Paget's disease. The neoplastic cells contain mucin, which is stained dark red by a special stain *(arrow)*.

Chapter 7

ADRENAL

ANATOMY AND NORMAL HISTOLOGY

In adults, the right adrenal gland is flattened and triangular and the left is elongate and semilunar. A normal adrenal gland weighs 4 to 5 g and is enclosed within a thin fibrous capsule. The principal components of the gland are the cortex and the medulla. The cortex is golden yellow, convoluted, and about 2 mm thick; it surrounds the gray-tan medulla.

Microscopically, the adult cortex consists of three zones. The zona glomerulosa lies beneath the capsule. It is thin, indistinct, and focally incomplete, consisting of cells with minimal eosinophilic cytoplasm and small, round, dark nuclei. It blends smoothly with the underlying zona fasciculata, which consists of long columns of large cells with pale vacuolated cytoplasm (Fig. 7–1). The zona reticularis lies innermost and consists of short anastomosing cords of eosinophilic cells. Zona fasciculata and zona reticularis are richly supplied with sinusoids and capillaries. The medulla comprises about 10% of adrenal mass (Fig. 7–2). It is composed of polyhedral cells with granular basophilic cytoplasm, uniform round-to-oval nuclei, and inconspicuous nucleoli, arranged in nests and short cords intermingled with numerous capillaries.

The focus in this chapter is on pathologic conditions that may require surgical intervention, as well as non-surgical conditions with which the urologist should be familiar. The discussion is separated as follows: general or global disorders of the entire gland, disorders of the adrenal cortex, and disorders of the adrenal medulla.

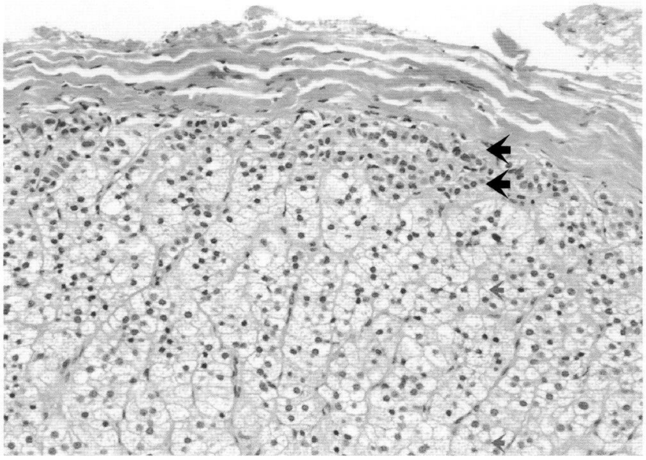

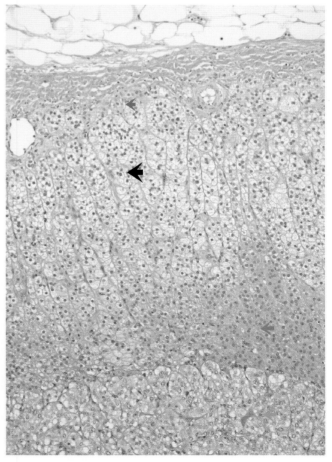

FIGURE 7–1 ▌█▐▐ Normal histology. Fibrous capsule is at top. Immediately beneath is the thin, incomplete, and inconspicuous zona glomerulosa, made up of cells with dark eosinophilic cytoplasm *(black arrows)*, overlying long columns of pale cells composing the zona fasciculata *(blue arrows)*.

FIGURE 7–2 ▌█▐▐ Normal histology. Section showing zona glomerulosa *(blue arrow)*, zona fasciculata *(black arrow)*, zona reticularis *(red arrow)*, and medulla *(green arrow)*.

Several images in this chapter are courtesy of Mayo Clinic Foundation, Rochester, MN.

GLOBAL DISORDERS
OF THE ADRENAL GLAND

ADRENAL HETEROTOPIA

Embryonic adrenal tissue is located near the urogenital ridge. Co-migration of adrenal and urogenital ridge tissue occurs with surprising frequency. Up to one third of patients have heterotopic adrenal tissue near the celiac axis, frequently composed of both cortical and medullary tissue. Adrenal cortical rests associated with descent of gonadal structures may occur in the broad ligament, in the spermatic cord (see Fig. 5–3), adjacent to the testis, and within the testis or ovary. Intrarenal (subcapsular) adrenal tissue is sometimes present and may be a source of diagnostic uncertainty intraoperatively—for example, during assessment of a donor kidney for transplantation (Fig. 7–3). Heterotopic adrenal tissue also arises in the lung, placenta, cranial dura mater, liver, and spinal canal. Rarely, hyperplastic nodules develop in heterotopic adrenal tissue.

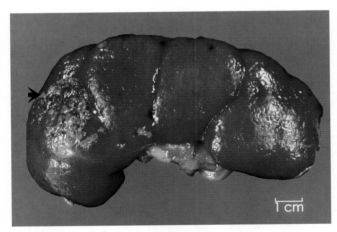

FIGURE 7–3 ▮▮ ▮▮   Heterotopic adrenal cortical tissue, appearing as an area of golden yellow irregularity in the renal cortex *(arrow)*.

ADRENAL CYSTS

Adrenal cysts may be encountered in patients of virtually any age, but most occur in patients between 40 and 60 years of age, most of whom are female. Most cysts are small incidental autopsy findings, but cysts containing several liters of fluid have been reported.

Adrenal cysts have multiple causes. Most adrenal cysts (about 85%) result from hemorrhage in normal or abnormal adrenals and are designated "pseudocysts" or "endothelial cysts," depending on whether an endothelial lining is present (Fig. 7–4). Causes include vascular malformations and metastatic cancer. About 7% are parasitic in origin, usually secondary to echinococcus infestation. About 9% of adrenal cysts have an epithelial lining, some of which originate from cystic change in entrapped mesothelium or in heterotopic urogenital tissue; others arise in association with adrenal adenoma, adrenal carcinoma, or pheochromocytoma.

ADRENAL INVOLVEMENT BY INFECTIONS

Infection by *Mycobacterium tuberculosis* results in enlargement of the adrenal, with extensive caseous necrosis. Extensive caseous necrosis of the adrenal may also result from dissemination of histoplasmosis, blastomycosis, and coccidioidomycosis. Granulomas usually do not occur in the adrenal, possibly because local corticosteroids alter the immune response.

The adrenal gland may show striking pathologic changes related to the abrupt, rapid, and often fatal course of *Waterhouse-Friderichsen syndrome*, a disorder associated with systemic effects of fulminant meningococcal or streptococcal infection. Adrenal enlargement due to hemorrhage is common (Fig. 7–5). Sinusoidal fibrin deposits, coagulative necrosis, and hemorrhage in and around the adrenal are usually present.

Bacterial adrenal abscess usually arises from infection of adrenal hematoma in neonates by *Escherichia coli*, group B *Streptococcus*, or *Bacteroides*. Malakoplakia of the adrenal gland has also been reported.

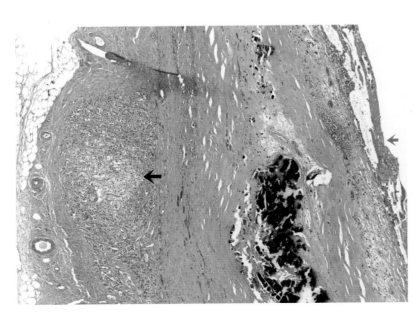

FIGURE 7–4 ▮▮ ▮▮   Adrenal cyst. From left, section includes fat, adrenal cortex *(black arrow)*, and a fibrous cyst wall with coarse calcifications. Cyst lumen is at right *(red arrow* indicates the amorphous material lining the cyst cavity). Immunostains did not demonstrate any epithelial or endothelial lining cells.

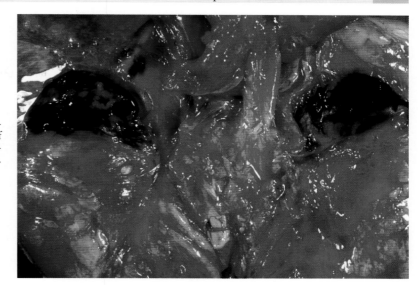

FIGURE 7–5   I ∎ I I   Adrenal glands at autopsy (posterior aspect of retroperitoneum) in a patient who died of meningococcal septicemia complicated by Waterhouse-Friderichsen syndrome. Both adrenals are hemorrhagic. (Courtesy of Raymond Redline, MD, Cleveland, OH.)

ADRENAL HEMORRHAGE

Adrenal hemorrhage may occur in postoperative or postpartum status, steroid or adrenocorticotropic hormone (ACTH) administration, coagulation disorders, metastatic malignancy, cardiac disease, thromboembolic disease, and sepsis, including Waterhouse-Friderichsen syndrome. Adrenal hematoma is occasionally noted in newborns after difficult delivery, causing concern for the possibility of adrenal tumor (Fig. 7–6). Hematoma more often involves the right adrenal.

DISORDERS OF THE ADRENAL CORTEX

ADRENAL CORTICAL HYPERPLASIA

Diffuse and Nodular Hyperplasia

Cortical hyperplasia is defined as a non-neoplastic increase in the number of cortical cells. It is usually bilateral and may be diffuse, nodular, or both. Hyperplasia may be accompanied by features of eucorticalism, hypercortisolism, hyperaldosteronism, or virilization.

Nodularity of the cortex is commonly observed at surgery and at autopsy. Multiple nodules are noted in 1.5% to 2.9% of autopsies. Nodules are heterogeneous; some are hyperplastic micronodules or macronodules, whereas others are neoplastic, such as adenoma arising in a background of hyperplastic change. Making this distinction may be virtually impossible. Localized cortical ischemia with secondary regeneration and hyperplasia may account for some instances of nodularity. Advancing age, hypertension, and diabetes mellitus are associated with increased incidence of nodularity. However, most patients with cortical nodularity have normal adrenal function.

Nodular adrenal glands contain multiple (and usually bilateral) discrete or confluent nodules that can be greater than 2.0 cm. in diameter (Fig. 7–7). Extrusion of the nodules into surrounding fat is common.

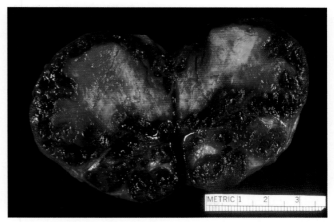

FIGURE 7–6   I ∎ I I   Organizing hematoma. This lesion can mimic neuroblastoma clinically and radiologically in a neonate following difficult delivery.

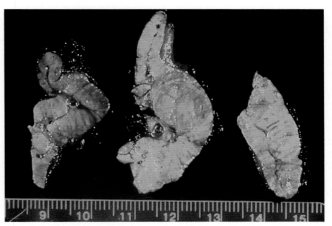

FIGURE 7–7   I ∎ I I   Diffuse and nodular cortical hyperplasia. The cortex shows diffuse irregular thickening and focal nodularity.

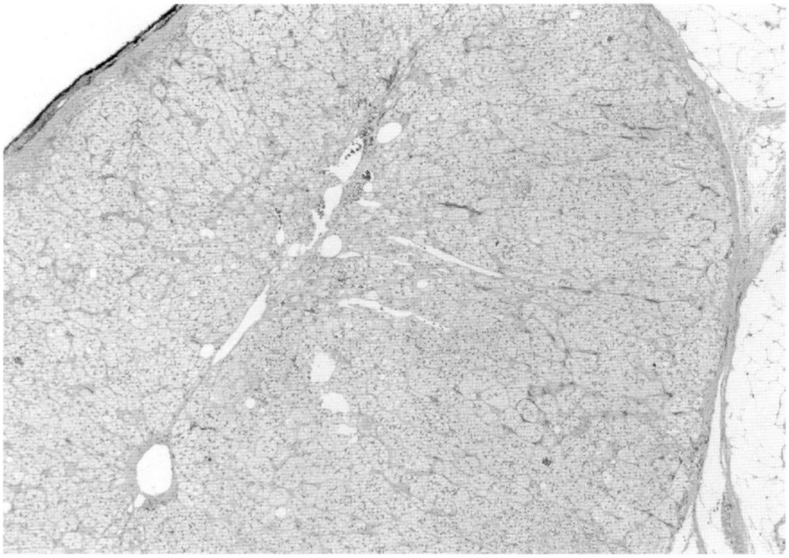

FIGURE 7–8 ▌▌▌ Cortical hyperplasia. The zona fasciculata is markedly expanded (compare with Fig. 7–2). No medullary tissue is present in this section.

Some nodules are composed only of cortical tissue, whereas others show fibrosis, cyst formation, fatty change, myeloid metaplasia, or, rarely, osseous metaplastic change. The cells within the nodules contain abundant cytoplasm, which may be vacuolated or eosinophilic. The cells are arranged in nests, sheets, cords or ribbons, and, sometimes, glands (Fig. 7–8).

Pigmented Cortical Nodule

Pigmented cortical nodules ranging from 0.1 to 1.5 cm in diameter are present in up to 37% of adrenals at autopsy. Most of these nodules are solitary, but they may be multiple and bilateral. The cells comprising these nodules contain granular brown pigment that is probably lipofuscin, a degenerative cellular product. The significance of pigmented cortical nodule is uncertain, but it is probably within the spectrum of nodular hyperplasia.

Cortical Hyperplasia with Hypercortisolism

Several processes result in hyperplasia of the adrenal cortex associated with excess production of cortisol. The most common of these is overproduction of ACTH by pituitary disorders *(Cushing's disease)*, including pituitary adenoma and hyperplasia of ACTH-producing cells. Less common disorders in this category are *ectopic production of ACTH and ectopic production of corticotropin-releasing factor (CRF)*. In these disorders, the adrenal gland is a "target organ." In contrast, autonomous cortical hyperfunction characterizes *macronodular hyperplasia with marked adrenal enlargement and primary pigmented nodular adrenocortical disease.*

In 80% to 90% of cases of Cushing's disease the adrenals are modestly enlarged, weighing up to 12 g, with diffuse and/or micronodular hyperplasia of lipid-rich vacuolated cells and lipid-depleted cells with eosinophilic cytoplasm. In 10% to 20%, the adrenals are larger, averaging 16 g, and have multiple nodules up to 5 cm in diameter (macronodular hyperplasia). The nodules merge with the adjacent hyperplastic cortex.

Approximately 15% of adult cases of Cushing's syndrome (clinical hypercortisolism unrelated to pituitary disease) result from *ectopic production of ACTH or CRF* by various neuroendocrine tumors. The pathologic findings are similar to those seen in cases of Cushing's disease.

Macronodular hyperplasia with marked adrenal enlargement is characterized by marked increase in the size of both adrenal glands with nonsuppressible hypercortisolism, without clinical, radiologic, or biochemical evidence of pituitary disease, suggesting autonomous adrenal cortical hyperfunction. The etiology of this rare disorder is unknown. Men are affected more often than women, and the average patient age is around 50 years. Combined weight of the adrenals ranges from 60 to 180 g. The adrenals appear bosselated, with multiple golden-yellow cortical nodules up to 3.8 cm in diameter. The nodules are microscopically similar to those noted in micronodular hyperplasia, sometimes with the addition of large vacuolated "balloon cells" and "pseudoglands." Extension of cortical cells into surrounding fat is often observed.

Primary pigmented adrenocortical disease (PPNAD) is another form of autonomous adrenal cortical hyperfunction. In this disorder, the adrenals may be stimulated by an immunoglobulin product of autoimmune dysfunction. Autosomal dominant inheritance is evident in half the cases, and, in these cases, other abnormalities may be present, including cardiac myxoma, mucocutaneous pigmentation, and large cell calcifying Sertoli cell tumor of the testis. PPNAD affects young persons and is more common in females. Some patients present with constant or episodic hypercortisolism, whereas others have no abnormal findings. The pituitary glands are normal. The adrenals are usually of normal size and are studded with black nodules that are mostly less than 0.3 cm in diameter but may be as large as 3 cm. Microscopically, the nodules are circumscribed but unencapsulated. They tend to congregate at the corticomedullary junction. The nodules consist of vacuolated lipid-rich cells and densely eosinophilic lipid-depleted cells. Variable amounts of intracellular lipofuscin are present, accounting for the pigmentation noted grossly.

ADRENAL CORTICAL ADENOMA

This is a benign neoplasm derived from cortical cells, usually solitary and unilateral, and more frequent in women. Adenomas commonly secrete excessive steroids, resulting in hypertension, Cushing's syndrome, virilization, or feminization. A small percentage of adenomas do not secrete enough steroids to produce clinical manifestations.

Adrenal Cortical Adenoma with Hypercortisolism

Most adrenal cortical adenomas associated with Cushing's syndrome are less than 6 cm in diameter (average 3.6 cm) and weigh less than 40 g. Adenomas are typically yellow or golden yellow, but some have widespread brown or black discoloration and are called *black adenomas*. Adenomas are circumscribed but unencapsulated. Small areas of hemorrhage, fibrosis, or cystic degeneration may be present (Fig. 7–9).

Tumor cells are arranged in nests or short cords. Most cells contain abundant lipid and are pale staining (Fig. 7–10). Minor components of smaller cells with dense eosinophilic cytoplasm are usually present. In some adenomas, large pale "balloon cells" or clusters of spindle cells are seen. Cell nuclei are fairly uniform, with inconspicuous nucleoli. Mitotic figures are infrequent, and necrosis is unusual (Fig. 7–11).

There is considerable overlap between the pathologic findings in cortical adenoma and hyperplastic macronodule. Cortical tissue adjacent to an adrenal cortical adenoma is usually atrophic, rather than hyperplastic.

Black adenoma is rare and is associated with hypercortisolism or hyperaldosteronism. In contrast to usual

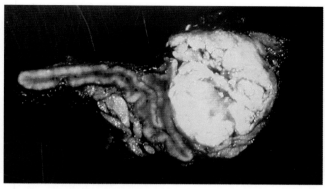

FIGURE 7–9 |▌|| Cortical adenoma. Note that the uninvolved cortex is of normal thickness, in contrast to the findings in Figure 7–7.

adenoma, black adenoma consists predominantly of lipid-poor cells with dark eosinophilic cytoplasm that often contains abundant lipofuscin, imparting the dark color of the tumor.

Adrenal Cortical Adenoma with Hyperaldosteronism (Aldosteronoma)

Aldosteronoma is usually unilateral and solitary, with a median diameter of 1.7 cm. Nearly all weigh less than 10 g. Most are bright yellow or yellow-orange and sharply circumscribed, with a fibrous pseudocapsule of variable thickness (Fig. 7–12). Cystic degeneration or hemorrhage may be seen in larger tumors.

Tumor cells are arranged in nests, cords, or interconnecting ribbons, with an extensive network of small blood vessels. Tumors are composed of a mixture of large vacuolated lipid-rich cells, smaller cells with dark eosinophilic cytoplasm, and "hybrid cells" with lightly eosinophilic cytoplasm.

FIGURE 7–10 |▌|| Cortical adenoma. Normal adrenal is at lower left. The adenoma forms an unencapsulated expansile nodule on the right. Its interface with normal adrenal is outlined by *black arrows*.

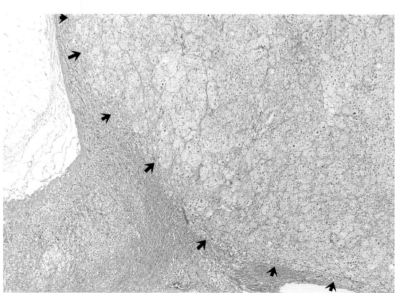

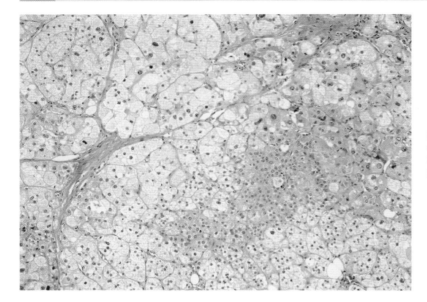

FIGURE 7–11 ▮▮▮▮ Cortical adenoma. Cells of the adenoma vary considerably in size; in this example, numerous "balloon cells" with copious cytoplasm are present.

Spironolactone bodies are sometimes seen in normal zona glomerulosa cells, or in the cells of aldosteronoma, in patients treated with spironolactone. They are laminated pink cytoplasmic inclusions, 2 to 12 μm in diameter, surrounded by a clear halo.

ADRENAL CORTICAL CARCINOMA

This cancer is derived from cells of the adrenal cortex. Estimated incidence is about one case per million people per year. Tumor development is associated with loss of heterozygosity in chromosomes 11, 13, and/or 17. The tumor can occur in patients of any age, but most patients are between 30 and 50 years old. Gender and side distribution are approximately equal. In a minority of cases, features of Cushing's syndrome, hypertension, virilization, or feminization are present.

Cortical carcinoma averages 12 to 16 cm in diameter, and most weigh between 500 and 1200 g. Tumors appear bosselated and consist of tan to yellow-orange nodules intersected by thick fibrous bands. Areas of necrosis, hemorrhage, and cystic degeneration are commonly present (Fig. 7–13). Extension of tumor into surrounding tissues or into large veins may be noted.

Tumor cells form broad elongate cords, thin parallel ribbons, sheets, or nests. Most tumors have areas of necrosis, which may be extensive (Fig. 7–14). Tumor cells may have abundant lipid-rich pale cytoplasm or moderate amounts of dark eosinophilic cytoplasm. Cell membranes are prominent. Spindle cells may be present. Nuclear atypia may be marked, and mitotic figures are usually found readily (Fig. 7–15).

The distinction between cortical adenoma and carcinoma may be difficult. Large size, extensive necrosis, more than six mitotic figures per 50 high-power fields, atypical mitotic figures, and vascular invasion are indica-

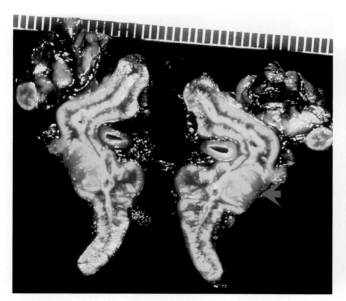

FIGURE 7–12 ▮▮▮▮ Aldosteronoma. As in this case, most are small and well circumscribed *(red arrow)*.

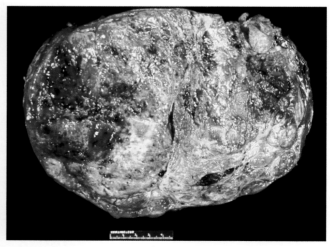

FIGURE 7–13 ▮▮▮▮ Cortical carcinoma. The tumor is large, with widespread hemorrhage, necrosis, and cystic degeneration. (Courtesy of Beverly Dahms, MD, Cleveland, OH.)

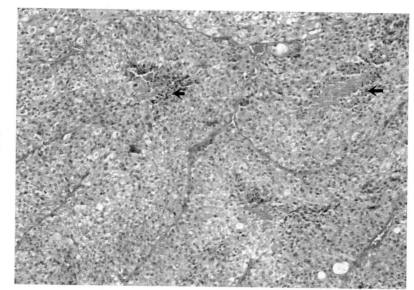

FIGURE 7–14 ▐▪▐▐ Cortical carcinoma. Tumor cells form cords and nests; several areas of necrosis are evident (*black arrows*).

tive of malignancy. Tumor invasion into an adjacent organ is observed only in malignant neoplasms. In some instances the ultimate diagnosis is determined by the patient's clinical course.

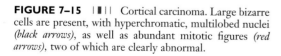

TABLE 7–1	

STAGING SYSTEM FOR ADRENAL CORTICAL CARCINOMA

T1	Tumor 5 cm or less, noninvasive
T2	Tumor larger than 5 cm, noninvasive
T3	Tumor of any size, locally invasive, not involving adjacent organs
T4	Tumor of any size, invading adjacent organs
N0	Negative regional lymph nodes
N1	Positive regional lymph nodes
M0	No distant metastases
M1	Distant metastases

From Lack EE: Atlas of Tumor Pathology, Third Series, Fascicle 19. Tumors of the Adrenal Gland and Extra-Adrenal Paraganglia. Washington, DC, Armed Forces Institute of Pathology.

The staging system that has been proposed for adrenal cortical carcinoma is shown in Table 7–1.

DISORDERS OF THE ADRENAL MEDULLA

ADRENAL MEDULLARY HYPERPLASIA

Adrenal medullary hyperplasia (AMH) is often a component of multiple endocrine neoplasia (MEN) syndromes types IIa and IIb and is considered a precursor of pheochromocytoma in these syndromes. Pheochromocytoma arises in 30% to 50% of patients with MEN type II and is bilateral and/or multifocal in 60% to 70%; malignant pheochromocytoma afflicts approximately 5% of patients with these syndromes.

Medullary hyperplasia may be diffuse, nodular, or both. It may be present in one or both glands. The adrenal gland is modestly enlarged, with expansion of the medulla by sheets and unencapsulated nodules of

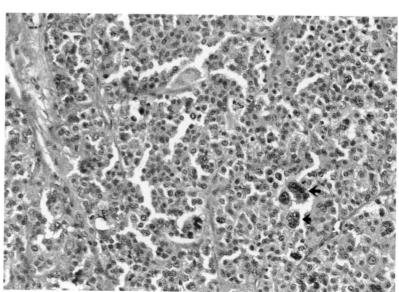

FIGURE 7–15 ▐▪▐▐ Cortical carcinoma. Large bizarre cells are present, with hyperchromatic, multilobed nuclei (*black arrows*), as well as abundant mitotic figures (*red arrows*), two of which are clearly abnormal.

chromaffin cells with eosinophilic cytoplasm. The cells are arranged in nests or trabeculae. They exhibit nuclear pleomorphism, hyperchromasia, and moderate mitotic activity. Eosinophilic "hyaline globules" may be present in some cells.

A large nodule of medullary hyperplasia is microscopically indistinguishable from a small pheochromocytoma. A nodule 1 cm or larger is considered a pheochromocytoma.

PHEOCHROMOCYTOMA

The adrenal medulla is one component of the sympathoadrenal neuroendocrine system. It is integrated with the paraganglionic cells of the sympathetic nervous system (SNS). Paraganglionic cells (chromaffin cells) are neuroendocrine cells. They develop adjacent to true ganglion cells, which are derived from neuroblasts. Paraganglionic cells and neuroblasts originate from the neural crest but follow separate paths of differentiation. Paraganglionic cells are the progenitors of adrenal medullary hyperplasia and paraganglioma; neuroblasts are the progenitors of neuroblastoma, ganglioneuroblastoma, ganglioneuroma, schwannoma, malignant peripheral nerve sheath tumor, and neurofibroma.

Pheochromocytoma is a paraganglioma derived from chromaffin cells in a specific anatomic site—the adrenal medulla. However, the term *pheochromocytoma* is commonly applied to extra-adrenal tumors arising from cells of the sympathoadrenal neuroendocrine system—tumors that are more appropriately designated "extra-adrenal paraganglioma." Because adrenal and extra-adrenal paraganglioma are pathologically indistinguishable, the only significant difference is that extra-adrenal retroperitoneal paraganglioma has a greater potential for malignancy than its adrenal counterpart.

Pheochromocytoma is rare in adults and very rare in children, and a large proportion are incidental autopsy findings. Peak incidence for pheochromocytoma is in the fifth decade. Males and females are affected with about equal frequency. Excluding familial cases, 5% are bilateral and 5% to 10% are extra-adrenal. More than half of familial cases are bilateral.

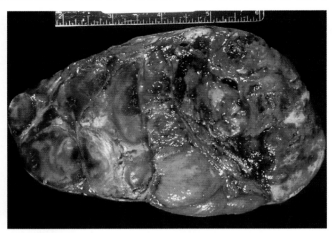

FIGURE 7–17 ||| Pheochromocytoma. This tumor is large and nodular, with widespread hemorrhage and necrosis. These findings are associated with malignancy.

Pheochromocytoma is round to oval and sharply circumscribed but unencapsulated. It averages 3 to 5 cm in diameter and weighs 75 to 100 g. It is tan, brown, or gray-white and may have areas of hemorrhage or cystic degeneration (Fig. 7–16). Malignant tumors may invade surrounding structures or large veins and weigh up to 800 g (Fig. 7–17).

Microscopically, tumor cells form nests ("zellballen"), cords, ribbons, or sheets (Fig. 7–18). Cells are round or polygonal, with plentiful cytoplasm that may be lightly eosinophilic, basophilic, purple, or lavender (Fig. 7–19). Intracytoplasmic "hyaline globules" are often noted. Nuclei are usually round to oval with small nucleoli. Marked nuclear atypia and hyperchromasia, focal necrosis, and increased mitotic activity are noted in some tumors (Fig. 7–20). Nuclear atypia is not predictive of malignant behavior, however.

Up to 14% of pheochromocytomas are malignant. The incidence of maligancy is low in children and higher in extra-adrenal intra-abdominal paraganglioma.

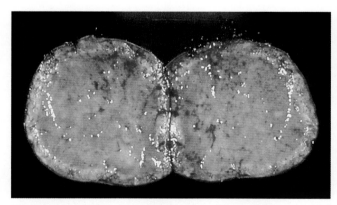

FIGURE 7–16 ||| Pheochromocytoma. The medulla is expanded by the neoplasm, which is surrounded by residual normal golden-yellow cortex.

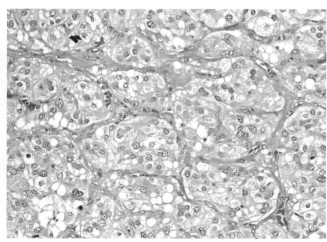

FIGURE 7–18 ||| Pheochromocytoma. Tumor cells arranged in nests ("zellballen").

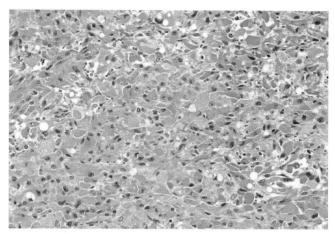

FIGURE 7–19 I▋II Pheochromocytoma. Tumor cells arranged in a sheet. Cytoplasmic staining is variable; in this example, the cytoplasm is darkly basophilic.

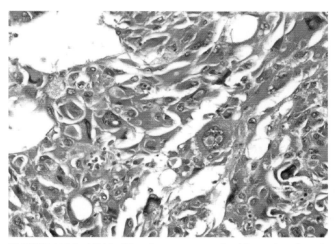

FIGURE 7–20 I▋II Pheochromocytoma. In this section there is marked nuclear atypia, a finding that is often noted in pheochromocytoma. This finding in pheochromocytoma is not independently predictive of malignant behavior.

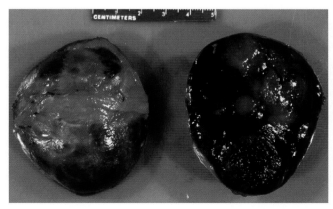

FIGURE 7–21 I▋II Neuroblastoma. Tumor is diffusely hemorrhagic, with a focus of necrosis and punctate calcification.

Features associated with malignancy include large size, local invasion, coarse tumor nodularity, mitotic activity, widespread necrosis, and lack of intracellular hyaline globules. Documentation of metastatic tumor is proof of malignancy.

Extra-adrenal intra-abdominal paraganglioma arises close to the adrenal, renal hilum, infrarenal aorta, iliac vessels, and urinary bladder. It may also arise in kidney, urethra, prostate gland, or spermatic cord. Most are solitary, and most occur in patients between 20 and 50 years old, with about equal gender distribution.

Average size is about 10 cm. The pathologic findings are indistinguishable from those of adrenal paraganglioma (pheochromocytoma). Up to 50% are malignant.

Urinary bladder paraganglioma occurs with about equal frequency in men and women, with an average age of 41 years. Symptoms include headache and sweating associated with voiding, sustained or intermittent hypertension, and intermittent gross hematuria. Most bladder paragangliomas are located in the trigone, and most are solitary. Tumors are usually less than 2 cm in diameter. The pathologic findings are similar to those of paraganglioma elsewhere. Up to 14% are malignant.

NEUROBLASTOMA AND GANGLIONEUROBLASTOMA

These neoplasms are derived from neuroblasts of the sympathetic nervous system. They differ from one another in that ganglioneuroblastoma has a component of ganglion cells and sometimes Schwann cells.

Neuroblastoma and ganglioneuroblastoma collectively are the fourth most common malignancy in childhood. Most occur in patients younger than 4 years old (median age 2 years) and are rare in patients more than 10 years old. Males and females are equally affected. The adrenal is the most common site of origin (38%), followed by extra-adrenal abdominal sites (30%). Other primary sites include the thorax, neck, and pelvis. "In situ neuroblastoma" in the adrenal is common in infancy, but most of these lesions (and a small number of fully developed neuroblastomas) regress or mature spontaneously.

Neuroblastoma usually forms a solitary circumscribed ovoid or multinodular mass, which may be more than 10 cm in diameter (Fig. 7–21). It may invade local structures or large veins. It is a soft, bulging, gray-white to tan tumor with a variable degree of hemorrhage, necrosis, and cystic degeneration.

Neuroblastoma is composed of sheets of "small round blue cells" with minimal cytoplasm (Fig. 7–22). Neuronal processes impart a pale pink fibrillar background (Fig. 7–23). Discrete clusters of neuronal processes surrounded by tumor cells produce distinctive "Homer Wright rosettes" (Fig. 7–24). Nuclei are round and fairly uniform, with inconspicuous nucleoli and stippled chromatin. Most tumors show stromal hemorrhage, necrosis, and dystrophic calcification.

Ganglioneuroblastoma also presents as an ovoid or multinodular mass (Figs. 7–25 and 7–26). In addition to the findings noted earlier, it contains ganglion cells with eccentrically located large nuclei, prominent nucleoli and

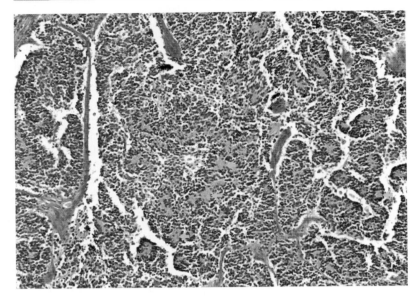

FIGURE 7–22 ▏▌▏▏ Neuroblastoma. Sheets of small dark blue cells, intersected by fibrous strands. Numerous Homer Wright rosettes are present *(yellow arrows).*

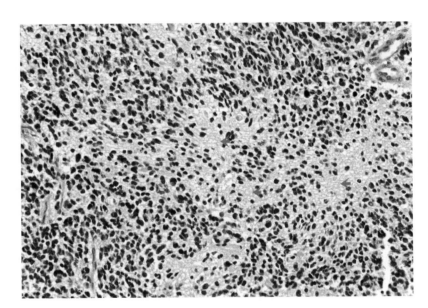

FIGURE 7–23 ▏▌▏▏ Neuroblastoma. The filamentous background consists of neurofibrillary strands, collectively called "neuropil" *(red arrows).*

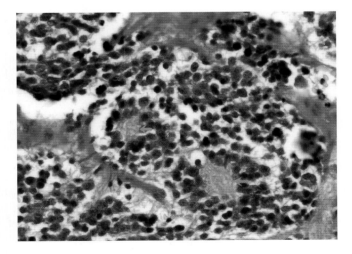

FIGURE 7–24 ▏▌▏▏ Homer Wright rosettes in neuroblastoma, consisting of small aggregates of neuropil surrounded by tumor cells *(green arrows).*

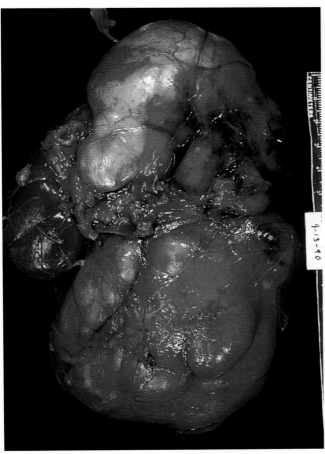

FIGURE 7–25   ▮▮▮   Ganglioneuroblastoma. This large multinodular tumor dwarfs the adjacent kidney, visible on the left. (Courtesy of Beverly Dahms, MD, Cleveland, OH.)

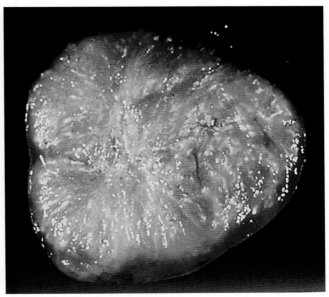

FIGURE 7–26   ▮▮▮   Cut surface of ganglioneuroblastoma. Necrosis is present but limited in distribution.

copious dark eosinophilic cytoplasm, and cells with schwannian differentiation (Figs. 7–27 and 7–28).

Prognosis for neuroblastoma and ganglioneuroblastoma is linked to age at diagnosis, microscopic findings, and tumor stage. Prognostic algorithms have been developed, and patients are assigned to "low-risk" or "high-risk" groups for treatment purposes. The details of these risk assessment protocols are available elsewhere. Several staging systems have been proposed for neuroblastoma.

FIGURE 7–27   ▮▮▮   Ganglioneuroblastoma. On the right, small clusters of neuroblastoma cells are present *(green arrows)*. On the left is a small aggregate of mature ganglion cells *(black arrows)*, surrounded by spindly cells with schwannian differentiation *(yellow arrows)*.

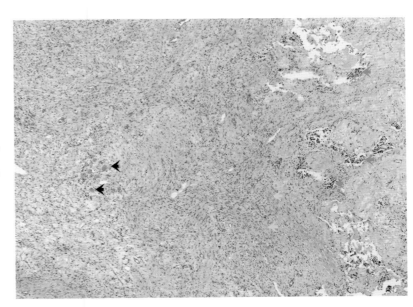

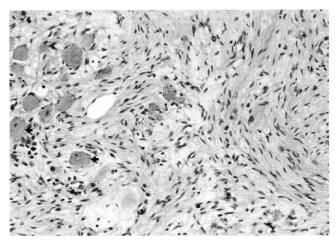

FIGURE 7–28 ▮▊▮▮ Ganglioneuroblastoma. Ganglion cells are on the left *(black arrows)*, and spindly schwannian cells are on the right.

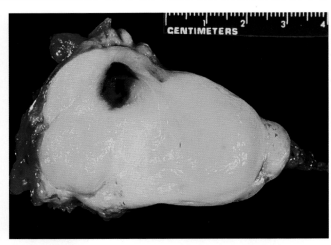

FIGURE 7–29 ▮▊▮▮ Ganglioneuroma. An area of cystic degeneration is present. (Courtesy of Beverly Dahms, MD, Cleveland, OH.)

The International Staging System is presented in Table 7–2 in abbreviated form.

TABLE 7–2
INTERNATIONAL STAGING SYSTEM FOR NEUROBLASTOMA

Stage I	Localized tumor, completely excised, ipsilateral and contralateral lymph nodes negative
Stage IIA	Unilateral tumor, incompletely excised, ipsilateral and contralateral lymph nodes negative
Stage IIB	Unilateral tumor, completely or incompletely excised, positive ipsilateral lymph nodes, negative contralateral lymph nodes
Stage III	Tumor crosses midline, with or without lymph node metastases; or unilateral tumor with contralateral lymph nodes positive
Stage IV	Tumor metastases to distant lymph nodes or other distant sites, except as defined in stage IV-S
Stage IV-S	Unilateral tumor, completely or incompletely excised, ipsilateral and contralateral lymph nodes negative, with metastases limited to liver, skin, and/or bone marrow

From Lack EE: Atlas of Tumor Pathology, Third Series, Fascicle 19. Tumors of the Adrenal Gland and Extra-Adrenal Paraganglia. Washington, DC, Armed Forces Institute of Pathology.

Assessment of cytogenetic alterations has provided much useful prognostic information in neuroblastoma. *NMYC* amplification, chromosome 1 copy number, 1p deletion, and DNA ploidy are examples of prognostic parameters that are being used to stratify patients into therapeutic protocols.

GANGLIONEUROMA

This is a benign neural neoplasm. Most occur in patients older than age 7 years, usually in the posterior mediastinum or retroperitoneum and infrequently in the adrenal. Some represent maturation of preexisting neuroblastoma, but the majority arise de novo.

Ganglioneuroma is typically smooth, gray-white or tan-yellow, well circumscribed, and rubbery, averaging about 8 cm in diameter (Fig. 7–29). It is composed of ganglion cells and Schwann cells in varying proportions. Schwann cells form intersecting fascicles, often in a loose myxoid stroma. Necrosis, mitotic figures, and cellular atypia are absent.

OTHER TUMORS OF THE ADRENALS

MYELOLIPOMA

Myelolipoma is a benign tumor predominantly occurring in the adrenal in patients averaging 50 years of age. Most are discovered incidentally. Side and gender distribution are about equal. Myelolipoma may originate as an embryonal rest of hematopoietic tissue or may represent metaplasia of cortical or stromal cells.

Myelolipoma is usually unilateral and solitary, varying in size up to 34 cm and weighing up to 5900 g. It is smooth, well circumscribed, and yellow to red-brown, depending on the amount of adipose or myeloid tissue present (Fig. 7–30). Microscopically, it is composed of mature adipose tissue and hematopoietic tissue, including myeloid and erythroid cells and megakaryocytes (trilinear hematopoiesis) (Fig. 7–31). Trabeculae of bone may be present.

RARE AND UNUSUAL PRIMARY ADRENAL NEOPLASMS

Tumors rarely arising in the adrenal include melanoma, lymphoma, adenomatoid tumor, gonadal stromal tumor, primitive neuroectodermal tumor, nephroblastoma, and a variety of benign and malignant soft tissue tumors (Fig. 7–32). These tumors are morphologically and biologically similar to their counterparts in more traditional sites.

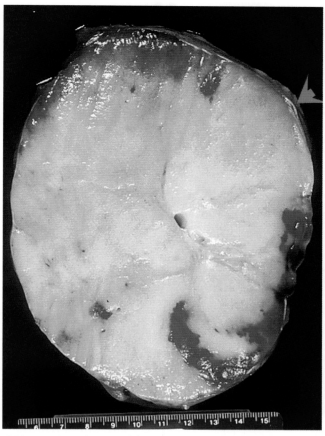

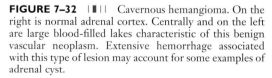

FIGURE 7–30   Myelolipoma. Tumor resembles mature fat with focal hemorrhage. A thin rim of adrenal cortex is visible at the periphery of the tumor *(arrow)*.

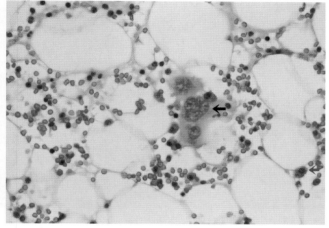

FIGURE 7–31   Myelolipoma. Mature fat cells predominate. Located centrally are megakaryocytes with multilobed nuclei *(black arrow)*. Other hematopoietic precursor cells are also present *(blue arrow)*.

FIGURE 7–32   Cavernous hemangioma. On the right is normal adrenal cortex. Centrally and on the left are large blood-filled lakes characteristic of this benign vascular neoplasm. Extensive hemorrhage associated with this type of lesion may account for some examples of adrenal cyst.

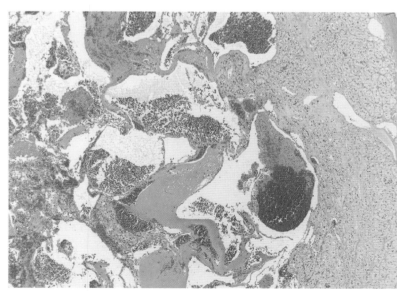

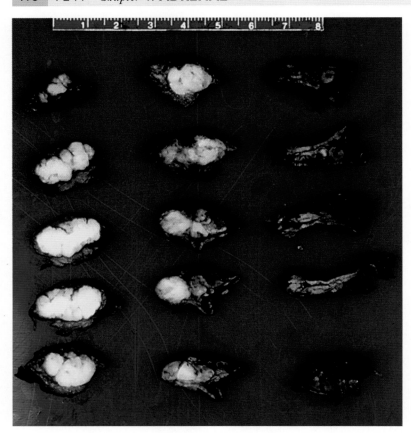

FIGURE 7–33 ▐▮▐▐ Adrenal metastasis of mixed germ cell tumor of testis. The adrenal mass lesion persisted after chemotherapy, prompting adrenalectomy. No residual viable germ cell tumor was identified microscopically.

ADRENAL METASTASES

The most common adrenal tumor is metastatic cancer from another site. Adrenal metastases are noted in about one fourth of patients dying of carcinoma. The three most common primary sites are breast, lung, and kidney. Adrenal metastases are bilateral in 40% of cases. The adrenals are also involved secondarily in up to 25% of cases of systemic lymphoma. Sarcomas rarely metastasize to the adrenals.

Adrenal metastases lack the orange-yellow color typical of cortical neoplasms (Figs. 7–33 and 7–34). Metastatic melanoma may appear brown or black. Metastases from lung, liver, or kidney may simulate cortical carcinoma microscopically.

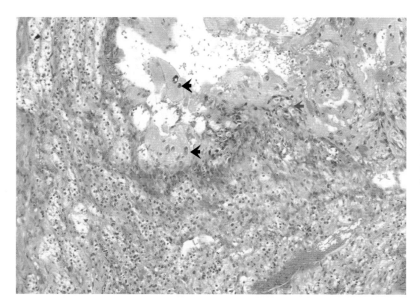

FIGURE 7–34 ▐▮▐▐ Adrenal metastasis of testicular choriocarcinoma. A blood-filled space is present centrally at the top; at its periphery are cytotrophoblasts (*blue arrow*) and multinucleated syncytiotrophoblasts (*black arrows*), cells characteristic of this cancer.

Selected References

Bostwick DG, Dundore PA. Biopsy Pathology of the Prostate. London: Chapman and Hall Medical, 1997.

Bostwick DG, Eble JN. Urologic Surgical Pathology. St. Louis: Mosby-Yearbook, 1997

Bostwick DG, Lopez-Beltran A. Bladder Biopsy Interpretation. New York: United Pathologists Press, 1999.

Foster CS, Bostwick DG. Pathology of the Prostate. Philadelphia: W. B. Saunders Co., 1998.

Lack EE. Atlas of Tumor Pathology, Third Series, Fascicle 19. Tumors of the Adrenal Gland and Extra-Adrenal Paraganglia. Washington, D.C.: Armed Forces Institute of Pathology, 1997.

Ro JY, Grignon DJ, Amin MB, Ayala A. Atlas of Surgical Pathology of the Male Reproductive Tract. Philadelphia: W. B. Saunders Co., 1997.

Ulbright TM, Amin MB, Young RH. Atlas of Tumor Pathology, Third Series, Fascicle 25. Tumors of the Testis, Adnexa, Spermatic Cord, and Scrotum. Washington, D.C.: Armed Forces Institute of Pathology, 1999.

Young RH, Srigley JR, Amin MB, Ulbright TM, Cubilla AL. Atlas of Tumor Pathology, Third Series, Fascicle 28. Tumors of the Prostate Gland, Seminal Vesicles, Male Urethra, and Penis. Washington, D.C.: Armed Forces Institute of Pathology, 2000.

Index

Note: Page numbers followed by f refer to figures; those followed by t refer to tables.

A

Abscess(es)
  adrenal, 186
  testicular, in bacterial orchitis, 126, 126f
Acquired immunodeficiency syndrome
      (AIDS), epididymitis with, 156
ACTH
  in adrenal cortical hyperplasia, 188
  in adrenogenital syndrome, 124
Adenocarcinoma
  bladder, 63, 63f, 64f
    clear cell, 63, 64f
    enteric type, 63, 63f
    mixed, 63
    mucinous, 63, 63f
    signet-ring, 63, 63f
  epididymal, 164
  of renal pelvis or ureter, 79
  of seminal vesicles, 119, 120f
  prostate, 98–102, 99f–105f
    atrophic pattern of, 110, 110f
    cancer volume and, 115
    detected by prostate-specific antigen, 114
    DNA ploidy and, 115
    extraprostatic extension of, 113, 114f
    genetic instability in, 115
    Gleason grading of, 102f–105f, 102–103,
        105
    gross pathology of, 98–99, 99f
    histologic variants of, 105f–110f, 105–110
    immunohistochemistry of, 101f,
        101–102, 102f
    location of, 115
    lymph node metastases in, 113
    microscopic features of, 99, 100f, 101f
    perineural invasion of, 99, 101f, 115
    positive surgical margins and, 114–115
    predictive factors in, 113–115, 114f, 114t
    staging of, 114t
    treatment changes in, 111–113, 112f, 113f
    "vanishing cancer" phenomenon in, 112,
        115
    vascular/lymphatic invasion of, 99, 101f,
        115
    with neuroendocrine differentiation, 107,
        108f
    with vaculolated cytoplasm, 106–107,
        107f
  urachal, 63–64, 64f
  urethral, 73, 74f
    clear cell, 74f
  urothelial, 79
Adenofibroma, nephrogenic, 12–13
Adenoid cystic/basal cell carcinoma, of
      prostate, 109–110, 110f
Adenoma
  adrenal cortical, 189f, 189–190, 190f
    black, 189
    vs. adrenal cortical carcinoma, 190–191

Adenoma (Continued)
    with hyperaldosteronism, 189–190, 190f
    with hypercortisolism, 189, 189f, 190f
  basal cell, of prostate, 92–93, 93f
  metanephric, 12, 13f
  renal, 11, 11f
  villous, of bladder, 50, 51f
Adenomatoid tumor, paratesticular, 160, 160f
Adenosis, of prostate
  atypical, 93–94, 94f
  sclerosing, 94–95, 95f
Adenosquamous carcinoma, of prostate, 108,
      109f
Adrenal gland
  anatomy and histology of, 185, 185f
  cortex of
    adenoma of, 189f, 189–190, 190f
    carcinoma of, 190f, 190–191, 191f, 191t
    disorders of, 187f–191f, 187–191
    heterotopic tissue of, 153, 153f, 186, 186f
    hyperplasia of, 187f, 187–188, 188f
  cysts of, 186, 186f
  global disorders of, 186f, 186–187, 187f
  hematoma of, 187
  hemorrhage and, 187, 187f
  heterotopia of, 153, 153f, 186, 186f
  infection of, 186, 187f
  medulla of
    disorders of, 191–196, 192f–196f
    ganglioneuroblastoma of, 193, 195, 195f,
        196f, 196t
    ganglioneuroma of, 196, 196f
    hyperplasia of, 191–192
    neuroblastoma of, 193, 193f, 194f, 195,
        196t
    pheochromocytoma of, 192f, 192–193,
        193f
  metastases to, 198, 198f
  myelolipoma of, 196, 197f
  neoplasms of, rare and unusual, 196, 197f
Adrenocortical rest(s), 186
  testicular, 122, 124
Adrenogenital syndrome, testicular "tumor"
      of, 124, 124f
Adult polycystic kidney disease, 3f, 3–4, 4f
Aldosteronoma, 190f, 189–190
Amyloidosis
  of bladder, 49, 49f
  of seminal vesicles, 118, 119f
  of urethra, 73
Anaplasia, in Wilms' tumor, 29, 29f
Androgen deprivation therapy, for prostatic
      adenocarcinoma, 111–112, 112f
Androgen insensitivity syndrome, Sertoli cell
      tumor and, 142
Angiomyolipoma, renal, 24, 24f, 25f
Angiosarcoma, of bladder, 67, 68f
Appendix epididymis, 151f, 153
  torsion of, 159

Appendix testis, 151f, 153
  torsion of, 159
Atrophic carcinoma, of prostate, 110, 110f
Atrophy, prostatic, 89, 90f, 91, 91f
Atypical adenomatous hyperplasia, of prostate,
      93–94, 94f

B

Bacille Calmette-Guérin
  granulomatous cystitis and, 42, 42f
  granulomatous prostatitis and, 85–86, 86
Bacterial prostatitis, acute, 84, 85f
Balanitis
  plasma cell, 168, 169f
  Zoon's, 168, 169f
Balanitis xerotica obliterans, 168–169, 169f
Basal cell adenoma, of prostate, 92–93, 93f
Basal cell carcinoma
  penile, 179, 179f
  scrotal, 182–183
Basal cell hyperplasia, of prostate, 91–93, 92f
  atypical, 93, 93f
Basal cell/adenoid cystic carcinoma, of
      prostate, 109–110, 110f
Basaloid carcinoma, of penis, 178
Bellini's ducts, 1
Benign prostatic hyperplasia, 88–89, 89f, 90f
Black adenoma, 189
Bladder
  adenocarcinoma of, urachal and
      nonurachal, 63f, 63–64, 64f
  anatomy and histology of, 33–34, 34f
  benign lesions of, 48–50, 49f–51f, 65f,
      65–66
  carcinoma in situ of, 51–53, 52f, 53f
  carcinoma of, 53f–62f, 53–63
  congenital anomalies of, 34, 35f–37f, 37
  exstrophy of, 37, 37f
  granular cell tumor of, 66
  hemangioma of, 66
  inflammatory conditions of
    miscellaneous, 43, 43f–46f, 45
    reactive, 37–43, 38f–43f, 45, 46f
    urothelial hyperplasia and, 45, 46f
  leiomyoma of, 65, 65f
  leukemia of, 69
  lymphoma of, 67–68, 69f
  melanoma of, 69, 69f, 70f
  metastases to, 70
  neoplasm(s) of
    adenocarcinoma as, 63f, 63–64, 64f
    hematopoietic malignant, 67–69, 69f
    miscellaneous, 69f, 69–70, 70f
    sarcomas as, 66f, 66–67, 67f
    soft tissue, benign, 65f, 65–66
    urothelial, 51f–62f, 51–63
  neurofibroma of, 66
  pheochromocytoma (paraganglioma) of,
      69–70, 70f, 193

Bladder *(Continued)*
    plasmacytoma of, 69
    urothelial changes in, 45, 46f–48f, 47
Blastema, in Wilms' tumor, 28f, 29
Bone-metastasizing renal tumor, of childhood,
        31, 31f
Bowenoid papulosis, 175–176, 176f
Bowen's disease, 174
Buboes, lymph node, in lymphogranuloma
        venereum, 172
Buck's fascia, 167, 168f

C
Calcification
    in chronic epididymitis, 156
    in large cell Sertoli cell tumor, 145, 145f
    in paratesticular region, 159, 159f
    of seminal vesicles, 119
Calcinosis, scrotal, idiopathic, 182, 182f
Calculus formation, in paratesticular region, 159
Calyx, renal, 1, 2f
Carcinoembryonic antigen reactivity, in ductal
        carcinoma, 105
Carcinoid tumor
    prostate, 107–108, 108f
    renal, 23, 23f
Carcinoma
    of adrenal cortex, 190f, 190–191, 191f
        staging of, 191t
        vs. adrenal cortical adenoma, 190–191
    of rete testis, 146, 147f
    of ureter or renal pelvis, 77f, 77–78, 78f
Carcinoma in situ
    bladder, 51–53, 52f, 53f
    squamous cell, penile, 174–176, 175f, 176f
    urothelial, 51–53, 52f, 53f, 77, 77f
Carcinosarcoma, of prostate, 109, 109f, 110f
Carney's syndrome, Sertoli cell tumor and,
        142, 145
Caruncle, urethral, 72, 72f
Caseous necrosis, in renal tuberculosis, 11, 11f
Chancre, syphilitic, 171–172, 172f
Chancroid, 172
Children
    renal tumors in, 27–32, 28f–32f
    rhabdomyosarcoma in, 66f, 66–67, 67f,
        162–163
Chlamydia trachomatis
    epididymitis due to, 156
    in lymphogranuloma venereum, 172
Cholesteatoma, 76
Choriocarcinoma, 138–139, 139f
    testicular, adrenal metastases of, 198f
Chromaffin cells, 192
Chromophobe renal cell carcinoma, 19–20, 20f
Clear cell adenocarcinoma
    bladder, 63, 64f
    urethral, 74f
Clear cell cribriform hyperplasia, of prostate,
        92, 92f
Clear cell renal cell carcinoma
    classification of, 14
    conventional, 14f, 14–15, 15f
    Fuhrman Nuclear Grading System for, 15,
        16f
    multilocular cystic, 15, 18f
Clear cell sarcoma, of kidney, 31, 31f
Collecting duct carcinoma, 20–21, 21f, 22f
    low-grade, 21, 21f, 22f
Colloid carcinoma, of prostate, 106, 106f
Condyloma acuminatum, 172f, 172–173, 173f
    urethral, 73
Cortical hyperplasia
    diffuse and nodular, 187f, 187–188, 188f
    with hypercortisolism, 188

Corticotropin-releasing factor, ectopic
        production of, 188
Cortisol, excess
    adrenal cortical adenoma with, 189, 189f,
        190f
    adrenal cortical hyperplasia with, 188–189
Cowper's glands, histology of, 83, 84f
Cribriform hyperplasia, of prostate, 92, 92f
Cryoablation therapy, for prostatic
        adenocarcinoma, pathologic
        interpretation of, 113, 113f
Cryptorchidism, testis in, 129, 130f
Crystalloids, of prostatic adenocarcinoma, 99,
        100f
Cushing's disease, 188
Cyclophosphamide, hemorrhagic cystitis due
        to, 39, 39f
Cyst(s)
    adrenal, 186, 186f
    dermoid, 137–138
        of paratesticular region and spermatic
            cord, 155
    epidermoid
        of paratesticular region, 155
        of penis, 173, 174f
        of testis, 124, 125f
    epididymal, 154, 154f
        acquired (spermatocele), 155, 155f
    in acquired cystic kidney disease, 6, 6f
    in polycystic kidney disease, 3f, 3–4, 4f
    in renal multicystic dysplastic conditions, 5,
        5f
    meatal, urethral, 72, 73f
    median raphe, 174, 174f
    mesothelial, of paratesticular region, 155
    mucous, 173
    penile, 173–174, 174f
    prostate, 95–96, 96f
    seminal vesicle, 119
    simple cortical, of kidney, 7, 7f
    urachal
        blind, 36f, 37
        classification of, 36f
Cystadenoma, papillary, of epididymis,
        160–161, 161f
Cystic fibrosis, testicular adnexae involvement
        in, 154
Cystic nephroma, 13, 13f, 14f
Cystic partially differentiated
        nephroblastoma, 29, 29f
Cystitis, 37
    acute, 39
    bullous, 40
    chronic, 39f, 39–40, 40f
        reactive urothelial changes in, 45
        squamous metaplasia and, 47
    denuding, 53
    emphysematous, 39
    encrusted, 40, 40f
    eosinophilic, 44f, 45
    follicular, 39, 39f
    granulomatous, 41–43, 42, 43f
    hemorrhagic, due to cyclophosphamide
        therapy, 39, 39f
    interstitial, of bladder, 43, 43f, 45
    papillary-polypoid, 40, 40f
    radiation, 43, 44f, 45
    tuberculous, 41
Cystitis cystica, 37, 38f
Cystitis glandularis
    intestinal, 38, 38f
    typical, 37–38, 38f
Cystosarcoma phyllodes, of prostate,
        116–117, 118f
Cytomegalovirus, epididymitis with, 156

D
Dermoid cyst, 137–138
    of paratesticular region and spermatic cord,
        155
Dialysis, acquired cystic kidney disease and, 6,
        6f
Diverticulum
    paraureteral, 75
    ureteral, 75, 75f
    urethral, 71f, 71–72, 72f
DNA ploidy, in prostate cancer, 115
Donovan bodies, 172
Donovanosis, 172
Ductal (endometrioid) adenocarcinoma, of
        prostate, 105f, 105–106, 106f
Ductus deferens, anatomy of, 152–153
Dysplasia, severe, of penis, 174

E
Ectopic kidney. *See also* Kidney.
    crossed, 2
    simple (inferior), 2
    superior, 2
Ectopic prostate, 48, 120. *See also* Prostate.
Efferent ductule(s)
    anatomy of, 151f, 152, 152f
    spermatocele of, 155, 155f
Embryonal carcinoma, of testis, 133–135,
        134f, 135f
Embryonic remnants, torsion of, 159
Endocervicosis, of bladder, 49–50, 50f
Endodermal sinus tumors, of testis, 135, 135f,
        136f
Endometrioid carcinoma, of prostate, 105,
        105f, 106, 106f
Endometriosis, bladder involvement in, 49, 50f
Endothelial cysts, adrenal, 186
Eosinophilic cystitis, 44f, 45
Epidermoid cyst
    of paratesticular region, 155
    of penis, 173, 174f
    of testis, 124, 125f
Epididymal cyst, 154, 154f
    acquired (spermatocele), 155, 155f
Epididymis
    adenocarcinoma of, 164
    adenomatoid tumor of, 160, 160f
    anatomy of, 152
    inflammatory and fibrous pseudotumor of,
        161–162, 162f
    papillary cystadenoma of, 160–161, 161f
Epididymitis
    acute, 156, 156f
    bacterial, 125, 126f
    bacterial vs. chlamydial, 156, 157t
    chronic, 156–157, 157f
    viral, 156
    xanthogranulomatous, 156
Epididymitis nodosa, 156
Epididymo-orchitis
    granulomatous, 127, 127f
    tuberculous, 127, 127f
    viral, 126–127
Epithelium
    prostatic, 81, 82f
    renal neoplasms of
        benign, 11f–14f, 11–13
        malignant, 14f–22f, 14–21. *See also* Renal
            cell carcinoma.
Erythroplasia of Queyrat, 174
Exstrophy, bladder, 37, 37f

F
Fat necrosis, scrotal, 182
Ferrein, medullary rays of, 1, 1f

Fibroepithelial polyp, 48, 79, 79f
Fibroma
    of prostate, 115
    paratesticular, 161
Fibrosarcoma, paratesticular, 163
Fibrosis, nonspecific paratesticular, 161
Fibrous histiocytoma, malignant,
        paratesticular, 163
Fibrous histiosarcoma, malignant, of bladder,
        67, 68f
Fibrous pseudotumor, paratesticular, 161–162,
        162f
Foamy gland carcinoma, of prostate, 106–107,
        107f
Foreskin
    balanitis xerotica obliterans of, 168–169,
        169f
Fungi, chronic epididymitis due to, 157
Funiculitis, 158

G
Ganglioneuroblastoma, 193, 195, 195f, 196f
    staging of, 196t
Ganglioneuroma, 196, 196f
Genetic instability, in prostate cancer, 115
Germ cell(s), primordial, 121, 122f
Germ cell aplasia, testis in, 129, 129f
Germ cell neoplasm(s)
    histiogenesis of, 131
    incidence of, 129
    intratubular, 131–140
        choriocarcinoma as, 138–139, 139f
            adrenal metastases of, 198f
        embryonal carcinoma as, 133–135, 134f,
            135f
        embryonal type with, 132, 132f
        endodermal sinus tumor as, 135, 135f,
            136f
        extragonadal, 139–140, 140f
        histiogenesis of, 131
        mixed, 139, 139f, 140f
            adrenal metastases of, 198f
        paratesticular, 164
        regressed ("burnt-out") testicular,
            139–140, 140f, 141f
        seminoma as, 132–133, 133f, 134f
        teratoma as
            immature, 137, 137f, 138f
            in adults, 135, 137f, 137–138, 138f
            in prepubertal males, 142
        unclassified, 131–132, 132f
        with no invasive component, 131–132
        yolk sac tumor as, 135, 135f, 136f
            in prepubertal males, 141–142
    non-intratubular, 140–142
    paratesticular, 164
    risk factors for, 129, 131
    spermatocytic seminoma as, 140–141, 141f
    staging of, 131t
Glans penis. *See also* Penis.
    anatomy and histology of, 167, 167f
    balanitis xerotica obliterans of, 168–169, 169f
Gleason grading system, of prostatic
        adenocarcinoma, 102f–105f,
        102–103, 105
Glomerulus(i), of kidney, 1, 1f, 2f
Gonadal stromal tumor, 162
Gonadoblastoma, 146, 146f
Gonocytes, 121
Granular cell tumor, bladder, 66
Granulation tissue, in xanthogranulomatous
        pyelonephrosis, 9
Granuloma(s)
    bladder, postsurgical, 42f, 42–43, 43f
    in testicular sarcoidosis, 127, 128f

Granuloma(s) *(Continued)*
    meconium, 158–159
    sperm, 157, 158f
    tuberculous, of testis, 127, 127f
Granuloma inguinale, penile ulcers with, 172
Granulomatous cystitis, 41–43, 42f–43f
    iatrogenic, 42, 42f
Granulomatous inflammation, chronic
        epididymitis and, 157
Granulomatous orchitis, idiopathic, 127, 127f,
        128f
Granulomatous prostatitis, 85f–87f, 85–86
    bacille Calmette-Guérin-induced, 85–86,
        86f
    idiopathic, 85, 85f
    infectious, 86
    other forms of, 86, 87f
    postsurgical, 86, 87f

H
Hemangioma
    bladder, 66
    cavernous, of adrenal, 197f
    renal, 25–26
    scrotal, 184f
    testicular, 148f
Hematocele, 154, 155f
Hematoma, adrenal, 187
Hematopoietic tumors
    bladder, 67–69, 69f
    paratesticular, 164–165
    penile, 180f, 181
    testicular, 146–147, 147f, 148f
Hemorrhage
    adrenal involvement in, 187, 187f
    renal angiomyolipoma and, 24
    testicular, 125
Hemorrhagic cystitis, due to
        cyclophosphamide therapy, 39, 39f
Herpes simplex virus, penile ulcers with,
        170–171, 171f
Hidradenitis suppurativa, 181, 182f
Histiocytoma, malignant fibrous
    paratesticular, 163
    renal, 27
HMB45, immunostaining for
    in bladder melanoma, 69
    in renal angiomyolipoma, 24, 27
Homer Wright rosettes, 193, 194f
Hot water balloon thermotherapy, for
        prostatic adenocarcinoma,
        pathologic interpretation of, 113
Hunner's ulcer, of bladder, 43, 43f
Hydatid of Morgagni, 153
Hydrocele, 154, 155f
    well-differentiated papillary mesothelioma
        and, 160, 160f
Hyperaldosteronism, adrenal cortical
        adenoma with, 189–190, 190f
Hypercortisolism
    adrenal cortical adenoma and, 189, 189f,
        190f
    adrenal cortical hyperplasia with, 188
Hyperplasia
    of adrenal cortex, 187f, 187–188, 188f
    of adrenal medulla, 191–192
    of prostate, 88–95, 89f–96f. *See also*
        Prostate, hyperplasia of.
    urothelial, 45, 46f
Hyperthermia
    microwave, for prostatic adenocarcinoma,
        113
    ultrasound, for prostatic adenocarcinoma,
        pathologic interpretation of, 113
Hypospermatogenesis, testis in, 128, 129f

I
Immunofluorescence technique, 172
Immunohistochemistry, of prostatic
        adenocarcinoma, 101f, 101–102,
        102f
Infantile polycystic kidney disease, 4, 4f
Infection(s)
    adrenal involvement in, 186, 187f
    bladder, malakoplakia and, 40, 40f, 41f
    penile nodules and warty lesions related to,
        172f–174f, 172–173
    penile ulceration related to, 170f, 170–172,
        171f
Infertility, testes in, 127–129, 129f
Inflammatory disorders
    of kidney, 7f–11f, 7–11
    of paratesticular region, 156–159
    of penis, 168–170, 169f, 170f
    of prostate, 83–86, 84f–87f
    of prostatic urethra, 120
    of scrotum, meconium-induced, 158–159
    of spermatic cord, 158
Inflammatory myofibroblastic tumor, of
        prostate, 115–116
Inflammatory pseudotumor
    of bladder, 45, 46f
    of paratesticular region, 161–162
    of prostate, 115–116
Interstitial cell tumor, renomedullary, 25, 25f
Interstitial cystitis, 43, 43f, 45
Intestinal metaplasia, of bladder mucosa, 38,
        39f

J
Juxtaglomerular cell tumor (reninoma), 25,
        25f, 26f

K
Kaposi's sarcoma, penile, 180f, 181
Keratin 34bE12, immunoreactivity to
    in basal cell hyperplasia of prostate, 92, 92f
    in benign prostatic epithelium, 81, 82f
    in prostatic adenocarcinoma, 101, 101f
    in prostatic intraepithelial neoplasia, 97, 97f
    in sclerosing adenosis, 95
Keratin markers, for urothelial carcinoma, 61,
        61f
Kidney. *See also* Renal *entries.*
    absence of, 1
    anatomy of, 1, 1f
    clear cell sarcoma of, 31, 31f
    congenital disorders of, 1–3
        ectopic, 2, 153
            crossed, 2
            simple (inferior), 2
            superior, 2
        horseshoe, 2–3, 3f
        hypoplasia of, 1
        supernumerary, 2
    cystic diseases of, 3f–7f, 3–7
        acquired, 6, 6f
        dysplastic, 4f, 4–6, 5f
        hereditary, 3f, 3–4, 4f
        miscellaneous, 6f, 6–7, 7f
    duplex collecting system of, segmental
        dysplasia of, 5, 6f
    inflammatory condition(s) of, 7f–11f, 7–11
        malakoplakia as, 10
        papillary necrosis as, 7–9, 9f
        pyelonephritis as, 7f–10f, 7–8
        tuberculosis as, 10–11, 11f
    medullary sponge, 6–7
    neoplasm(s) of
        benign epithelial, 11f–14f, 11–13
        in children, 27–32, 28f–32f

Kidney (*Continued*)
malignant epithelial, 14f–22f, 14–21.
See also Renal cell carcinoma.
neuroendocrine, 23, 23f
rare, 27
soft tissue, 24f–26f, 24–27
rhabdoid tumor of, 31–32, 32f
tumors metastatic to, 27, 28f
Klinefelter's syndrome, testis in, 129, 130f

L

Lamina propria, of bladder, 33, 34f
Laser therapy, for prostatic adenocarcinoma,
pathologic interpretation of, 113
Leiomyoma
bladder, 65, 65f
paratesticular, 162, 162f
prostate, 115
renal, 26f, 26–27
ureteral or renal pelvic, 79
Leiomyosarcoma
bladder, 67f, 67–68, 68f
paratesticular, 163
prostate, 116, 117f
renal, 27
ureteral or renal pelvic, 79
Leukemia
bladder, 69
penile, 181
prostate, 118, 118f
testicular infiltrates with, 147
Leydig cell(s), 121, 122f
in cryptorchidism, 129, 130f
Leydig cell tumor, 142, 142f–144f
Lipogranuloma, of penis, 170, 170f
Lipoma
paratesticular, 159, 159f
renal, 27
Liposarcoma
spermatic cord, 162, 163f
Lymph node(s)
buboes of, in lymphogranuloma venereum,
172
in prostate cancer, 113
inguinal, metastases to, in scrotal
neoplasms, 182
Lymphangioma, renal, 26
Lymphogranuloma venereum, penile ulcers
with, 172
Lymphoma
bladder, 67–68, 69f
malignant
of prostate, 117–118, 118f
paratesticular, 164–165
penile, 180f, 181
renal, 27, 27f, 28f
testicular, 146, 147f

M

Macronodular hyperplasia
with adrenal enlargement, 188
Malakoplakia
bladder, 40, 40f, 41f
epididymal, 157
prostatic, 86, 87f
renal, 10
testicular, 126, 127f
ureteral or renal pelvic, 76
urethral, 73
Maturation arrest, testicular, 128–129, 129f
Meconium-induced inflammation, of scrotum,
158–159
Median raphe cyst, of penis, 174, 174f
Medullary sponge kidney, 6–7
Megaureter, primary, 75
Melanin-like pigment, in prostate, 81, 82f

Melanoma
bladder, 69, 69f
penile, 179, 180f, 181
urethral, 73, 74f
Melanosis, penile, 167, 168f
Mesoblastic nephroma, 29, 30f, 31
Mesonephric collecting tubule, vestigial
caudal, 153
Mesonephros, 121
Mesothelial cyst, of paratesticular region, 155
Mesothelioma
benign papillary
of tunica vaginalis, 160, 160f
malignant
paratesticular, 163–164, 164f
Mesothelium (tunica vaginalis), 121, 121f
Metaplasia
prostatic, 86, 88, 88f
prostatic urethral, 120
Metaplastic carcinoma, prostatic, 109, 109f,
110f
Metastases
from prostate, immunohistochemical
staining for, 101, 101f, 102f
to adrenal, 198, 198f
to bladder, 70
to kidney, 27, 28f
to paratesticular region, 164f, 165
to penis, 181, 181f
to renal pelvis or ureter, 79
to scrotum, 184
to testis, 148f, 148–149, 149f
Michaelis-Gutmann bodies, 10, 40, 87f
Microwave hyperthermia, for prostatic
adenocarcinoma, pathologic
interpretation of, 113
Mixed germ cell tumor, 139, 139f, 140f
Molluscum contagiosum, 173, 173f, 174f
Mucin, luminal, of prostatic adenocarcinoma,
99, 100f
Mucinous adenocarcinoma
of bladder, 63, 63f
of prostate, 106, 106f
Mucinous metaplasia, of prostate, 88, 88f
Mucous cyst, of penis, 173
Müllerian remnants, in paratesticular region,
153, 154
Multiple endocrine neoplasia (MEN)
syndromes, 191
Multiple myeloma, testicular plasmacytoma
and, 146–147, 148f
Myelolipoma, adrenal, 196, 197f
Myofibroblastic tumor
of prostate
inflammatory, 115–116
postsurgical, 115

N

Neisseria gonorrhoeae, epididymitis due to, 156
Nephroblastoma, 27, 28f, 29
cystic partially differentiated, 29, 29f
Nephrogenic adenofibroma, 12–13
Nephrogenic metaplasia
in urethral diverticulum, 71, 71f
of bladder, 47, 47f, 48f
of prostate, 88
of ureter or renal pelvis, 76
of urethra, 72, 73f
Nephrolithiasis, medullary sponge kidney
and, 6
Nephroma
cystic, 13, 13f, 14f
mesoblastic, 29, 30f, 31
Nephron, of kidney, 1
Neuroblastoma, 193, 193f, 194f, 195
staging of, 196t

Neuroectodermal tumor (extraskeletal
Ewing's sarcoma), 163
Neuroendocrine carcinoma, of prostate, 107,
108f
Neuroendocrine cells, of prostatic epithelium,
81, 82f
Neuroendocrine renal neoplasms, 23, 23f
Neurofibroma, bladder, 66
Nodular hyperplasia
of adrenal gland, 141, 141f
of prostate, 88–89, 89f, 90f
Nodule(s)
adrenal
in adrenal nodular hyperplasia, 187f,
187–188, 188f
pigmented, 188
in splenogonadal fusion, 122, 123f
in xanthogranulomatous pyelonephrosis, 9,
9f
of ectopic adrenocortical tissue, 122, 124
penile, infection-related, 172–173
postoperative spindle cell
of bladder, 45, 45f
of prostate, 115

O

Oncocytoma, 11–12, 12f
Orchitis, 125–126, 126f, 127f
bacterial, 125–127, 126f
idiopathic granulomatous, 127, 127f, 128f
syphilitic, 127
Organ of Giraldés, 154
Organ of Haller, 154

P

Paget's disease, scrotal, 183, 183f, 184f
Papilla(ae), of kidney, 1, 2f
Papillary adenoma, 11f
Papillary carcinoma, of penis, 178
Papillary cystadenoma, of epididymis,
160–161, 161f
Papillary mesothelioma, well-differentiated, of
tunica vaginalis, 160, 160f
Papillary necrosis, of kidney, 9, 9f
Papillary renal cell carcinoma, 18f, 18–19, 19f
Papillary urothelial carcinoma, 54–56
grade 1, 55f, 56, 56f
grade 2, 55f, 56–57, 57f
grade 3, 57f, 57–58, 58f
staging of, 58, 58f, 58t, 59f
Papilloma, urothelial, 53f, 53–54, 54f, 77
inverted, 54, 54f, 55f, 77
Paradidymis, 54
Paraganglioma (pheochromocytoma)
extra-adrenal, 192f, 192–193, 193f
intra-abdominal, 193
urinary bladder, 69–70, 70f, 193
of prostate, 116, 116f
Paraganglionic cells, 192
Paratesticular region. *See also* Epididymis;
Spermatic cord; Tunics, testicular.
anatomy of, 151f, 151–153, 152f
congenital anomalies of, 153f, 153–154, 154f
embryology of, 151, 151f
metastases of, 164f, 165
neoplasms of, 159–165
benign, 159f–162f, 159–162
malignant, 162–165, 163f, 164f
pseudotumors in, 159–162
non-neoplastic diseases of, 154–159
calculi and calcification of, 159
celes and cysts of, 154–156
inflammatory and reactive diseases of,
156–159
torsion of embryonic remnants and, 159
Paraureteral diverticulum, 75

Penis
  anatomy and histology of, 167, 167f, 168f
  cysts of, 173–174, 174f
  inflammatory disorders of, 168–170, 169f, 170f
  melanosis of, 167, 168f
  neoplasm(s) of
    basal cell carcinoma as, 179, 179f
    hematopoietic, 180f, 181
    leukemia as, 181
    lymphoma as, 180f, 181, 181f
    melanoma as, 179, 180f, 181
    metastatic to, 181, 181f
    rare, 179, 179f–181f, 181
    sarcoma as, 180f, 181
    squamous cell carcinoma as, 176f–178f, 176–179
    squamous cell carcinoma in situ as, 174–176, 175f, 176f
  nodules and warty lesions of
    infection-related, 172f–174f, 172–173
  ulceration of, infection-related, 170f, 170–172, 171f
Periorchitis
  chronic, 161
  meconium, 159
  nodular fibrous, 161
  pseudofibromatous, 161
  reactive, 161
Peutz-Jeghers syndrome, Sertoli cell tumor and, 142
Peyronie's disease, 169–170, 170f
Pheochromocytoma (paraganglioma)
  bladder, 69–70, 70f
  extra-adrenal, 192f, 192–193, 193f
  prostate, 116, 116f
Phyllodes tumor, of prostate, 116–117, 118f
Placental-like alkaline phosphatase, 132, 132f
Plasma cell balanitis, 168, 169f
Plasmacytoma
  bladder, 69
  testicular, 146–147, 148f
Polycystic kidney disease
  adult, 3f, 3–4, 4f
  infantile, 4, 4f
Polyp(s)
  benign, with prostatic-type epithelium, 120
  fibroepithelial
    bladder, 48
    ureteral, 79, 79f
    prostatic, 70, 71f
    urethral, 120
    congenital, 70, 71f
Postatrophic hyperplasia, of prostate, 91, 91f
Postoperative spindle cell nodule
  of bladder, 45, 45f
  of prostate, 115
Postsclerotic hyperplasia, of prostate, 89, 91, 91f
Postsurgical myofibroblastic tumor, of prostate, 115
Priapism, in penile metastases, 181
Primary megaureter, 75
Primary pigmented adrenocortical disease, 188–189
Prostate
  adenocarcinoma of, 98–102, 99f–105f
    extraprostatic extension of, 113, 114f
    grading of, 102f–105f, 102–103, 105
    histologic variants of, 105f–110f, 105–110
    predictive factors in, 113–115, 114f, 114t
    staging of, 114t
    treatment changes in, 111–113, 112f, 113f
  atrophy of, 89, 90f, 91, 91f
  atypical adenosis of, 93–94, 94f

Prostate *(Continued)*
  cysts of, 95–96, 96f
  ectopic, 48, 120
  histology of, 81, 81f, 82f
  hyperplasia of, 88–95, 89f–96f
    atypical adenomatous, 93–94, 94f
    basal cell, 91–93, 92f
      atypical, 93, 93f
    nodular (benign prostatic hyperplasia), 88–89, 89f, 90f
    postatrophic, 91, 91f
    postinflammatory, 89, 91, 91f
    postsclerotic, 89, 91, 91f
    stromal with atypical cells, 95, 96f
  inflammation of, 83–86, 84f–87f
  intraepithelial
    neoplasia of, 96–98, 97f, 98f
  leukemia of, 118
  malignant lymphoma of, 117–118, 118f
  metaplasia of, 86, 86f, 88f
  sclerosing adenosis of, 94–95, 95f
  soft tissue tumors of
    benign, 115–116, 116f
    malignant, 116–118, 117f, 118f
  urothelial carcinoma of, 111, 111f
Prostate-specific antigen, 81, 82f
  prostate adenocarcinoma detected by staging of, 114t
    staining for, 101, 101f, 102f
Prostatic acid phosphatase, 81
  in prostatic adenocarcinoma, 101–102
Prostatic intraepithelial neoplasia, 96–98, 97f, 98f
  clinical significance of, 98
  diagnostic criteria for, 97f, 97–98, 98f
  spread of, 98
Prostatic urethra, 119–120
  glandular and squamous metaplasia of, 120
  inflammation of, 120
  urethral polyp in, 70, 71, 120
  urothelial carcinoma involving, 111, 111f
Prostatitis
  acute bacterial, 84, 85f
  chronic abacterial, 84–85
  granulomatous, 85f–87f, 85–86
    bacille Calmette-Guérin-induced, 85, 86, 86f
    idiopathic, 85, 85f
    infectious, 86
    other forms of, 86, 87f
    postsurgical, 86, 87f
    xanthogranulomatous, 86, 87f
Psammoma bodies, in papillary renal cell carcinoma, 18
Pseudocyst(s). *See also* Cyst(s).
  adrenal, 186
Pseudotumor
  fibrous, of paratesticular region, 161–162, 162f
  inflammatory
    of bladder, 45, 46f
    of paratesticular region, 161–162
    of prostate, 115–116
Pyelitis cystica, 75
Pyelonephritis
  acute, 7, 7f, 8f
  chronic, 8, 8f, 9f
  emphysematous, 7, 7f
  xanthogranulomatous, 9f, 9–10, 10f
Pyonephrosis, 7, 8f

R
Radiation cystitis, 43, 44f, 45
Radiation therapy, for prostatic adenocarcinoma, pathologic interpretation of, 112f, 112–113

Renal. *See also* Kidney.
Renal agenesis, 1
Renal cell carcinoma
  chromophobe, 19–20, 20f
  classification of, 14
  clear cell
    conventional, 14f, 14–15, 15f
    Fuhrman Nuclear Grading System for, 15, 16f
    multilocular cystic, 15, 18f
  collecting duct, 20–21, 21f, 22f
    low-grade, 21, 21f, 22f
  papillary, 18f, 18–19, 19f
  renal medullary, 21, 22f
  staging of, 22t
  unclassified, 21
  with sarcomatoid features, 15, 17f
Renal cystic disease(s), 3f–7f, 3–7
  acquired, 6, 6f
  dysplastic, 4f, 4–6, 5f
  hereditary, 3f, 3–4, 4f
  miscellaneous, 6f, 6–7, 7f
Renal dysplasia, 4f, 4–6, 5f
  multicystic and aplastic, 5, 5f
  segmental, 5, 6f
  with lower urinary tract obstruction, 5, 6f
  with multiple malformation syndromes, 5–6
Renal medullary carcinoma, 21, 22f
Renal pelvis
  anatomy and histology of, 33, 33f
  congenital malformations of, 73, 75, 75f
  neoplasms of, 77f–79f, 77–79
    rare, 79
  non-neoplastic conditions of, 75f, 75–76, 76f
  soft tissue tumors of, 79, 79f
Renal sarcoma, 27
Reninoma (juxtaglomerular cell tumor), 25, 25f, 26f
Renomedullary interstitial cell tumor, 25, 25f
Rete testis, 121, 123f
  anatomy of, 152, 152f
  carcinoma of, 146, 147f
Retroperitoneal fibrosis, of ureter, 76, 76f
Rhabdoid tumor, of kidney, 31–32, 32f
Rhabdomyosarcoma
  arising from teratoma, 137, 137f
  bladder, 66f, 66–67, 67f
  paratesticular, 162–163
  prostatic, 116, 117f

S
S-100 protein, immunoreactivity to
  in bladder melanoma, 69
  in sclerosing adenosis, 95
Sarcoidosis
  epididymitis in, 157
  granulomatous, of testis, 127, 128f
Sarcoma(s)
  bladder, 67, 68f
  clear cell, of kidney, 31, 31f
  paratesticular, 163
  penile, 180f, 181
  prostatic, 117
  renal, 27, 31, 31f
  scrotal, 184
Sarcomatoid carcinoma
  of bladder, 59, 59f, 60f
  of penis, 178–179
  of prostate, 109, 109f, 110f
Schiller-Duval bodies, 135, 136f
Schistosomiasis, granulomatous cystitis with, 41, 42f
Sclerosing adenosis, of prostate, 94–95, 95f

Scrotum, 181–184
  anatomy of, 151–152
  neoplasm(s) of
    basal cell carcinoma as, 182–183
    benign soft tissue, 184, 184f
    metastases to, 184
    Paget's disease as, 183, 183f, 184f
    sarcoma as, 184
    squamous cell carcinoma as, 182, 183f
  non-neoplastic conditions of, 181–182
Seminal vesicles, 118–119, 119f, 120f
  adenocarcinoma of, 119, 120f
  amyloidosis of, 118, 119f
  calcification of, 119
  cysts of, 119
  histology of, 81, 83, 83f
  infection of, 118–119
  prostatic cancer involving, 119, 120f
Seminal vesiculitis, 119
Seminiferous tubules, 121–122, 122f
  inflammation of, 127
Seminoma, 132–133, 133f, 134f
  spermatocytic, 140–141, 141f
Senile seminal vesicle amyloidosis, 118, 119f
Sertoli cell(s), 121, 122f
Sertoli cell tumor, 142, 144f–145f, 145
  large cell calcifying, 145, 145f
  sclerosing, 145, 145f
Sertoli cell–only syndrome, testis in, 129, 129f
Sex cord tumors, testicular, 142, 142f–145f, 145–146
Sickle cell disease, renal medullary carcinoma and, 21, 22f
Signet-ring adenocarcinoma, of bladder, 63, 63f
Signet-ring cell carcinoma, of prostate, 107, 108f
Small cell carcinoma
  of bladder, 64–65, 65f
  of kidney, 23
  of prostate, 107–108, 108f
Smooth muscle neoplasms, of ureter or renal pelvis, 79
Soft tissue tumors
  paratesticular, benign, 162
  prostate
    benign, 115–116, 116f
    malignant, 116–118, 117f, 118f
  renal
    benign, 24f–26f, 24–26
    malignant, 26–27
  renal pelvic and ureteral, 79, 79f
  scrotal, benign, 184, 184f
  testicular, 148, 148f
Sperm granuloma, 157, 158f
Spermatic cord
  anatomy of, 152–153
  heterotopic adrenal cortical tissue in, 153, 153f
  inflammation of, 158
  liposarcoma of, 162, 163f
  non-neoplastic diseases of, 154–159
    celes and cysts of, 154–156
    inflammatory and reactive diseases of, 156–159
  pseudotumor of, inflammatory and fibrous, 161–162, 162f
  torsion of, testicular infarction with, 124–125, 125f
Spermatocele, 155, 155f
Spindle cell nodule, postoperative
  of bladder, 45, 45f
  of prostate, 115
Spironolactone bodies, 190
Splenogonadal fusion, 122, 123f, 153

Squamous cell carcinoma
  of bladder, 62f, 62–63
  of penis, 176f–178f, 176–179
    clinical features of, 176, 176f, 177f
    differentiation and grading of, 176–177, 177f
    etiology of, 176
    growth patterns of, 177–178
    staging of, 178, 178t
    subtypes of, 178f, 178–179, 179f
  of prostate, 108
  of renal pelvis or ureter, 79, 79f
  of scrotum, 182, 183f
  of urethra, 73, 73f
  of urethral diverticulum, 72, 72f
Squamous cell carcinoma in situ, penile, 174–176, 175f, 176f
Squamous intraepithelial lesion, high-grade, of penis, 174
Squamous metaplasia
  of bladder, 47, 47f
  of prostate, 86, 88, 88f
  of ureter or renal pelvis, 75–76
Streak gonads, 146, 146f
Stromal hyperplasia, with atypical cells, of prostate, 95, 96f
Stromal tumors, testicular, 142, 142f–145f, 145–146
Suture granuloma, of bladder, 43, 43f
Syphilis, penile ulcers with, 171–172, 172f
Syphilitic orchitis, 127

T
Teratoma (dermoid cyst)
  immature, 137, 137f, 138f
  in prepubertal males, 142
  of paratesticular region and spermatic cord, 156
  of testis, 135, 137f, 137–138, 138f
Testicular tunics
  anatomy of, 151–152, 152f
  fibrous proliferation of, 161–162, 162f
  inflammatory and fibrous pseudotumor of, 161–162, 162f
Testis, 121–149
  anatomy and histology of, 121f–123f, 121–122
  cryptorchid, 129, 130f
  embryology of, 121
  hemorrhage of, 124–125
  in infertility, 127–129, 129f, 130f
  infarction of, 124–125, 125f, 126f
  neoplasm(s) of, 129–149
    benign, 122–127, 123f–128f
    choriocarcinoma as, 138–139, 139f
      adrenal metastases of, 198f
    germ cell, 129–142. *See also* Germ cell neoplasm(s).
    hematopoietic, 146–147, 147f, 148f
    metastatic, 148f, 148–149, 149f
    mixed germ cell/sex cord/stromal, 146, 146f
      adrenal metastases of, 198f
    rete testis carcinoma as, 146, 147f
    sex cord/stromal, 142, 142f–145f, 145–146
    soft tissue, 148, 148f
    WHO classification of, 129, 131t
  "streak," 146, 146f
  "tumor" of, of adrenogenital syndrome, 124, 124f
Thyroidization, in chronic pyelonephritis, 8, 9f
Torsion, of embryonic remnants, 159
Trigone, female, 34f

Tuberculosis
  adrenal involvement in, 186
  chronic epididymitis and, 118f, 156–157, 157f
  granulomatous prostatitis and, 86, 86f
  renal, 10–11, 11f
Tuberculous cystitis, 41
Tuberous sclerosis, renal angiomyolipoma and, 24
Tumor(s). *See named tumor; e.g.,* Wilms' tumor; *specific neoplasm.*
Tunic(s), testicular
  anatomy of, 151–152
  fibrous proliferation of, 161–162
  inflammatory and fibrous pseudotumor of, 161–162, 162f
Tunica albuginea, 167, 168f
Tunica vaginalis, 121, 121f
  meconium-induced inflammation of, 158–159
  well-differentiated papillary mesothelioma of, 160, 160f

U
Ulcer(s)
  Hunner's, of bladder, 43, 43f
  penile, infection-related, 170f, 170–172, 171f
Ultrasound hyperthermia, for prostatic adenocarcinoma, pathologic interpretation of, 113
Umbilicourachal sinus, 35f, 37
Urachus
  adenocarcinoma of, 63–64, 64f
  alternating sinus of, 34, 35f, 37
  anomalies of, 34, 35f–37f, 37
  completely patent, 34, 35f, 37
  incompletely patent, 36f, 37, 37f
Ureter(s)
  anatomy and histology of, 33, 34f
  congenital malformations of, 73–75, 75f
  epithelial neoplasms of
    benign epithelial, 77
    malignant, 77f, 77–79, 78f
  fibroepithelial polyps of, 79, 79f
  metastases to, 79
  neoplasms of, 77f, 77–79, 78f
    rare, 79
    staging of, 78t
  non-neoplastic conditions of, 75f, 75–76, 76f
  soft tissue tumors of, 79, 79f
Ureteral diverticulum, 75, 75f
Ureteritis cystica, 75, 75f
Ureterocele, 75, 75f
Ureteropelvic junction obstruction
  chronic pyelonephritis and, 8, 8f
  congenital, 75
Urethra
  anatomy and histology of, 33–34
  caruncle of, 72, 72f
  congenital polyp of, 70, 71f
  diverticulum of, 71f, 71–72, 72f
  malignant tumors of, 73, 73f, 74f
  meatal cyst of, 72, 73f
  non-neoplastic disorders of, 70–73, 71f–74f
  posterior valves of, 73, 74f
  prostatic, 119–120
    glandular and squamous metaplasia of, 120
    inflammation of, 119–120
    polyps of, 71, 71f, 120
    urothelial carcinoma involving, 111, 111f
Urethral valves, posterior, 73, 74f

Urinary tract obstruction, renal dysplasia
  associated with, 5, 6f
Urothelial carcinoma, 54–62
  adenocarcinoma as, 79
  diagnosis of, 55
  grading of, 55f–58f, 56–58
  lymphoepithelioma-like, 61, 61f
  metastatic to penis, 181, 181f
  metastatic to ureters, 79
  nonpapillary variants of, 56, 59, 59f–62f,
    61–62
  of prostate and prostatic urethra, 111, 111f
  of ureters and renal pelvis, 77f, 77–78, 78f
  papillary, 54–58, 55f–58f
  presenting signs of, 54–55
  sarcomatoid, 59, 59f–60f
  squamous cell, 62f, 62–63, 79, 79f
  staging of, 58, 58f–59f, 58t, 78t
Urothelium
  anatomy and histology of, 33, 34f
  carcinoma in situ of, 51–53, 52f–53f
  dysplasia of, 51, 51f
  hyperplasia of, 45, 46f
  metaplasia of, 47, 47f, 48f
  neoplasms of, 51f–62f, 51–63
  reactive changes in, 37–43, 38f–43f, 45, 46f

V
Vaginalitis, meconium, 158–159
Varicocele, 154–155, 155f
Vas deferens
  anatomy of, 152–153
  inflammation of, 157–158, 158f
Vasa aberrantia, 154
Vasitis, 157
Vasitis nodosa, 157–158, 158f
Verrucous carcinoma, of penis, 178, 178f, 179f
Verumontanum mucosal gland hyperplasia,
  88, 90f
Vesicourachal sinus, 35f, 37, 37f
Vesicoureteric reflux, 75
  chronic pyelonephritis and, 8, 8f
Villous adenoma, of bladder, 50, 51f
Viral epididymo-orchitis, 126–127
Von Brunn's nests, 33, 37, 38f, 53f
Von Hansemann histiocytes, 10
Von Recklinghausen's disease, bladder
  neurofibroma with, 66

W
Walthard rest, 154
Warthin-Starry stain, 171
Warty (condylomatous) carcinoma, of penis, 178

Warty lesions, penile, infection-related,
  172f–174f, 172–173
Waterhouse-Friderichsen syndrome, adrenal
  involvement in, 186, 187f
Wegener's granulomatosis, granulomatous
  prostatitis with, 86, 87f
WHO classification
  of testicular neoplasms, 129, 131t
  of urothelial tumors, 56–58
Wilms' tumor, 27, 28f, 29
  anaplasia in, 29, 29f
Wolffian remnants, in paratesticular region,
  153, 154

X
Xanthoma, prostatic, 86, 87

Y
Yolk sac tumor
  in postpubertal males, 135, 135f, 136f
  in prepubertal males, 141–142

Z
Zellballen, 69, 192, 192f
Zinner's syndrome, 119
Zoon's balanitis, 168, 169f